THE
CHANGE
BEFORE
THE
CHANGE

Praise for *The Change Before The Change*

'A tour de force that may become the benchmark in its field ... Dr Laura Corio tells you everything you need to know about the years before menopause, anticipates your questions, and answers them in warm, accessible language.' **Lee Ellen Morrone, M.D., The Mount Sinai Medical Center**

'A must read for every woman who wants to take control of her hormonal destiny.' **Barry Sears, Ph.D., author of *The Zone***

THE CHANGE BEFORE THE CHANGE

Everything you need to know to stay
healthy in the decade before menopause

DR LAURA E. CORIO AND LINDA G. KAHN

PIATKUS

Visit the Piatkus website!

Piatkus publishes a wide range of best-selling fiction and non-fiction, including books on health, mind, body & spirit, sex, self-help, cookery, biography and the paranormal.

If you want to:
- read descriptions of our popular titles
- buy our books over the Internet
- take advantage of our special offers
- enter our monthly competition
- learn more about your favourite Piatkus authors

VISIT OUR WEBSITE AT: www.piatkus.co.uk

This edition first published in Great Britain in 2002 by
Piatkus Books Ltd
5 Windmill Street
London W1T 2JA
e-mail: info@piatkus.co.uk

This new edition published 2005

The moral rights of the authors have been asserted

a catalogue record for this book is available from the British Library

ISBN 0 7499 2619 8

This book has been printed on paper manufactured with respect for the environment using wood from managed sustainable resources

Printed & bound in Great Britain by
William Clowes Ltd, Beccles, Suffolk

To my parents, who taught me about love,
caring for people, and striving to be the best.

Over the past two decades I have seen thousands of women through their perimenopausal years. Throughout this book, I have drawn on the stories they have generously shared with me to illustrate the vast range of symptoms and experiences that characterize this transition. Many of the case histories you will read are composites. When I have based examples on particular patients, I have changed their names and distinguishing features in order to protect their privacy.

At the end of each chapter of this book is a discussion of treatment options, including vitamins, minerals, foods, herbs, phytoestrogens, and hormone preparations that can be used to alleviate particular symptoms. These recommendations are not a prescription, and you should not implement any of these strategies without first consulting your physician. I have included them because I believe the best patient is an educated patient—the more informed you are, the better you will be able to collaborate with your doctor to come up with a treatment plan that suits your individual needs.

The American edition of this book has been adapted for the British market: the names of drugs, medical terms and procedures have been changed to their UK equivalents. We are indebted to Dr. Danny Tucker, MBBS, MRCOG for his advice on this aspect of the book, and to Tony Stephenson of the Imperial Cancer Research Foundation for his input on Chapter 10.

CONTENTS

Woman to Woman

I love being a doctor. In particular, I love being a women's doctor. In twenty years as a board-certified physician specializing in obstetrics and gynaecology, I've seen thousands of patients, from teenagers to great-grandmothers. A typical day might include counseling one woman about getting pregnant and prescribing birth control for the next, figuring out why one patient is bleeding all the time and why another hasn't seen a period for months, treating some women for diseases and helping others avoid them, scanning bones, doing biopsies, and perhaps even delivering a baby or two. Whatever the immediate concern, I make it my business to spend time getting to know my patients—not just their bodies, but their thoughts and feelings as well—and explaining what's going on with them physically. It's my strong belief that understanding your own body and working with a doctor who understands you as a whole person are the keys to maintaining lifelong emotional, psychological, and physical well-being.

Back when I was a medical student—one of only 10 women in a class of 110—topics such as PMS and menopause were simply not discussed. In fact, the entire concept of gender-specific medicine didn't yet exist. When we learned about heart disease, for example, all the information came from studies of men; it was assumed that women's bodies were the same, just smaller. In those days it didn't even cross my mind to question this exclusively male orientation. After all, I was expected to be "one of the guys." What an awakening it was to encounter women's health issues in the flesh when I hung out my shingle and began practicing real medicine!

I'll never forget how, in those early days, a patient came in complaining of terrible premenstrual symptoms. I just nodded my head and took notes, although I hadn't a clue what to tell her. After hours, I ran to the medical library and read everything I could find on the subject. The next day I put together a PMS handout detailing vitamins and minerals to take and foods to avoid. Over the years I've expanded this handout into an entire PMS-prevention plan.

Today, my focus has shifted to a new topic, one probably never dreamed about—and certainly never spoken about—by my medical school professors: perimenopause. About ten years ago I noticed that a lot of my patients in their forties were reporting similar symptoms: irregular bleeding, hot flushes, palpitations, mood swings, headaches, insomnia, memory loss, vaginal itching and dryness, lack of libido, dry skin and hair, weight gain. After a few years of these complaints, they'd come in and say, "All done!" They'd stopped having their periods and had entered menopause. Clearly their bodies were going through a major transition in those years leading up to menopause. Once again, I hit the library. I discovered that contrary to the prevailing wisdom, which says that your hormones shift *after* menopause, serious hormone fluctuations take place *long before* you stop bleeding that can cause a multitude of often debilitating symptoms. In fact, most women find their symptoms are at their worst during perimenopause; after menopause they begin to feel better.

When you think about it, this makes perfect sense. The human body isn't like a light switch that turns on and off at a flick. It's a complex organism that changes over time. Perimenopause is the perfectly natural, gradual transition from menstruation to menopause, the period in which your ovarian function winds down and your hormones readjust to meet the needs of your post-reproductive life.

Losing your period is one of the *last* signs that this transition has taken place. Most of the other elements of menopause—physical, sexual, and psychological—kick in several years earlier. Although the average age of menopause is 51, most women begin feeling the effects of their declining oestrogen levels between 45 and 47, although perimenopause can occur as early as 35 or as late as 55. Now I've made it a routine part of my practice to introduce the topic of perimenopause with all my patients over the age of 35. During their regular exam, I ask whether they've experienced any of the typical symptoms. More often than not, especially with patients in their forties, the answer is,

"Why yes, I have. But I figured it was just stress or middle age and there wasn't anything I could do about it."

This kind of resigned attitude drives me crazy. There's no need to be a martyr! Practically every week new studies are showing that simply incorporating particular vitamins, minerals, herbs, and foods into your diet and making certain lifestyle adjustments can counter many of the annoying, uncomfortable, and sometimes painful effects of perimenopause. If those approaches don't work, there's an enormous range of hormone preparations to choose from. With the help of your doctor, you should be able to control your symptoms rather than let them control you.

Even though more and more doctors are recognizing and treating perimenopause these days, there are still some with their heads in the sand. As recently as a year ago I received a referral from a psychiatrist I know. The patient had come to her because when the patient told her former gynaecologist about her symptoms, she said that because she was still getting her periods her problem wasn't physical—she was stressed out and needed to see a shrink. It turned out there was nothing wrong with her head; she was in full-blown perimenopause!

One of the reasons it has taken so long for perimenopause to be acknowledged is that unlike menopause itself, there's no red flag to tell you it's taking place. The signs of perimenopause vary widely from woman to woman. Some feel as if an alien is inhabiting their bodies, whereas others sail right through it. Blood tests of your hormone levels can give a clue as to whether you're in perimenopause, but they're not definitive. Rather, diagnosis is based on a number of intangible assessments that can only be made when your gynaecologist takes the time to discuss a broad range of changes you may be experiencing in your quality of life—time too many doctors cannot or will not spend.

For me, taking the time to talk with my patients is critical to giving them good care. It's also what makes being a doctor so rewarding for me. I often find my patients have much to teach me—"If you listen, you will learn," I always say. In fact, it was a patient who more than ten years ago introduced me to natural hormones, which are now the treatment of choice for many of my perimenopausal patients. She had been living in California, where she started taking natural hormones. When she moved to New York and began seeing me, she told me about them, but I was a bit skeptical. To convince me of their merit, she brought me a stack of medical articles explaining the benefits of natural hormones over synthetic ones. After reading the literature, I began to prescribe natural oestrogen and progesterone to other patients and soon became a convert.

Now the range of available hormonal treatments for peri-menopause has increased even more. In addition to natural hormones, the advent of low-dose oestrogens has transformed the way I treat my perimenopausal patients. Only one-sixth the strength of oral contra-ceptives, they are powerful enough to alleviate most perimenopausal symptoms and can be taken long-term without putting your breasts, uterus, and ovaries at risk. A wave of new hormone patches, gels, creams, and suppositories is also enabling me to tailor treatments even more specifically to my patients' medical needs.

Ideally, finding relief for your perimenopausal symptoms should be a collaboration between you and your doctor. My heart sinks when women come in complaining of this symptom and that symptom and just want to be "fixed." Your body is not a car that you simply take to the shop for a new set of spark plugs. It's a complicated, fascinating or-ganism that should command your full interest and attention.

Because perimenopausal symptoms are so varied, treatment has to be highly individualized. Some women do beautifully on just vita-mins, herbs, and phytoestrogens, others need natural hormones, and still others need synthetics. Also, because perimenopause is a time when your hormones are in constant flux, your treatment may need to be adjusted several times over the course of your transition. Good communication with your doctor and a willingness to make healthy lifestyle changes are essential.

As of the year 2000, fifty million American women—one-third of the female population—are of perimenopausal or menopausal age. Unlike our mothers, we don't have to suffer in silence. We're no longer embarrassed to admit that, yes, our hormones *do* affect how we think and feel. In our forties and fifties we're just reaching our peak perfor-mance, and there's no reason why we shouldn't be feeling great. Whether we're busy at the job, raising children we postponed having in order to get our careers off the ground, taking care of aging parents, or juggling all at once, we can't afford to be dragging around, losing our concentration, and worrying about hot flushes.

The aim of this book is to provide you with the information you need to take charge of your perimenopause. I'm not only going to tell you what changes you may expect during this transition, but I will explain why those changes are taking place biologically. With this level of understanding, you'll be able to make better choices among the treatment options available today, as well as the ones poised to flood the market in the next few years.

Part I of this book deals with the many different symptoms of perimenopause, beginning with the most common—menstrual irregularities. In each case I'll explain exactly what's going on in your body and suggest treatments that have proven successful for my patients and that you may want to discuss with your own doctor. There's also a chapter on how perimenopause affects fertility. As more and more of my patients are postponing motherhood to further their careers, I'm spending a lot of time counseling women about the challenges of getting pregnant during perimenopause.

Part II focuses on the relationship between perimenopause and the long-term health of your bones, heart, breasts, reproductive organs, and thyroid. Perimenopause is the ideal time to take stock of your physical condition and make a concrete commitment to doing all you can now to reduce your risk of illness in the future.

In each chapter you'll find specific advice about state-of-the-art medical treatments, supplements, and herbs that have been proven—both by research and in my own experience—to work best, and lifestyle and dietary factors that the traditional "just pop a pill" approach often neglects. All of this culminates in Chapter 13 with my prescription for a healthy perimenopause, including general recommendations about diet, exercise, and vitamin and mineral supplements. For easy reference, there are separate appendices summing up information found throughout the book on herbs, phytoestrogens, hormones, and screening tests.

Far too many women dread the first signs of "the change" and struggle to get through their perimenopausal years. With good healthcare and self-care, it doesn't have to be that way. Rather, this time of life should be a celebration of our prime in which we enjoy our power, revel in our achievements, and look and feel as positive and energetic as we can.

Part One

BEFORE THE CHANGE

CHAPTER 1

How Do I Know If I'm in Perimenopause?

There was a huge snowstorm raging outside, and we'd been receiving cancellation calls all day. So I was surprised to open the door to one of our examining rooms and find Marian perched on the end of the table. Marian started seeing me twelve years ago, when she was single and living in the city. A husband and two children later, she now lived in the suburbs but still remained a loyal patient.

"Why didn't you reschedule?" I asked. "You took your life in your hands driving all the way in from Long Island."

"I couldn't wait another day, Dr. Corio," she replied.

"What's wrong?"

"What isn't? I feel like my whole body is falling apart—in fact, it doesn't even feel like my own body anymore!" Marian went on to list a host of symptoms: migraines, hot flushes, insomnia, dry itchy skin, urinary tract infections, irregular periods, and decreased libido. "Poor Skip," she continued, referring to her sweetheart of a husband. "My moods have been all over the place and I haven't let him touch me in weeks. He's been really understanding, but I know that for both our sakes I can't put off dealing with this any longer."

"Well, Marian—how old are you now?" I glanced down at her chart. "Forty-three? It sounds to me as if you may be in perimenopause."

"You're kidding!" she responded. "But my mother didn't go through menopause until she was 50."

"And you may not, either. Perimenopause can begin up to a decade before menopause," I reminded her. "When was your last period?"

"About three weeks ago."

"And how was it? Longer or shorter than usual? Heavier or lighter?"

"A little heavier and longer than normal. And I had wicked PMS—my breasts were killing me and I had really bad cramps. I told Skip he should buy some stock in Neurofen. It was like being a teenager all over again."

"Funny you should say that," I said, "because in some ways peri-menopause is the mirror image of puberty. One of the reasons you're experiencing irregular periods, mood swings, and PMS is that after twenty years of relative stability, your hormones are beginning to fluc-tuate again. In your case, it's because your body is winding down its reproductive life; in a teenager's, it's because her body is winding up."

"Lovely," Marian said, rolling her eyes. "But if I'm reliving those happy teenage years, how come I have no sex drive?"

"Because perimenopause is like puberty in reverse. Although your oestrogen levels are bouncing around, they're basically on their way down, whereas a teenager's are basically on their way up. Your skin is getting drier; a teenager's gets oilier."

"So is there anything I can do to feel like a human being again, or do I just have to wait this out?"

"Of course there are things you can do—why should you suffer?" We went on to discuss a myriad of options, from vitamin and mineral supplements to herbs and foods she could try to relieve her various symptoms. "Before you leave today I'd like to write you a prescription for blood testing to check your oestrogen, progesterone, and testos-terone levels," I added. "This is the perfect time because you're in the middle of the second half of your cycle. If these levels are no longer in the normal range and your symptoms aren't improving with just the complementary treatments, we can talk about the possibility of adding a low dose of hormones."

"I can't tell you how relieved I am to know I'm not completely falling apart!" Marian sighed as she leaned back on the table so I could begin her physical examination. "It was definitely worth braving the hazards of the Long Island Expressway to see you today."

CHECKLIST OF PERIMENOPAUSAL SYMPTOMS

Every woman experiences perimenopause differently. Some have virtually no symptoms; others have every one in the book. Because the range of symptoms is so diverse, many women don't make the connection with perimenopause and either suffer in silence or run from one specialist to another looking for cures. If you are experiencing any of the following, ask your gynaecologist if he or she thinks you may be in perimenopause.

- irregular periods
- PMS symptoms—bloating, cramps, breast tenderness
- hot flushes and night sweats
- insomnia and fatigue
- heart palpitations
- mood swings and irritability
- migraine headaches
- memory problems
- fuzzy thinking or inability to concentrate
- dry, itchy, irritated skin
- dry or thinning hair
- brittle nails
- weight gain, especially around the middle
- vaginal dryness or itchiness
- pain with intercourse
- loss of interest in sex
- vaginal infections
- urinary tract infections
- frequent urination or stress incontinence
- joint pain
- irritable bowel syndrome

WHAT'S HAPPENING TO MY BODY?

Perimenopause is a transitional time between your childbearing and post-childbearing years. Basically, your ovaries, the organs that sponsor your reproductive life, are signing off. Once stuffed with as many as

6 to 7 million follicles (sacs that contain immature eggs), they now have many fewer, and the ones that remain are no longer in peak condition. Your ovaries are therefore producing less and less of the sex hormones needed to help those follicles mature.

Sex hormones don't only affect the stimulation and release *(ovulation)* of mature follicles, however. There are receptors for oestrogen, progesterone, and testosterone in virtually all your tissues. That's why when you're in perimenopause you'll not only notice that your periods are becoming irregular, but you'll probably also experience other symptoms in seemingly unrelated parts of your body.

The swan song of your ovaries is often not a graceful "adieu." Rather, they tend to try to make several comebacks before their final exit, resulting in sometimes wild fluctuations in hormone levels. Overall, however, the changes in your hormone levels occur in three stages:

1. During the first phase of perimenopause your progesterone level declines, leaving you in a state of oestrogen dominance. You might feel like you're constantly in PMS, with bloating, cramps, mood swings, and tender breasts. My patients describe it as feeling like their period is coming every day.

2. During the second phase your oestrogen level also declines, leading to such symptoms as hot flushes, memory problems, heart palpitations, migraine headaches, and vaginal dryness. Patients with these symptoms often are up all night and feel like they're losing their minds.

3. The third phase, or late perimenopause, sets in when oestrogen and progesterone levels decline to near menopausal levels. At this point many of your symptoms may recede, although you may continue to experience some, such as hot flushes, well into your menopausal years.

To fully understand the changes your body is going through in perimenopause, you need to have a grasp of what your ovaries have been doing up to now. Although I'm sure you learned the basics in high school biology, if you're like most of my patients you probably could use a refresher course. It's especially important to be familiar with the key hormones involved in the menstrual cycle: oestrogen, progesterone, follicle-stimulating hormone (FSH), luteinizing hormone (LH), gonadotropin-releasing hormone (GnRH), and testosterone. It is when their levels change that you experience perimenopausal symptoms. So sharpen your Number 2 pencils and read on!

THE MENSTRUAL CYCLE 101

At least ten times a week my perimenopausal patients ask questions that cause me to whip out a piece of paper and sketch the three phases of the menstrual cycle—the follicular phase, ovulation, and the luteal phase—and explain the hormones that control them.

The day you begin to bleed is called day 1. If you have a 28-day cycle, you ovulate on day 14, right in the middle. From day 1 to ovulation is called the *follicular phase.* From ovulation to the first day of your next period is called the *luteal phase.* The length of your cycle depends on the length of your follicular phase. For instance, if you have a 28-day cycle,

VARIATIONS IN CYCLE LENGTH
In normal cycles, the luteal phase is always 14 days.

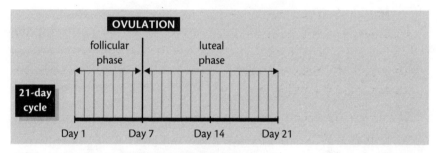

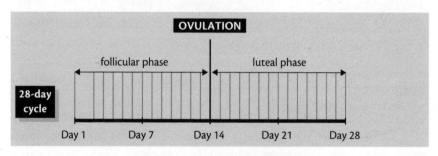

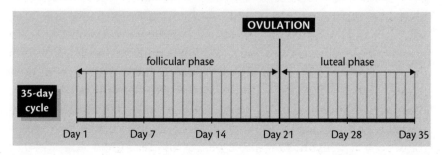

your follicular phase is 14 days; if you have a 21-day cycle, your follicular phase is only 7 days; if you have a 35-day cycle, your follicular phase could be as long as 21 days. In a normal cycle your luteal phase should remain constant at 14 days. In perimenopause, however, it can shorten or even disappear altogether if you're not ovulating.

Follicular Phase

Your body's main aim during the follicular phase of your cycle is to produce enough oestrogen to mature the egg in your follicle. At the beginning of your menstrual cycle, your oestrogen levels are low. Detecting this, the hypothalamus gland in your brain releases gonadotropin-releasing hormone (GnRH). This stimulates the pituitary gland, also in the brain, to release follicle-stimulating hormone (FSH). As its name implies, FSH stimulates follicles to begin developing and producing oestrogen.

By the end of the follicular phase, your ovaries are producing not only high levels of oestrogen but male hormones (androgens) such as androstenedione and testosterone as well. My normally-cycling patients tell me they feel great at this time of the month—energetic, outgoing, creative, and clear-thinking.

By contrast, perimenopausal women who do not ovulate get stuck in the follicular phase, building up more and more unopposed oestrogen. This oestrogen dominance makes them feel horrible—they become bloated, their breasts hurt, they get cramps, and their moods fluctuate wildly.

Ovulation

When the oestrogen circulating in your bloodstream reaches a critical level, it stimulates your pituitary to release a surge of luteinizing hormone (LH). The subsequent LH peak lasts 48 to 50 hours. Your ovaries release an egg approximately 24 to 36 hours after the oestrogen peak and 10 to 12 hours after the LH peak. Ovulation kits measure LH, indicating the optimal time to have intercourse if you want to conceive.

LH stimulates your ovaries to *luteinize*, or convert cholesterol into progesterone. Along with LH and FSH, progesterone stimulates breakdown of the tissue supporting the follicular wall. The wall becomes thinner and thinner until the follicle ruptures and the egg is released.

Progesterone also raises your basal body temperature, which is why, if you take your temperature at the same time each day, you'll notice a rise when you're ovulating and thus are most fertile. (See Chapter 7 for a discussion of how to use a basal body thermometer to track ovulation.)

You'll probably find yourself in a romantic mood around the time you ovulate. This is because the high androgen levels reached at the end of the follicular phase stimulate the libido. So you may experience a wave of lust right around the time your ovaries are releasing a mature egg—Mother Nature's way of ensuring the continuity of the species. In addition to feeling sexy, my patients tell me that around the time they ovulate they feel open to being cared for emotionally and physically, content, and energetic.

Luteal Phase

In the first week or so after ovulation, your body is preparing to support a possible pregnancy. The follicle cells left behind after the egg has been released reorganize to form the *corpus luteum*, which continues to pump out progesterone. (The name, which means "yellow body," refers to *lutein*, the yellow pigment these cells fill up with.)

High levels of progesterone prevent more follicles from developing and keep your uterine lining plush. Without a certain amount of circulating progesterone, your uterine lining will not be able to sustain a fertilized egg. This is why perimenopausal women, whose progesterone levels may be falling, are susceptible to spontaneous miscarriage in the first trimester of pregnancy. To get them through this time, I often monitor progesterone levels and, if needed, prescribe natural progesterone supplements for the first eleven weeks of pregnancy. The corpus luteum also produces oestrogen and a protein called inhibin. Oestrogen, progesterone, and inhibin together send a message to the brain to suppress GnRH, FSH, and LH secretion.

If fertilization occurs, the embryo will produce a hormone called human chorionic gonadotropin (HCG). HCG signals the corpus luteum to continue producing oestrogen and progesterone, ensuring that you don't menstruate and shed your uterine lining. However, if an egg has not been fertilized by eight days after ovulation, your ovaries begin to prepare for the next cycle. Your oestrogen, progesterone, and inhibin levels fall, allowing GnRH and FSH to rise again. The corpus

---

How Do I Know If I'm Ovulating?

Besides using an ovulation kit or a basal body thermometer, you can occasionally rely on your body to give you a signal that you're ovulating. Although some women don't feel anything at all, others say they feel a sharp pelvic pain, like a hard pinch, and notice spotting in the middle of their cycles. Known as mittelschmerz (German for "middle pain"), these symptoms are common and perfectly normal signs of ovulation.

---

luteum self-destructs, and without the hormonal support it provides, your uterine lining collapses. You get your period just as new follicles are being stimulated, and the cycle begins all over again.

For some women, the luteal phase can be rough. They may feel nervous, anxious, irritable, lethargic, depressed, bloated, hungry, crampy, and weepy—in other words, they may suffer premenstrual syndrome (PMS).

Patients often ask me whether they're feeling lousy because they have PMS or because they're in perimenopause. The key here is that perimenopausal symptoms occur throughout your cycle, while PMS symptoms occur in the second half and improve when you get your period.

IS THERE A TEST TO SHOW IF I'M IN PERIMENOPAUSE?

My patients would love to have a way of confirming that they're in perimenopause. The test for menopause is clear-cut: twelve months without a period, or FSH and LH in the menopausal range. Unfortunately, however, there's no sure-fire method to identify perimenopause. The best way for your doctor to determine whether you're in perimenopause is to take a thorough medical history, reviewing all your symptoms, and perform a physical examination. A blood test to check the levels of the hormones listed in the table on page 17 can confirm your doctor's diagnosis but should not be relied upon 100 percent.

Why not? Because perimenopause is characterized by hormonal fluctuations, so a blood test of your hormones could indicate normal levels even if you're in the throes of the transition. But the same test

HORMONE LEVELS BEFORE, DURING, AND AFTER MENOPAUSE

performed next month could show your hormones to be completely out of whack. Reading these tests is like looking at a still from a movie. They can never give you a true sense of what's happening. I use them, but I interpret them guardedly.

The reason your hormone levels may swing in and out of the normal range in perimenopause is that they are determined by the condition of the particular follicle that matures each month. If you happen to release a healthy egg, your circulating oestrogen, progesterone, FSH, LH, and inhibin levels will be normal; if instead you release a worn-out egg, your hormone levels will be in the perimenopausal range.

Of all these hormones, inhibin is the most sensitive marker of follicular health. But as of yet, there is no known way to measure inhibin levels. Instead, we measure circulating FSH levels, because without adequate inhibin, FSH is released in greater than normal amounts. In other words, as your inhibin goes down, your FSH goes up.

To determine a patient's FSH level, I take a blood sample on the third day of her cycle. This also tells me her levels of oestradiol—one of the three main kinds of oestrogen your body produces—and LH. To

THE THREE FORMS OF OESTROGEN

Oestrogen is really an umbrella term. Each of its three major types plays a distinct role in the body.

Oestradiol (E$_2$). Oestradiol is the predominant form of oestrogen circulating in your body from menarche to menopause, and therefore the one that we test when we do hormone studies. There are oestradiol receptors on virtually every cell in your body—not just your reproductive organs—including your brain, skin, hair, heart, liver, blood vessels, bones, breasts, vagina, bladder, colon, uterus, and thyroid gland. Oestradiol affects more than 400 of your bodily functions. That is why when you enter perimenopause and your oestradiol levels begin to fluctuate and eventually decline, you may experience a wide range of physical, mental, and emotional symptoms. Although 95 percent of your circulating oestradiol is produced by the ovaries during your reproductive years, it is also produced in small amounts by fat cells. Fat cells become your most significant source of oestradiol after menopause.

Oestrone (E$_1$). Oestrone, a weaker oestrogen, is the main form of oestrogen after menopause. It is produced in fat cells from the male hormone androstenedione. Obese women of any age have high levels of oestrone. During your reproductive years, your ovaries and liver produce small amounts of oestrone from oestradiol. After menopause, some of your oestrone is converted to oestradiol, but it amounts to much less than you had premenopausally.

Oestriol (E$_3$). Oestriol is only produced in significant amounts by the placenta during pregnancy, when levels skyrocket. The reason pregnant women glow and have thick, lustrous hair is because oestriol receptors are mostly found in skin, hair, and vaginal tissue. The weakest form of oestrogen, oestriol is one-third as potent as oestradiol and does not appear to affect the bones, breast, brain, heart, and other organs the way oestradiol does. When you're not pregnant, your liver produces small amounts of oestriol from oestrone.

find out her serum level of progesterone, I take blood either ten days after she's ovulated or four days before she expects her next period.

Saliva testing of hormone levels is possible but not widely available. It is simple and painless: all you need to do is to spit into a test tube during the second half of your cycle (around days 20 to 23 of a 28-day cycle). The drawback of saliva testing is that at present it can only be used to measure oestrogen, progesterone, and testosterone levels, not FSH or LH.

READING THE TEST RESULTS

	NORMAL	MENOPAUSAL
Serum FSH (day 3)	2.5 to 18 mIU/ml	.18 to 153 mIU/ml
Serum LH (day 3)	1.5 to 15 mIU/ml	16 to 65 mIU/ml
Serum oestradiol (day 3)	24 to 190 pg/ml	less than 36 pg/ml
Serum progesterone (day 24)	4 to 28 ng/ml	0 to 0.7 ng/ml
Saliva oestradiol (day 20 to 23)	0.5 to 5.0 pg/ml	less than 1.5 pg/ml
Saliva progesterone (day 20 to 23)	0.1 to 0.5 ng/ml	less than 0.05 ng/ml
Saliva testosterone (day 20 to 23)	13 to 37 pg/ml (age 40 to 49)	12 to 34 pg/ml (age 50 to 59)

OTHER IMPORTANT HORMONES TO HAVE CHECKED IN PERIMENOPAUSE

While I'm testing blood levels of the reproductive hormones, I always check TSH (thyroid-stimulating hormone), free T_4 (thyroid hormone), and prolactin levels, as well. As you'll learn in Chapter 12, thyroid disease often sets in when women reach their forties and early fifties, and it can affect the menstrual cycle in a way that mimics perimenopause. If thyroid disease is a culprit, your periods should return to normal as soon as it's treated.

Prolactin is a hormone normally produced by the pituitary gland during lactation. Elevated prolactin levels in a non-pregnant woman can indicate a pituitary adenoma—a benign tumor of the pituitary gland, which has been associated with abnormal bleeding patterns. If this is the case, it can be treated with medication.

And then there's testosterone. "You've got to be kidding!" my patients often respond. "Isn't that the male hormone? I don't produce testosterone." Surprise—you do! In fact, your body makes two male hormones, testosterone and androstenedione, albeit in much lower levels than men. Twenty-five percent of testosterone and 50 percent of androstenedione are made in the ovaries, which continue to produce testosterone until five years after menopause. Another 25 percent of testosterone and the remaining 50 percent of androstenedione come from the adrenal glands. A full 50 percent of your testosterone is converted from androstenedione in cells dispersed all over your body.

In perimenopause, testosterone can decrease, remain unchanged, or increase. Fluctuating testosterone levels can contribute to certain perimenopausal symptoms, and taking testosterone supplements can often provide relief.

TREATING YOUR PERIMENOPAUSAL SYMPTOMS

In this chapter I've given a brief overview of the major hormonal players in the drama of your reproductive life and how their waxing and waning can cause perimenopausal symptoms. You will hear more about them throughout this book. To treat these symptoms I usually recommend complementary approaches first, such as vitamins, minerals, herbs, and changes in diet and lifestyle. Each chapter provides details of the specific supplements and dosages that work best for each condition.

Here I'd like to preview two other important options: phytoestrogens and hormones.

Phytoestrogens

Phytoestrogens are plant-derived compounds that bind to oestrogen receptors in the body. These weak oestrogen mimics—phytoestrogens are only $1/1,000^{th}$ to $1/10,000^{th}$ as potent as your body's own oestrogen—can act as natural supplements when your ovarian supply begins to decline in perimenopause.

There are three major types of phytoestrogens. *Isoflavones,* which include genistein and daidzein, are found in high concentrations in soybeans and soy products as well as in lentils, chickpeas, and red clover. *Lignans* are especially abundant in flaxseed and are also present in many fruits and vegetables as well as cereals. *Coumestans* can be obtained from bean sprouts and alfalfa.

Soy is particularly rich in phytoestrogens, which is why it's getting so much press these days. Tofu, soy nuts, and soy milk are excellent sources not only of soy protein and isoflavones, but of calcium as well. Soy foods can help moderate a wide range of perimenopausal symptoms.

I always recommend getting your phytoestrogens through food, not from pills or powders. The protein in soy is necessary to activate the isoflavones. Isoflavone supplements that lack soy protein do not have any effect.

Hormone Supplements

If a perimenopausal patient isn't getting enough relief from diet, herbs, and phytoestrogens, we sit down and have a chat about hormone replacement therapy. She usually has one of three reactions: "Give me the drugs—anything to make me feel better," "Do you have something natural instead of that synthetic stuff made from horses' urine?" or "Forget about it—I refuse to take hormones under any condition." Even if she is dead-set against hormone replacement, I persist, because few women are aware of the multitude of products available these days, including low-dose and natural prescriptions.

Depending on your medical and family history, your symptoms, and your personal preferences, you can choose from a wide array of available doses and combinations of oestrogen, progesterone, and testosterone. And you don't always have to take a pill—in addition to oral hormone replacement therapy, there are transdermal patches and gels as well as vaginal creams.

It wasn't until recently that hormone replacement therapy was even an option for women who hadn't yet entered menopause. I still see patients who have been refused hormones by other physicians who won't treat them because they are still menstruating. However, there is no biological reason to wait. Perimenopause may actually be the ideal time to start hormone supplements. Not only can hormones relieve perimenopausal symptoms, but they also provide a broad array of long-term health benefits.

Low-dose oral contraceptives are a great choice for perimenopausal women. In addition to providing birth control, they even out hormone levels, thereby minimizing many of the symptoms that can arise when your oestrogen levels start fluctuating. Birth control pills can also reduce your risk of a variety of diseases. Physicians used to stop prescribing oral contraceptives by age 35 because we didn't know enough about their long-term effects, but today we are comfortable

---

WHAT DO I MEAN BY NATURAL?

A natural hormone—also known as a *bioidentical* hormone—is a substance that is identical to a hormone that is made in the human body. It does not necessarily mean that the hormone is derived from plants. Natural hormones may be made in a lab from a plant extract, to be sure, but they may also be made from other chemicals—the source is unimportant. The point is that they are exactly like what's in your body, so that when your body metabolizes them, the breakdown products are familiar to your body as well.

Synthetic hormones, by contrast, are different from the hormones your body produces. Again, the source is unimportant—synthetic hormones can be cooked up in a lab, isolated from pregnant mares' urine (hence Premarin), or even extracted from plants. Regardless of their origin, they are not bioidentical to the hormones your body produces, so when they are metabolized, you are exposed to a host of foreign molecules that may cause unpleasant side effects. These breakdown products may even be harmful to your health.

Appendix C lists currently available natural and synthetic hormones by brand name.

---

recommending them up until menopause, and then switching to hormone replacement therapy.

Standard hormone replacement therapy contains a combination of an oestrogen and a progestogen, both of which can be either synthetic or natural.

Another important new option is provided by the increased availability of *natural hormones*. Natural forms of oestrogen, progesterone, and testosterone can often be used instead of the standard synthetics, although it should be noted some patients respond better to synthetics.

I am not a strong advocate of synthetic hormones, such as the widely prescribed Premarin and Provera. They are not the same as those found in the body and are therefore tolerated less well. They cause more side effects than natural hormones do and may even be detrimental to your health. Think about it: Doesn't it make more sense to put something back in your body that is chemically the same as what you're used to, rather than some foreign compound that may not be close to anything found in human biology? There's a big drop-out rate from hormone replacement therapy with synthetic hormones—primarily because women don't like the way it makes them feel. They hate the weight gain, the bloating, and the mood swings. Most of my patients who take natural hormones tell me that they feel great: they can maintain or even lose weight, and they're even-tempered—basically, they feel the way they felt before they entered perimenopause.

The first step toward making a decision about hormone replacement therapy is to have a conversation with your doctor in which, together, you evaluate the risks and benefits in relation to your individual health needs. Every woman's situation is unique, and there's no right or wrong answer. The important thing right now is to have this initial conversation and begin thinking about your options. Even if you decide not to try hormone replacement therapy today, you can always revisit the subject in the future.

CHAPTER 2

The First Sign: Menstrual Irregularities

The other day I got to the office after spending the morning at the hospital on the labor floor and had phone messages from four of my perimenopausal patients. One, a 49-year-old who had been having irregular cycles for the past four months, told me she'd been bleeding and spotting for two months straight. Another, 51 years old, had been taking natural progesterone for five months to control her heavy periods and now wasn't getting her period at all. A 52-year-old patient who had been experiencing normal periods on natural progesterone cream called to say she hadn't bled in 40 days. And a 50-year-old with fibroids whom I'd put on low-dose hormone replacement therapy was now getting heavy periods less than three weeks apart.

One of the surest signs you're in perimenopause, according to my patients, is that your once-predictable period is now "all over the place." While 90 percent of women have regular menstrual cycles up to age 40, only 10 percent are regular by age 50. In fact, perimenopausal women have a higher rate of irregularity than any group besides teenagers.

Contrary to popular belief, most women's periods don't just evaporate the day they enter menopause. Rather, menstruation winds down gradually. As I explained in Chapter 1, during perimenopause your ovaries produce fewer and weaker follicles until, eventually, they stop ovulating once and for all. Only 12 percent of women just wake up one day and never have another period. The other 88 percent notice fluctuations in their cycle as their ovaries lose steam: their cycles are longer or shorter than usual, heavier or lighter, or characterized by intermittent spotting.

Fluctuations in your cycle are usually nothing to worry about, but you should keep track of them because in certain circumstances they may indicate a potential for other problems. Usually I recommend that my perimenopausal patients keep a bleeding chart, like the one on page 26, for at least three months on which they note every day that they bleed and whether the flow is heavy, moderate, light, or merely spotty. That way, when they come in for their appointments we have concrete information that can help me figure out what's going on with their hormones.

WHAT CHANGES IN MY PERIOD CAN I EXPECT?

It's hard to make too many generalizations about perimenopausal bleeding patterns because each woman's experience is unique and the variety of possible changes is virtually limitless. You may skip a few periods and then bleed for two weeks straight, or you may have many light periods very close together. Over the course of your perimenopause, your bleeding pattern may shift as well. The factors that determine the fate of your menstrual cycle are (1) whether or not you're still ovulating, and (2) your hormone levels.

In early perimenopause most women are still ovulating. One of the first changes you might notice is the shortening of your menstrual cycle from an average of 28 to 30 days to an average of 21 to 24 days. During this time the first half of your cycle, the follicular phase, is shrinking from an average of 14 days to just 10. Your ovaries are becoming less sensitive to FSH (follicle-stimulating hormone), so your pituitary gland has to pump out more to get a response. This high FSH level makes you ovulate sooner than before. Shortening of the second half of your cycle, the luteal phase, may follow later in perimenopause because the less healthy follicles that remain will produce defective corpus luteums. In the end stage of perimenopause, when your ovaries run out of eggs, you'll stop ovulating altogether and your cycles will lengthen and ultimately cease.

A study of 500 perimenopausal women found that they generally experienced one of three overall bleeding patterns. Twelve percent had sudden cessation of their periods. Seventy percent reported infrequent

Patient _____

Address _____

Phone _____

MENSTRUAL RECORD CHART

Year Month	1	2	3	4	5	6	7	8	9	10	11	12	13	14	15	16	17	18	19	20	21	22	23	24	25	26	27	28	29	30	31	No. of days from start of period to beginning of next	Breast Exam Done (✓)
January																																	
February																																	
March																																	
April																																	
May																																	
June																																	
July																																	
August																																	
September																																	
October																																	
November																																	
December																																	

TYPE — X Normal
OF — O Exceptionally light
FLOW — ■ Exceptionally heavy
— S Spotting

Don't forget to have this chart with you when you call or visit your doctor.

Dr. _____

WHAT'S THAT WORD ON MY CHART?

AMENORRHOEA—no period for more than 60 days

HYPERMENORRHOEA—frequent periods, less than 21 days apart

HYPOMENORRHOEA—light periods or spotting

MENORRHAGIA—very heavy periods or flooding

METRORRHAGIA—irregular bleeding between periods

OLIGOMENORRHOEA—infrequent periods, more than 36 days apart

periods and/or lighter periods or spotting. The remaining 18 percent had more frequent periods, irregular bleeding between periods, and/or very heavy periods or flooding. Each of these patterns reflects specific changes in levels of oestrogen and progesterone triggered by the condition of the ovarian follicle.

Following are stories about three of my patients, Mary Ann, Elizabeth, and Jackie, who illustrate these three common patterns. If you don't see your own pattern precisely reflected in any of them, don't worry. There are countless variations on these themes. And you may find that you've shifted from one pattern to another over the course of your perimenopause; that's also perfectly normal. Every woman's experience is different, which is why you need to work with your doctor to devise a treatment strategy that takes into account your individual symptoms, hormone levels, and bleeding pattern. You may have to change your treatment strategy several times during your perimenopause to accommodate your shifting hormones.

MARY ANN—SUDDEN CESSATION OF PERIODS

Mary Ann is the consummate professional. A partner in an established law firm, she's always punctual for her visits, dressed in either a navy blue or gray tailored suit. Over the past seven years I've learned a little bit about her life: she's single, has never had children, exercises religiously, and is a health-food nut—but smokes half a pack of cigarettes a day. Although her wire-thin frame belies her 44 years, her skin is lined and her fingers stained from nicotine. High strung and introverted, she's a loner, although occasionally a man passes through her life, in which case she always uses condoms.

After exchanging greetings, I asked her if anything had changed since our last visit a year ago.

"Well, I haven't had a period for seven months," she responded matter-of-factly.

"Any staining or spotting?" I queried.

"No, not a drop."

"And how do you feel?"

"Perfectly fine, Dr. C.," she answered.

I asked whether she was undergoing any unusual stress in her job or her personal life that might be causing her to skip periods. She said no. Was she exercising more than usual, or had she changed eating habits? Again, no. I checked her weight, and although it was extremely low for her height, it was the same as it had been since I'd known her.

"I figured I was in menopause, although it seems a little early," she said, stepping off the scale.

"Menopause does occur about a year and a half earlier in women who smoke," I explained, "but you could just be in perimenopause."

I examined her carefully, especially her thyroid gland, and, during the internal exam, feeling for cysts on her ovaries that could be causing her amenorrhoea, but they were normal. When I was done, I told her I wanted to do some blood tests to check her hormone levels and to make sure she wasn't pregnant. "Fine," she said, "although I can assure you that I'm *not* pregnant!"

Two days later I called her with the blood test results. Her TSH, free T_4, and prolactin levels were normal and her HCG (human chorionic gonadotropin) was negative—she wasn't pregnant. Her FSH was 26 mlU/ml, elevated and in the menopausal range; her oestradiol was 40 pg/ml, in the normal range; and at 10 mlU/ml her LH was normal. The clincher was her progesterone, which, at 0.1 ng/ml, indicated that she was no longer ovulating.

"It looks like perimenopause," I told her, "so you may still get your period. Call me in two months and let me know what's happening."

Two months later she phoned. No period, no spotting—nothing. I had her come in for another set of blood tests. The results of this second round showed FSH in the menopausal range (46 mlU/ml), elevated LH (30 mlU/ml), low oestradiol (20 pg/ml), and low progesterone. Sure enough, Mary Ann had entered menopause—in her usual efficient, no-nonsense way.

WHEN YOUR PERIODS JUST STOP. It is not uncommon for a perimenopausal patient to tell me she hasn't had a period in six months. My only concern in this situation is that she may be producing unopposed oestrogen, which puts her at risk for uterine, breast, ovarian, and colon cancer. So blood tests, especially of oestradiol levels, are always in order. If the patient's oestradiol level is low, then she's entering menopause and doesn't have to worry. If it's high, she needs to take natural progesterone to balance out the excess oestrogen.

The most likely explanation for not getting your period is anovulation, which may signal perimenopause but may also occur for other reasons. Over the past couple of years I've had three different patients in their forties tell me they haven't had a period in more than two months and thought they were in menopause. None of them had any menopausal symptoms. When I worked up their blood, lo and behold, they weren't even in perimenopause, much less menopause. For some reason their hypothalamus glands had shut down and they were not producing any oestrogen or progesterone *(hypothalamic amenorrhoea)*. On questioning them, I found that each was under a significant amount of stress—divorce, relocating, taking care of sick parents—that had caused them to stop menstruating.

ELIZABETH—INFREQUENT, LIGHT PERIODS

I always look forward to appointments with Elizabeth. Even though we now only see each other at her annual exam, we've developed a great relationship over the fifteen years that she's been my patient. Indeed, she was one of my first private clients, and I delivered both of her children, Tom, now age 10, and Katie, age 7. Elizabeth is one of these terrific, dynamic, together women who manages to juggle running her own small business designing dried floral arrangements, volunteering at her kids' schools, and maintaining a lively social life with her husband, Andrew, a real estate developer. Not only that, but she looks great, with thick wavy brown hair, clear skin, and a strong, compact body.

After a warm greeting and a few minutes catching up with each other's lives, we got down to business. "I have to tell you, Laura, I had a little scare recently," she said with a conspiratorial grin.

"What do you mean?" Elizabeth had always been a conscientious diaphragm user, replacing it every other year. Nevertheless, accidents can happen—overall, the diaphragm's efficacy is 95 percent, meaning 5 out of 100 women using it do become pregnant.

"Well, I had a few periods pretty close together—around 26 days—then missed a period altogether, and then a couple of weeks after I was supposed to get it I had a little spotting. I took a pregnancy test and it was negative, but I didn't really believe it until I got a real period about four weeks after that."

"And how long ago did this happen?" I asked.

"Approximately 40 days ago. That was my most recent period. I'm actually about 10 days overdue for my next one. It's really annoying—I always have to walk around with tampons because I never know when to expect it."

"Do you feel like it's coming?"

"Well, I feel premenstrual all the time—my breasts are sore and I'm bloated—but that's been the case pretty much continuously since this whole thing started, except when I was actually bleeding—another reason I initially thought I was pregnant."

"When you did have your period, was it normal?" I queried.

"Maybe a couple of days short," Elizabeth answered. By now my probing had made her a little anxious. "Is there something I should be worried about, Laura?"

"Probably not," I reassured her. "My guess is that you're entering perimenopause."

"Oh my gosh, I can't believe I never thought of that!" she responded. Now age 47, Elizabeth had heard my spiel on perimenopause a good ten times, so she was familiar with the concept.

I did a full exam and noticed that her breasts were indeed swollen and lumpy, but her uterus, ovaries, and thyroid were all normal. When it was over, I handed her a preprinted index-sized card. "I want you to keep a bleeding record and come back to see me in three months. You should have a period within 60 days. In the meantime, keep track of any other changes you may notice, like hot flushes, insomnia, and vaginal dryness. And, of course, call me if anything shifts dramatically or you begin experiencing severe bleeding or cramping.

"Also, when you do get your next period," I continued, "I want you to stop in for a blood test on the third day of bleeding so we can check your thyroid and prolactin to make sure everything is normal and look at your hormone levels to see where you're at. In the meantime, start taking a multivitamin, vitamin D, natural vitamin E, and a calcium/magnesium supplement daily."

"Yes, ma'am!" she replied with a salute. I gave her a hug and wished her well.

Elizabeth came in a week later, on the third day of her cycle, and had blood drawn. I called her immediately upon receiving the results. Her LH level was fine, her oestradiol was low, and her FSH was slightly elevated, which I explained could indicate the hormonal fluctuations of perimenopause. Her TSH, free T_4, and prolactin levels were normal and she wasn't pregnant.

At her next appointment Elizabeth gave me a big smile when I entered the examining room, but I noticed that her face looked a little drawn. "So, how are you feeling?" I asked.

"Pretty good," she responded with slightly less than her usual gusto.

"Let's take a look at your bleeding chart."

Elizabeth handed me her menstrual record, meticulously filled out. She had gotten her period four days after our last visit—two weeks late—and it was shorter and lighter than normal. She hadn't had any bleeding since then.

Patient: *Elizabeth Jones* Phone _____

Address _____

MENSTRUAL RECORD CHART

Year	Month	1	2	3	4	5	6	7	8	9	10	11	12	13	14	15	16	17	18	19	20	21	22	23	24	25	26	27	28	29	30	31	No. of days from start of period to beginning of next	Breast Exam Done (✓)
	January																																	
	February																																	
	March																																	
	April																				X	X	X	X	O									
	May																																	
	June	O	O	O																														
	July																																	
	August																																	
	September																																	
	October																																	
	November																																	
	December																																	

TYPE OF FLOW
X Normal
O Exceptionally light
■ Exceptionally heavy
S Spotting

Don't forget to have this chart with you when you call or visit your doctor.

Dr. _____

"This looks perfectly normal for a woman going through peri-menopause," I reassured her. "Your last period was more than 60 days ago, so let's take another look at your hormone levels and see if anything has changed."

We drew blood and when the results came back, her FSH was still elevated, her oestradiol still low, and she had low progesterone, indicating that she had stopped ovulating.

"You have several choices," I said to her. "At your last visit you told me that you were feeling bloated and premenstrual all the time. This means that even though your oestrogen level is low, you're still producing more oestrogen than progesterone. You could tough it out, because it looks like you're on your way to menopause. But if you want relief from your symptoms, I suggest either taking natural progesterone in a pill or a cream, or low-dose birth control pills. I can also give you a list of vitamins, herbs, and foods to incorporate into your diet to help regulate your oestrogen levels and control your perimenopausal symptoms."

"I don't want to take pills right now. I think I'll go with the cream and the herbs," she replied.

"Okay, then. First, take ¼ teaspoon of 5 percent progesterone cream and rub it on your body twice a day, always changing the sites, starting on day 10 of your period and continuing until you begin to bleed. This should even out your symptoms and make you feel normal, not premenstrual all the time. Second, in addition to your daily multivitamin, vitamin E, and calcium/magnesium supplement, I want you to pick up some evening primrose oil. It'll really help with your breast soreness and bloating. Try to take 1,000 to 2,000 mg a day. And call me in the next couple of months to let me know how things are going."

Elizabeth called in two months. "That progesterone cream and evening primrose oil are working great. Thank you so much—I never felt better!"

WHEN YOUR PERIODS BECOME SCANTY. You may experience light or infrequent periods in either anovulatory or ovulatory cycles. If you're not ovulating, the weak follicles remaining in your ovaries are not producing adequate oestrogen to build up your uterine lining during the follicular phase, so there is little or nothing to shed when the time eventually comes. You may experience spotting in ovulatory cycles if the corpus luteum is defective, producing only low levels of oestrogen and progesterone.

JACKIE—FREQUENT, HEAVY PERIODS

My nurse buzzed me in my office. She had a patient on the line who had been bleeding for two weeks straight. "Have her come in immediately," I said. "This could be a problem."

Later that afternoon Jackie arrived. Slightly heavyset with wisps of graying hair escaping her barrettes, she normally exuded a relaxed earthiness. Jackie had been coming to me for two years, after the doctor she'd been seeing for most of her life retired. Married to a history professor with two college-age children, she had gotten her real estate license around the time I met her and now, at age 49, was thriving in her new career.

But the minute I entered the examining room I could tell something was wrong. Normally rosy and ebullient, Jackie was white as a sheet with deep circles under her eyes. Even her lips were pale.

"So you've been bleeding for two weeks?" I began.

"And my last period was two weeks before this one," she added. "Dr. Corio, I'm worn out."

I ran through my litany of questions and discovered that in the last year her cycles had been very erratic: occasionally she had experienced normal 28-day intervals, but she'd also had spotting in between periods. Now her periods were coming less than 21 days apart and she was bleeding very heavily, often passing clots.

"I'm going through a tampon sometimes every ten minutes," she told me. "At night I wear a super-plus and a maxi pad, and I still have to get up three or four times to change them. The worst is that I don't know when to expect my period anymore. We were having dinner in a restaurant recently and all of a sudden I was pouring blood—all over my white pants!"

When I asked whether she was on any medication, she reminded me that she took Synthroid because her thyroid functioning was low. I asked her when her thyroid was last tested and she said her internist had checked it a month ago and it was normal. I then took her vitals: her blood pressure was low, only 90/50, and her pulse was rapid, 100 beats per minute, a sign of a low blood count. Upon exam, her thyroid gland felt normal, as did her ovaries, although her uterus was slightly enlarged, possibly due to fibroids.

"Jackie, I'd like to do a biopsy of your uterus today," I said, "removing just a small sample of tissue to make sure everything is okay. It takes about ten seconds. You'll feel crampy while it's being done, but the cramps will pass and you'll be able to walk out of here like every other patient."

"Do I really need to have it, Dr. Corio?" she asked. I detected a note of fear in her voice.

"In anyone who bleeds as much as you are, I'm very concerned about pre-cancer of the uterus. You're in perimenopause and it looks as if you're making much too much oestrogen and no progesterone. That kind of imbalance is extremely dangerous.

"At the very least," I continued, "you could have fibroids that need to be taken care of." I explained that fully one-third of women who have symptoms like hers—extremely heavy and prolonged bleeding, breakthrough bleeding, or two or three periods less than 21 days apart—suffer a physical problem such as fibroids, polyps, or adenomyosis (endometriosis of the uterus).

I performed the endometrial biopsy, which is technically known as a Pipelle, removing a tiny amount of Jackie's endometrial tissue. This small sample enables me to detect pre-cancer or cancer of the uterus in a patient.

"I'm also going to need to take some blood," I said when the Pipelle was finished. "In addition to your hormone levels, I want to check your red blood cell count and ferritin level. I'm fairly certain you're anaemic—one of the reasons you're so pale and weak. In fact, I'd like you to start taking iron pills twice a day immediately along with your regular vitamin regimen."

"Any special brand?"

"No, although you may want to try slow-releasing iron if you're prone to constipation." I then proceeded to outline ways she could introduce more iron into her diet.

Before we were through, I recommended she have a transvaginal sonogram to rule out any physical problem that could be causing her excessive bleeding such as fibroids, polyps, adenomyosis, or cancer.

If a woman experiences bleeding between her periods and has polyps, she may need a full-fledged dilation and curettage (D&C). (For more on fibroids, endometriosis, adenomyosis, and uterine polyps, see Chapter 11.)

"Call me in the morning for the results of your blood tests," I said when we were through. "And don't worry," I added, touching her arm, "we'll have this under control in no time."

The next morning I received the results of Jackie's blood tests: HCG negative; TSH, free T_4, and prolactin normal; FSH 20 mlU/ml, slightly high; and LH normal. Her oestradiol was way up, as I suspected—160 pg/ml, and her progesterone was nonexistent. She was also anaemic.

I called Jackie with the results and explained that she was indeed in perimenopause and that she had stopped ovulating, so she was producing unopposed oestrogen. To balance it, I prescribed natural oral micronized progesterone, 200 mg in the morning, 200 mg in the evening, for 14 days starting immediately.

The next day I got the results of her Pipelle. I told Jackie she needed to come in to talk to me. When she arrived at the office, I explained that her biopsy showed simple hyperplasia without atypia, a worrisome condition of the uterus. She drew in her breath. "But by continuing the natural progesterone for three months straight without a break, I think we can counteract the effects of the unopposed oestrogen and bring your tissue back to normal."

"Okay, Dr. Corio," she responded bravely, but I could tell she was still frightened.

"Jackie, I've seen this problem a hundred times," I tried to reassure her. "We'll take another biopsy in a couple of months, after you've stopped the progesterone, and see how you're doing. Call me in a few weeks—I'd like to hear about your bleeding pattern." In the meantime, her transvaginal sonogram report came to my office and was normal.

Jackie's bleeding stopped about a week after she began the progesterone. She called when she'd finished the progesterone and told me she hadn't bled at all. I asked her to stay off the progesterone and return in two months so we could do a repeat biopsy.

"Well, you certainly look more like your old self," I commented when she returned. Her cheeks were pink and she looked well rested.

"I feel like my old self," she affirmed.

I did another Pipelle and took more blood for a red cell count. Both came back normal.

THE DANGER OF HEAVY, FREQUENT PERIODS

Always inform your doctor *immediately* if your periods are less than 21 days apart or significantly heavier or longer than normal, or if you have bleeding in between your periods. Whether or not you're ovulating, the excess oestrogen produced during the follicular phase when you experience heavy, frequent, or intermittent bleeding is opposed by little or no progesterone, putting you at high risk for breast, uterine, ovarian, and colon cancer. In one study, pre-cancerous or cancerous cell growths *(hyperplasia)* were found in 19 percent of women with these symptoms.

"Until you reach menopause," I told her over the phone, "I want to cycle you for the first ten days of every month on natural progesterone or put you on birth control pills to regulate your bleeding." I cautioned her to call me if any of her periods were shorter than 21 days or heavier or longer than normal—we didn't want this to reoccur.

Jackie chose to continue the natural progesterone. I told her to call me if she didn't get a period. When she came back to see me six months later she reported that she hadn't had a period in two months. We tested her hormone levels, and they showed she was now menopausal. We both breathed a sigh of relief.

WHEN YOU'RE BLEEDING TOO MUCH. If you've stopped ovulating, you may experience extremely heavy periods. This signals that you're undergoing only the follicular phase of your cycle, in which oestrogen levels rise. Because no follicle is being released, this may go on for longer than the normal 14 days and you may produce an excess of oestrogen, in turn stimulating an excess buildup of the uterine lining. When your oestrogen level finally drops, you'll experience heavy and prolonged bleeding.

Frequent, heavy, and intermittent bleeding may also occur if you ovulate but have weak corpus luteums that don't produce enough progesterone. In this case, both your follicular and luteal phases will be shortened, and you may experience heavy periods coming anywhere from a couple of days to a couple of weeks early. If your hormones are waxing and waning, every time your oestrogen and/or progesterone level drops you'll bleed, resulting in spotting or bleeding in between periods. This can occur whether or not you're ovulating.

WHEN SYMPTOMS SIGNAL TROUBLE

My rule of thumb is that if you're over age 35 and have any of the following symptoms, call your doctor immediately.

- if your periods are less than 21 days apart, from the first day of bleeding of one cycle to the first day of bleeding of the next cycle
- if your periods are extremely heavy (one pad or tampon an hour)
- if your periods are lasting longer than usual
- if you're having bleeding in between periods

In any of these cases, your doctor should perform an endometrial biopsy (Pipelle) and transvaginal sonogram to rule out pre-cancer of the uterus.

OTHER CAUSES OF ABNORMAL BLEEDING

Although by far the most common cause of abnormal vaginal bleeding during perimenopause is hormonal disorders, I always take a detailed medical history to rule out any other possible reasons for irregular bleeding. Pregnancy is the most obvious possible cause of skipped periods or spotting. And as I mentioned earlier, stress can cause you to stop menstruating as well.

Certain medications such as steroids, digoxin, psychotropic drugs, and anticholinergic drugs prescribed for neurological problems can affect the menstrual cycle, as can birth control pills, synthetic progesterone (progestogens) such as Norplant or Depo-Provera, or IUDs. Uterine lesions such as polyps, fibroids, adenomyosis (endometriosis in the uterus), and cancer may cause irregularities, as can diseases of the thyroid, liver, blood, and adrenal glands.

TREATMENT OPTIONS

The first strategies I suggest for minimizing any perimenopausal symptoms are a healthy diet and exercise (see Chapter 13 for details), a good multivitamin, natural vitamin E, vitamin D, and a calcium/

magnesium supplement daily. In addition, there are vitamins, herbs, foods, and natural and synthetic hormone products that alleviate particular bleeding problems. Medical and surgical treatments for abnormal bleeding are also available, although my preference is to try complementary approaches first, unless there's a physical problem.

Whichever approach they choose to take, my patients generally report back to me after two months how their symptoms are being controlled. Frequently we have to make adjustments to their treatment, but it is usually possible for patients to get relief from their abnormal perimenopausal bleeding.

Vitamins and Minerals

IRON. Anaemia is a concern in women who experience frequent and/or heavy periods. In addition to increasing iron intake in the diet, I recommend a daily iron supplement (28 mg). The ferrous sulphate form is best absorbed and should be taken alone on an empty stomach with vitamin C. Your doctor should check your red blood cell count and ferritin level periodically to see if you need to increase the dose. *Caution: only take iron if you have iron-deficiency anaemia, otherwise you might overload your liver.*

VITAMINS B_6 AND B_{12} AND FOLIC ACID. In addition to helping with anaemia, the B complex vitamins will enhance your mood if you are suffering premenstrual symptoms. The B vitamins elevate progesterone and suppress oestrogen, which is necessary if your periods are too heavy. If your multivitamin doesn't contain 50 to 100 mg B_6, 50 to 100 mcg B_{12}, and 400 mcg folic acid, take an additional supplement.

NATURAL VITAMIN E. Vitamin E is an antioxidant that can help protect against cancer. It is also an oestrogen inhibitor, helping to balance out the high levels of unopposed oestrogen that can put you at risk for cancer. Take 400 to 800 IU a day of natural vitamin E.

CALCIUM. Studies have shown that calcium reduces premenstrual symptoms; indeed, a new theory suggests that PMS may actually be caused by a calcium deficiency. I recommend 1,200 mg daily in two 600 mg doses.

MAGNESIUM. Magnesium is wonderful for relieving PMS symptoms as well—especially your chocolate craving. You should always take magnesium with calcium, as the two minerals depend on each other. To activate 1,200 mg calcium you need 600 mg magnesium. Also, taking magnesium with your calcium helps prevent constipation.

Herbs

I've found herbal treatments to be very effective with my perimenopausal patients. But before you try any of the following, consult your doctor. In some cases it may be okay to combine herbs, but in certain cases combinations can be dangerous. I also recommend taking tablets that have been made by a reputable manufacturer, as you want to be sure that you're getting the correct dose.

EVENING PRIMROSE OIL. This is my top pick for an herb to relieve menstrual problems. It contains gamma linoleic acid (GLA), a perfect omega-6 fatty acid for humans. GLA is a building block of prostaglandins, substances that increase hormone synthesis, therefore raising progesterone levels and helping with bleeding abnormalities, PMS symptoms, and menstrual pain. Take 1,000 to 3,000 mg daily.

BLACK COHOSH (REMIFEMIN). This herb has been used for centuries by the Algonquian Indians to treat gynaecological problems. A vasodilator, it is an excellent menstruation promoter. It also contains phytoestrogens, which alleviate a host of perimenopausal symptoms, including irregular and painful bleeding. Take one Remifemin pill in the morning and one in the evening.

CHASTEBERRY (VITEX). Used historically to regularize abnormal bleeding patterns, ease menopausal symptoms, and treat amenorrhoea, chasteberry raises LH levels—thereby raising progesterone levels and protecting against unopposed oestrogen. The recommended dose is 10 mg chasteberry seeds three times a day.

LIQUORICE (DGL). This may have steroidal effects and act as an antiinflammatory agent, like aspirin or ibuprofen, to reduce cramps and heavy bleeding. It also contains phytoestrogens and oestriol, a form of oestrogen, so it is generally beneficial to perimenopausal women. Take 500 mg daily, unless you have high blood pressure or kidney or liver disease, in which case you should steer clear.

Foods

Omega-3 fatty acids, which are found in dark-fleshed fish and flaxseed, have been shown to relieve menstrual pain. Try to eat 2 to 3 servings of fatty fish a week or 3 to 5 tablespoons (25 to 50 g) freshly ground flaxseed daily. Alternatively, you can take six 1,000 mg fish oil capsules a day.

Phytoestrogens

When patients come to me in full-blown perimenopause who have decreased oestrogen and progesterone levels and are experiencing shortened menstrual cycles (i.e., shortened luteal phases), I suggest they incorporate more soy products into their diets.

SOY. Soy contains isoflavones (a type of phytoestrogen or plant oestrogen), which lengthen the luteal phase (the second half of the cycle). As an added benefit, soy can alleviate other menopausal symptoms such as hot flushes and mood swings. Try to incorporate up to 50 mg soy isoflavones in your diet daily through food, not supplements or powders. In Appendix B you'll find a chart in which I delineate foods that are best for providing soy isoflavones.

By contrast, I tell patients with high oestrogen levels who are experiencing heavy bleeding, fibroids, or endometriosis to avoid soy, as it will only worsen their condition.

Medical Treatments

To regulate hormone levels and control abnormal bleeding, you may need to take medicine or supplements of progesterone and/or oestrogen. You have several options.

PROGESTERONE THERAPY. Natural progesterone counteracts the effects of excessive oestrogen in anovulatory women, relieving PMS symptoms and painful periods. Derived from Mexican wild yams and

soybeans, natural progesterone is the exact duplicate of the progesterone that occurs in the body, so is much easier to tolerate than synthetic progestogen supplements like Provera or Depo-Provera. I prefer
treating my patients with natural progesterone such as prescription 5
percent progesterone cream, oral micronized progesterone (OMP), or
progesterone suppositories.

LOW-DOSE BIRTH CONTROL PILLS. Containing 20 to 35 mcg oestrogen as well as synthetic progestogen, low-dose pills can reduce
menstrual blood flow by 60 percent in women with a normal uterus,
thereby regulating abnormal bleeding patterns and correcting iron-
deficiency anaemia. The pill can also alleviate perimenopausal symptoms such as painful or heavy periods, cramps, bloating, and breast
soreness. It will cause you to have lighter periods every 28 days
like clockwork, and it will reduce problems associated with fibroids
and endometriosis. Going on the pill will also prevent pregnancy
and reduce your risk of uterine, ovarian, and colon cancer—an added
bonus.

MEDICATED IUDS. Containing a slow-releasing progestogen, medicated IUDs are indicated for women with extremely heavy bleeding.
After one year of use, they have been shown to reduce blood loss by
97 percent.

**NONSTEROIDAL ANTI-INFLAMMATORY DRUGS OR ANTI-
PROSTAGLANDINS.** These drugs are often prescribed to reduce menstrual flow. Taking 500 mg of Ponstan (mefenamic acid) tablets twice a
day for three days beginning on the first day of the period has been
shown to reduce bleeding by 30 to 50 percent. Over-the-counter
anti-inflammatory agents to ask your doctor about include Advil,
Neurofen, or generic ibuprofen.

NATURAL OESTROGEN. If you have scanty periods, I recommend
natural oestrogen in order to stabilize your uterine lining. Along with
it, I always prescribe natural progesterone. There are a variety of natural oestrogen products—patches, creams, gels, and pills—on the market today (see Appendix C for a fuller description). Taking a low dose
of natural hormones may be enough to correct your bleeding until
you reach menopause.

KEEP IN MIND

Although abnormal bleeding is a common feature of the perimenopausal years, because this time of life coincides with an increased risk of certain diseases, you should report any changes in your cycle to your healthcare practitioner. In addition:

- Keep track of your periods with a menstrual chart (see page 26).
- Call your doctor if your periods are less than 21 days apart, or heavier or longer than usual, or if you experience bleeding between periods.
- Call your doctor if your periods are more than 60 days apart.
- Make sure your doctor is aware of any alternative treatments—vitamins, minerals, and/or herbs—you are taking to treat your perimenopausal symptoms.

ZOLADEX. A GnRH agonist, Zoladex is a medication that is given to stop your period for a length of time, making you essentially postmenopausal. I would advise using it if you have fibroids that are causing abnormal bleeding and making you anaemic. Not only will it shrink the fibroids, but it will also build up your blood count. The downside is that because it completely stops oestrogen and progesterone production in your body, it puts you at risk for osteoporosis. Therefore it shouldn't be used for longer than six months and should be prescribed along with a calcium/magnesium supplement. (See Chapter 11 for more on fibroids and Zoladex.)

Surgical Treatments

If your excessive bleeding cannot be controlled by any of the options already mentioned and your doctor has ruled out any organic pathology such as polyps, fibroids, adenomyosis, or cancer, then you have two remaining choices. *Hysterectomy*—surgical removal of the uterus—is the traditional, failsafe route. It can be performed vaginally, abdominally, or laparoscopically (through tiny incisions in the abdomen). Over the past few years a new form of laser surgery called *endometrial ablation* has gained popularity. In this case the surgeon burns off the endometrium, the lining of the uterus from which you bleed.

Endometrial ablation has an 80 to 90 percent success rate—not quite as good as hysterectomy, which is 100 percent effective. However, more and more women are choosing endometrial ablation because they have a reduced hospital stay, rapid recovery, and reduced postoperative discomfort owing to the fact that they have avoided major abdominal surgery. (For more on surgical treatment of gynaecological problems, see Chapter 11.)

CHAPTER 3

Can Somebody Open a Window?
Hot Flushes, Insomnia, and Other Joys

"I wake up in the middle of the night in a puddle of sweat. My head is so soaked that I have to blow-dry my hair! I change the sheets, change my nightgown, and by that time I'm so upset I can't get back to sleep."

"I went to the dentist and the hygienist asked me if I'd just come from the gym—my hair was all matted and my skin was all flushed."

"It was so embarrassing—I was wearing this beautiful silk blouse and all of a sudden it was drenched. Now I only wear cotton and always carry an extra shirt in my bag."

"I'm sitting in an important meeting with all these people and I'm sweating and turning purple and feel like everyone's looking at me."

Sound familiar? One of the most commonly reported symptoms of perimenopause, hot flushes affect up to 80 percent of women between the ages of 40 and 50, generally for between one and five years. While many women associate hot flushes with menopause, a full 75 percent of women experience hot flushes as early as five years *before* their periods stop, although hot flushes do become more frequent in later perimenopause.

Depending on the frequency and severity of your episodes, hot flushes can be a minor annoyance or a major issue. Some women can keep them under control simply by wearing layers of light clothes and avoiding triggers such as spicy foods. Others experience such overwhelming attacks that they develop anxiety and insomnia, leading to a whole host of other problems.

A hot flush can be a frightening experience, not only because your body seems to be totally out of control but also because the hot flush can occur at any time, in any place, with no predictable pattern or warning. Most of my patients with hot flushes find them extremely stressful, which to me is reason enough to seek relief. Who needs more stress, especially at our time of life? Overall, one-third of women get medical treatment for their hot flushes.

Hot flushes are closely related to two other common perimenopausal complaints, insomnia and heart palpitations, and my patients often come to me with at least two of the three. The common link is the brain: the hormones and chemicals it produces affect your temperature, your sleep cycle, and your heart rhythm. Worrying only makes these kinds of symptoms worse, because stress has a direct effect on brain chemistry. So in addition to recommending a variety of complementary and medical treatments, I find that educating my patients about what they're experiencing not only helps put their mind at ease but actually eases their symptoms.

WHAT EXACTLY IS A HOT FLUSH AND WHERE DOES IT COME FROM?

If you're lucky enough never to have had a hot flush, here's a description of what you're missing. A hot flush is a sensation of intense heat felt in your upper body, arms, and face that can last several seconds to several minutes, usually followed by profuse sweating and, sometimes, chills. The temperature of your skin becomes elevated by about 7 degrees, while your heart rate increases by 10 to 15 percent. Some women experience hot flushes only rarely, whereas others suffer episodes every 10 to 30 minutes. Some women sweat so much that they look like they've just taken a shower, whereas others hardly register that they're experiencing a hot flush until they realize they're wearing T-shirts to the office in January.

Hot flushes occur when the blood vessels dilate and constrict in an irregular pattern (vasomotor instability). They are frequently associated with nausea, heart palpitations, dizziness, numbness, and tingling in the arms, hands, and fingers. They're worse during times of stress and at night, when they can cause or contribute to an already existing case of perimenopausal insomnia. They can also exacerbate feelings of fatigue, irritability, panic, anxiety, and depression. While not life-threatening, hot flushes can wear you out physically, mentally, and emotionally— reason enough to take them seriously.

Although we still don't know what exactly triggers hot flushes, the prevailing wisdom is that they occur when fluctuating oestrogen levels in the brain throw the body's thermoregulatory system out of whack. Generally, your body has a set point temperature of around 98.6° F that is matched by your body's core temperature. Under certain circumstances your hypothalamus gland, the area in your brain that controls thermoregulation, changes that set point and produces chemical signals that tell your body to heat up or cool down.

For example, when your hypothalamus is exposed to a fever-causing agent, your set point is readjusted to a higher level. Until your body's core temperature heats up to this new level, you'll feel cold, which is why you get chills when you have a fever. Your blood vessels constrict in order to minimize heat loss, and you start shivering in order to warm yourself up.

During a hot flush, the exact opposite occurs. Low oestrogen causes your set point to drop suddenly, and to adjust your core temperature to this new level, your body must release heat. Your blood vessels will rise to the surface and dilate, causing your skin to flush and become warm. You also begin perspiring in order to cool yourself down.

Simple enough, right? Well, almost. The truth is that oestrogen doesn't just go knocking at the door of your hypothalamus saying, "Turn the thermostat down!" Other molecules, called neurotransmitters, actually mediate the message. Because these chemical messengers play such an important role in causing not only hot flushes, insomnia, and heart palpitations but also mood changes, memory loss, and other cognitive symptoms discussed in Chapter 4, I'd like to take a moment now to introduce some of them to you.

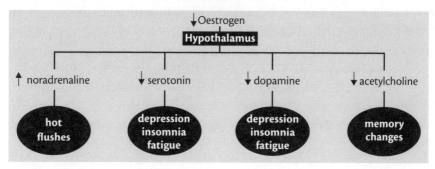

THE BRAIN/BODY CONNECTION

In response to declining oestrogen levels, the hypothalamus increases production of noradrenaline, but decreases production of three other key neurotransmitters.

THE WONDERFUL WORLD OF NEUROTRANSMITTERS

The brain is a fascinating, complex organ made up of billions of what Agatha Christie's fictional sleuth Hercule Poirot was fond of calling "little gray cells." These nerve cells, or neurons, are highly organized into networks that allow for the processing and storage of information. When they need to communicate with each other, either because they're taking in sensory data from the great outdoors or retrieving it so that you can act on it, they rely on chemical messengers called neurotransmitters. As the name implies, neurotransmitters transmit signals from one neuron to another.

The thermoregulatory center of the hypothalamus gland in the brain releases four different neurotransmitters. First and foremost in terms of hot flushes is *noradrenaline,* a stress hormone. When your oestrogen level declines, your hypothalamus steps up production of noradrenaline. Noradrenaline acts directly on your thermoregulatory center, helping to lower your set point and thereby causing a hot flush.

About one minute before the onset of a hot flush, you may experience an aura that gives you a little advance warning. Out of nowhere you may have a sense of anxiety or dread, feel suddenly weak, or experience an increased heart rate. All these stress symptoms are caused by the release of noradrenaline.

Serotonin and *dopamine,* neurotransmitters best known for affecting mood, are produced by the hypothalamus as well. In addition to their important emotional functions, both of these neurotransmitters are involved in the reproductive system and are affected by shifting oestrogen levels during perimenopause. When your oestrogen levels decline, your serotonin and dopamine levels do, too. Lowered levels of serotonin and dopamine can contribute to perimenopausal depression, insomnia, and fatigue.

Last but not least, *acetylcholine* is a neurotransmitter essential to establishing the neural networks in the brain early in life. Acetylcholine is critical for learning, memory, and spatial reasoning. Oestrogen helps maintain the production of acetylcholine, so when your oestrogen levels decline in perimenopause, so do your acetylcholine levels. Therefore, you may experience memory changes (see Chapter 4). Acetylcholine is derived from choline, one of the B complex vitamins.

WHEN A HOT FLUSH ISN'T PERIMENOPAUSE

Although it seems that hot flushes and menopause go hand in hand, you can have hot flushes at any time during your reproductive life. Women with chronic hormonal imbalances or who have severe PMS or who have just given birth may experience hot flushes, too. There are also numerous other conditions that can cause hot flushes, including thyroid disease, psychosomatic stress reactions, and fever, as well as some more uncommon yet serious medical conditions.

Recently a new patient, 41 years old, came to see me for a routine checkup. She mentioned that she was experiencing light but crampy periods and fairly severe hot flushes and asked whether I thought she was going into menopause. Listening to her medical history, I wasn't at all certain. An insulin-dependent diabetic since age 30, she also suffered from a metabolic disease called MELAS that was causing progressive cerebral degeneration. She was losing her hearing and had experienced several small strokelike episodes. I prescribed evening primrose oil and my vitamin regimen for her menstrual symptoms and told her I'd like to check her hormone levels on the third day of her period. The results were perfectly normal, making it difficult for me to diagnose perimenopause. My gut feeling was that most likely her hot flushes were related to her brain disorder, so I told her to check back with her neurologist to see if he agreed with me. He did. Nevertheless, because evening primrose oil influences the brain to boost hormone levels, she did experience relief from her symptoms.

Other diseases that may cause hot flushes include nonmalignant tumors of the gastrointestinal tract, ovaries, lungs, and thyroid gland. All these tumors produce serotonin, one of the neurotransmitters

DRUGS THAT MAY CAUSE HOT FLUSHES

Certain medications and drugs can cause hot flushes by influencing the thermoregulatory system in the brain. These include:

- vasodilators such as nitroglycerin and prostaglandins
- calcium channel blockers such as nifedipine, verapamil, and diltiazem
- anti-seizure medications such as phenytoin, Tegretol, and Valium
- morphine and other opiates
- recreational drugs such as amyl nitrite and butyl nitrite
- cholinergic drugs such as metrifonate and anthelminthic
- bromocriptine, used to treat Parkinson's disease and pituitary adenoma
- tamoxifen, used to treat breast cancer
- Evista, used to treat and prevent postmenopausal osteoporosis
- oral triamcinolone, used to treat psoriatic arthritis
- cyclosporine
- Clomid, used to treat infertility

produced by the hypothalamus. Serotonin imbalance probably causes the hot flushes associated with these conditions. Brain disorders or tumors, pancreatic islet-cell tumors, as well as malignant tumors of the thyroid and kidney, also cause hot flushes. In these cases, other chemical triggers are suspected to set off the reaction.

Because neurotransmitters are the major controllers of the thermoregulatory system, any condition that affects neurotransmitter levels or neural pathways can cause flushes. These include emotional and psychological conditions ranging from simple embarrassment to more severe anxiety disorders, as well as diseases such as Parkinson's and multiple sclerosis. Spinal cord injury, hypertension, and migraine headaches are also potential causes.

Alcohol, smoking, spicy foods, and food additives can all cause hot flushes. Even something as simple as drinking a hot beverage can trigger a thermoregulatory adjustment. Eating a big meal can set one off as digestion diverts blood to the abdomen, therefore raising the core body temperature. Hot tubs, overheated rooms, steamy weather, strenuous exercise, overdressing, and sleeping with too many blankets have the potential to precipitate hot flushes as well.

CAROL—THE EFFECTS OF ALCOHOL

Carol came to me for the first time about a year ago on the recommendation of her aunt, who's been a patient of mine for years. When I opened the examining-room door I encountered an extremely thin, extremely made-up woman. She was dressed conservatively yet expensively in a tailored olive-green pants suit and beige silk blouse.

After we'd introduced ourselves, she plunged right in. "Dr. Corio, I am miserable. I'm having these weird symptoms. My joints are killing me, I feel tired and weak, but the worst of it is these hot flushes."

"Why don't you give me some background on your health before we begin the exam," I said, taking a seat.

In eliciting her history, I found that she had "a bit of a problem" with alcohol. She had been drinking one to two bottles of wine a day for the past twenty years. She also revealed that she went to her internist a year ago and was diagnosed with hepatitis C.

"Have you ever gone to AA? Have you ever been able to stop drinking?" I asked.

"I've tried, but it just doesn't work for me," she answered.

Carol said she was 40 years old and had smoked a pack a day since she was 15. She was married, her husband was a consultant who worked sporadically, she didn't work, and they lived a leisurely life traveling to exotic places. I casually asked if her husband also drank.

"Yes," she replied, "but not like me."

"And how are your periods? Have you noticed any changes?"

"Yes, they're coming less frequently. They're sort of unpredictable."

Beneath Carol's make-up I could see the damage years of abuse had wreaked on her skin. Her eyes, too, were filled with pain. "I'm going to give you a thorough exam," I said, "then we'll do a full workup and then we'll do some tests to see if you're going through perimenopause. But Carol," I continued, "alcohol alone could explain your hot flushes."

Carol came in for her blood test on the third day of her next period. The results showed that her FSH was elevated at 26 mlU/ml, her LH was slightly elevated at 17 mlU/ml, and her oestrogen was slightly elevated at 78 mlU/ml. Her liver enzymes, predictably, were off the charts.

"It looks as if you're entering perimenopause," I told her, "but the reason your hot flushes are so bad is because on top of that the alcohol is giving you a double whammy."

"Is there nothing I can do?" she asked.

"Normally I prescribe oestrogen," I replied, "but with your liver disease, it's contraindicated. Because oestrogen is metabolized by the liver, if the liver is not functioning normally, the buildup could be dangerous. Ask your liver specialist if natural progesterone is okay, or Depo-Provera shots. Of course," I continued, "if there were any way you could curtail the drinking, you'd feel a lot better."

Before Carol left, I pleaded with her to see a rehabilitation physician I knew to try to get into recovery. "Here's his number," I said, handing her a slip of paper. "I'll call him as well so he'll expect your call. Please do this—I'm so very worried about you."

"Okay, Dr. Corio," Carol said. As soon as she left the room, I phoned the rehab center.

Carol's liver specialist gave her the go-ahead to try progesterone, and within a month Carol's hot flushes had improved. Unfortunately, she never called the rehab center, and today her alcoholism and liver disease are worse than ever.

FINDING RELIEF FROM HOT FLUSHES

Good news—you don't have to suffer in sweaty silence. My patients have come up with all kinds of ingenious ideas for handling hot flushes.

FOODS TO AVOID IF YOU'RE HAVING HOT FLUSHES

Food can be a major hot-flush trigger. Basically, if it's hot—temperature-wise or spice-wise—it'll make you flush. Certain chemicals in foods can also set you sweating. Steer clear of the following:

- spicy foods, especially those containing capsaicin, the active ingredient in chili peppers
- chocolate
- lemon
- hot liquids
- caffeinated beverages
- monosodium glutamate (MSG)
- sodium nitrate, found in cured meats such as hot dogs, bacon, salami, and ham
- sulphites, found in red wine, dried fruits, and cheddar cheese

One tells me she packs a battery-operated misting fan in her pocketbook and whips it out whenever she feels a flush coming on. Another has taken up yoga to reduce her stress level. A number of them are now into the layered look, because it allows them to peel off pieces of clothing when their temperature starts to rise. Sometimes simple lifestyle changes like these are all you need to keep hot flushes at bay.

If your hot flushes aren't responding to dietary and behavioral changes, there are a number of complementary and medical alternatives you can try. I usually start by recommending a regimen of vitamins, herbs, and exercise, and then if that doesn't work, move on to hormone supplements.

Vitamins

NATURAL VITAMIN E. In addition to being a powerful antioxidant, vitamin E prevents excess FSH and LH production. I recommend 400 to 800 IU natural vitamin E for hot flushes; but remember, it can take 2 to 6 weeks to be effective. Unfortunately, its effects wear off—sometimes it only works for a few months.

VITAMINS B$_6$, B$_{12}$, AND FOLIC ACID. Your body metabolizes B complex vitamins under stress, so it's especially important to maintain a sufficient level during this symptomatic time. In addition, vitamin B$_6$ raises your levels of acetylcholine, one of the neurotransmitters active in the thermoregulatory center, helping to protect against hot flushes. If your multivitamin doesn't contain 50 to 100 mg B$_6$, 50 to 100 mcg B$_{12}$, and 400 mcg folic acid, take an additional supplement.

Herbs

EVENING PRIMROSE OIL. I recommend trying 1,000 to 3,000 mg a day of evening primrose oil, which is rich in gamma linoleic acid (GLA), an omega-6 fatty acid that regulates hormone levels. Patients have reported back to me that it works in the short term, but eventually its effects diminish.

BLACK COHOSH (REMIFEMIN). This contains phytoestrogens and other compounds that act directly on the pituitary gland to suppress LH levels. It relieves hot flushes in 85 percent of patients within 6 to 8 weeks. I've had great success recommending one Remifemin pill in the morning and one at night.

Phytoestrogens

In Japan, where women eat a diet high in soybean products and ingest an average of 200 mg phytoestrogens a day, hot flushes are virtually unheard of. But when Japanese women move to the UK and adopt a Western diet with low intake of phytoestrogens, they report hot flushes and other perimenopausal symptoms nearly as often as native-born British women do. What's the difference? Soy!

SOY. Soybeans contain high amounts of isoflavones, particularly genistein and daidzein, plant-based oestrogens that mimic oestradiol. A recent study of 104 postmenopausal Italian women showed that a daily dose of 60 g soy protein (76 mg isoflavones) taken for 12 weeks reduced their hot flushes by 45 percent. To get relief from hot flushes, I recommend up to 50 mg isoflavones daily from food sources, not supplements or powders (see Appendix B).

Activities

EXERCISE. The burn of a good workout can also help alleviate the burn of hot flushes. The frequency of hot flushes may be affected by levels of circulating opiates, brain chemicals that increase feelings of vitality and are responsible for the "runner's high" some joggers experience. Decreasing oestrogen lowers your opiate levels, which in turn raise your noradrenaline and increase your hot flushes. To counteract this, vigorous aerobic exercise during perimenopause boosts your production of opiates.

A study of over 1,600 Swedish women found hot flushes to be only half as common among those who were physically active as among those in the control group. For this reason, as well as for weight maintenance and cardiovascular health, I recommend patients do at least 30 minutes of aerobic exercise three times a week. Try to schedule your exercise for early in the day or at lunchtime. Exercise should not be performed within five hours of bedtime or else it may contribute to insomnia, which I'll discuss in more detail shortly. Also, some women find that extremely vigorous exercise contributes to their hot flushes. If this is the case, don't stop exercising—just modify your routine.

SEX. There is a fascinating correlation between increased hot flushes and decreased sexual activity, suggesting that regular intercourse may actually protect against hot flushes. Unfortunately, sex may not be high on your list of priorities for reasons I'll discuss in Chapter 5. If you are feeling in the mood, however, go for it—doctor's orders!

Medical Treatments

CLONIDINE. Clonidine, which reduces noradrenaline levels in the brain, has been shown to reduce hot flushes by 50 percent. Although some doctors still recommend it, I don't because it is habit forming and sedating, and it causes undesirable side effects such as insomnia and dizziness.

OESTROGEN. For perimenopausal women, oestrogen is the number-one way to relieve hot flushes. As long as there are adequate oestrogen levels in your brain, your thermoregulatory system will keep running smoothly. A very good choice for perimenopausal women who have

HYSTERECTOMY AND HOT FLUSHES

Women who undergo hysterectomies and have their ovaries removed (surgical menopause) experience an acute drop in hormone levels and dramatic hot flushes. If you are willing to go on hormone replacement therapy immediately postoperatively, you may avoid hot flushes, especially if you take testosterone along with oestrogen supplements. If you undergo a hysterectomy but your ovaries are preserved, you should go through a normal perimenopause. In this case you may or may not experience hot flushes, but if you do they probably won't be as severe as they would be if you had your ovaries removed.

fluctuating oestrogen levels and do not want to go on full-fledged hormone replacement therapy is the *low-dose transdermal natural oestradiol patch*. The patch delivers 0.025 mg oestradiol and has been shown to work in 84 percent of cases. Another good choice is *low-dose birth control pills* (20 to 35 mcg oestrogen), because they not only provide contraception but also reduce symptoms such as hot flushes. *Standard oestrogen replacement therapy*, whether natural or synthetic, plus natural progesterone relieves hot flushes in 95 percent of cases.

PROGESTOGENS. In cases when I haven't been able to prescribe oestrogen, such as when a patient has breast or uterine cancer, I've treated hot flushes with progestogens and had very good results. Progestogens help stabilize the thermoregulatory set point. A 200 mg shot of Depo-Provera given intramuscularly every other month relieves 90 percent of hot flushes.

NATURAL PROGESTERONE. Progesterone stabilizes the neurotransmitters in the hypothalamus and suppresses both FSH and LH, thereby relieving hot flushes. Natural progesterone is only available as a suppository or injection in the UK.

TESTOSTERONE. Adding androgens such as testosterone to oestrogen therapy may relieve difficult-to-treat hot flushes. In the brain, testosterone is converted to oestradiol, thereby increasing an oestrogen supplement's potency right where you need it most. By adding testosterone to the mix, you therefore don't have to take such a high dose of oestrogen.

SELECTIVE SEROTONIN REUPTAKE INHIBITORS (SSRIS). SSRI antidepressants such as Seroxat, Prozac, Effexor, and Lustral may be an effective way to decrease hot flushes in patients who cannot take oestrogen. Recent studies on breast cancer survivors showed a 67 percent reduction in frequency and 75 percent reduction in severity of hot flushes among women taking Seroxat and similar improvements in women taking the other SSRIs. It seems that the optimal dose is half the amount normally used to treat depression.

INSOMNIA

One of the questions I routinely ask patients in their thirties and up is whether they have insomnia. "I haven't slept well for years" is the most common reply. And most of them are not just being facetious. Once you've had children and dealt with years of midnight feedings, bedwettings, and nightmares, you may find it difficult if not impossible to regain a normal sleeping pattern. Part of the problem may be that you're segueing directly from child-induced insomnia to midlife insomnia without having a chance to catch a good night's sleep in between.

There is some scientific debate about whether or not insomnia is a symptom of perimenopause. However, women who suffer hot flushes and have to get up two, three, or four times a night to change their soaking nightgowns and pillowcases would testify on the positive side. In addition, I've seen many patients without hot flushes whose sleep patterns changed for the worse when their FSH levels began to rise and then improved when they began hormone treatment, indicating a direct link between insomnia and perimenopause.

Alex, a 38-year-old patient of mine, is a perfect example. As I was walking out the door of the exam room after her routine annual visit, having finished talking with her, she said, "Oh, by the way, I forgot to tell you about an ongoing problem, Dr. C. I've been having this terrible insomnia and I've seen many doctors about it. In fact, I've had a total workup at the Columbia Presbyterian Sleep Disorders Clinic and they can't figure out why I can't sleep."

"Has anyone mentioned perimenopause to you?" I asked, shutting the door behind me again.

"Peri what?" she said, with a perplexed look on her face.

I took my seat once more and launched into my spiel about perimenopause. When I was through, I said, "Let's draw your blood on the third day of your period and see where you're at in terms of hormones. I know you're young, but we could be surprised."

Alex came back for her blood test, and the results were close to the menopausal range. "I think we may have figured out what's causing your insomnia. Maybe we should try some natural oestrogen and natural progesterone and see if you improve." Within two months Alex phoned to tell me her sleeping pattern had improved substantially.

Perimenopause aside, sleep disturbances generally increase with age. One-third of American adults—men as well as women—report trouble falling asleep or staying asleep, and as many as 17 percent of the adults in the United States are severe insomniacs. So when women report insomnia during their perimenopausal years, it's difficult to prove whether their condition is hormone related or merely a natural effect of the aging process.

Overall, however, women have higher rates of sleep disturbance than men in every stage of life. Women also show a dramatic increase in sleep problems in the perimenopausal years—increasing from about 36 percent reporting insomnia at age 30 to 50 percent at age 54, suggesting a connection. And recent research has identified biochemical pathways that may predispose perimenopausal women to insomnia.

Deep sleep is associated with the release of human growth hormone, which is produced by that very busy hypothalamus gland. Production of growth hormone peaks during adolescence—one of the reasons teenagers can sleep until noon or later; from then on, it's downhill. Most people begin to notice a deterioration in the quality of their sleep beginning in their late thirties; by their sixties, as circulating growth hormone levels approach zero, so does their experience of deep sleep. A common pattern of disturbed sleep includes taking longer to fall asleep—from an average of 8 to 10 minutes to up to half an hour—as well as one or more waking episodes lasting an hour or two during the night.

Without the restorative effects of sleep, we become vulnerable to illness. Shift workers, for example, have higher rates of gastrointestinal and cardiovascular disease as well as depression and infertility than does the general population. In addition, the effects of sleep deprivation impair memory and concentration—the reason why night-shift work and long-distance trucking are associated with increased risk of accidents—as well as causing anxiety and emotional volatility (see Chapter 4 for a fuller discussion).

A fascinating study of the metabolic effects of sleep deprivation on young men recently performed at the University of Chicago showed that sleep deprivation can actually hasten the aging process. Eleven young men were subjected to different amounts of sleep over sixteen consecutive nights. After six nights of being allowed to sleep only four hours per night, they showed signs of insulin resistance, a metabolic change that contributes to a host of serious health problems including obesity, hypertension, heart disease, and impaired kidney function (for more on insulin resistance, see Chapter 6). They also suffered memory problems because their brains were not absorbing enough glucose. After the subjects were allowed to stay in bed twelve hours a night for the next seven nights, during which they averaged more than nine hours of sleep, their metabolisms recovered.

Other hormonal changes can contribute to sleep problems as well. In women with hot-flush–related insomnia, waking episodes actually begin during the same immediate pre-flush period when they might experience an aura. Although most women think sweating and chills are what wakes them up, it seems that their insomnia is in fact a result of the same chemical changes in the brain that trigger the flush. In other words, they're waking up *before* they feel the heat. Studies have shown that when oestrogen is administered to control hot flushes, waking episodes decrease as well.

In addition, women often find themselves having to get up one or more times in the middle of the night to urinate, which prevents them from getting a good night's sleep. One reason for these urges may be that changes in the urinary tract caused by declining oestrogen levels can lead to frequent urination, a subject I'll discuss in detail in Chapter 5. Another theory suggests that the problem is not lowered oestrogen levels but an age-related disturbance in the antidiuretic hormone system in the brain, which normally suppresses the urge to urinate during sleep.

When I prescribe oestrogen supplements to perimenopausal women suffering mood changes, their insomnia often resolves itself as well. The reason most likely has to do with the neurotransmitter

---

WHEN YOU WISH YOU COULD SLEEP ALL DAY

Even if you're getting a good night's sleep, you may still feel fatigued. Many of my perimenopausal patients complain that they can hardly make it through the day. "I got my sons off to school this morning," one recently told me, "and then I just crawled back into bed." Hormones can help. I prescribed her a low-dose natural oestrogen patch and oral micronized progesterone, and within two weeks she said she was back to her old self.

---

dopamine, which increases when oestrogen levels go up and decreases in perimenopause, when oestrogen and human growth hormone levels go down. Dopamine affects the circadian rhythm, the internal clock that synchronizes bodily functions with the external environment. Depressed people, who, like perimenopausal women, have decreased circulating dopamine, also suffer sleep disturbances, particularly a pattern of early-morning awakening.

Patients often ask whether I recommend melatonin to help regulate their disturbed sleep patterns. I tell them it's very controversial, so I prefer not to. Melatonin, which also influences the body's circadian rhythm, is produced by the pineal gland in the brain when the eyes sense darkness approaching. As you age, you naturally produce less. Although melatonin supplements have been championed as a panacea for innumerable ills, including sleep disturbances ranging from jet lag to serious insomnia, scientists generally dismiss its curative properties as medically unfounded except in cases of jet lag.

MAUREEN—INSOMNIA AND HOT FLUSHES

"I can't take it anymore. I just can't take it."

I was sitting opposite Maureen, a longtime patient. A 48-year-old kindergarten teacher and mother of two young children, Maureen was generally an oasis of calm. In her dependable tartan skirts and flats, she was normally soft spoken and well groomed. On this day, however, she looked like a rag—completely wiped out. Her voice was shaking, her face was haggard, and her usually impeccable posture had deteriorated to a slump.

"Every night I get these awful waves of heat that wake me up every hour on the hour," she continued. "In the morning I feel like I've been fighting all night. I'm drenched, I'm anxious, I'm not myself. During the day I can't keep up with the kids at school, much less my own when I come home. Isn't there something you can give me to stop this flushing? I have to get some sleep, Doctor C. I have to get some sleep!"

"You poor thing!" I sympathized. "I'm going to check your thyroid, because if it's overactive it could be making you hot and anxious all the time." I palpated her thyroid gland, and it felt normal. "Are you on any medications, or have you changed your diet or routine in a way that may be causing you not to sleep?"

"No. What's causing me not to sleep is that I wake up every hour drenched with sweat," she replied with an uncharacteristic note of sarcasm.

"Okay," I said. "How are your periods?"

"Maybe a little shorter than usual, but basically regular—every 30, 31 days."

"I'd like to check your hormone levels. Even though your bleeding pattern hasn't changed, this crazy flushing makes me think you might be entering perimenopause. I want you to come for a blood test on the third day of your next period. In the meantime, let's talk about vitamins and herbs that can help control your hot flushes." I proceeded to tell her about black cohosh (Remifemin) and evening primrose oil, and I instructed her to take a natural vitamin E supplement and increase her intake of soy as well. "Until we know for sure that your oestrogen levels are decreased, I don't want to give you supplements, even though they work a lot faster than the herbs, which take a month to kick in."

Five days later Maureen came in for her blood test. The next day, just as I was reading the lab results, she phoned the office in tears. "Give me the drugs," she begged. "I can't go through another night of this."

"As I figured, your blood test showed elevated FSH and decreased oestrogen," I told her. "I'm going to put you on a low-dose natural oestrogen patch. Normally I don't prescribe oestrogen without progesterone in a woman who still has a uterus. But this is an extremely small amount of oestrogen—half the amount in normal oestrogen replacement therapy—and because you're still having regular cycles, your body is producing enough progesterone to balance it out. And keep up your herbs and vitamins."

A week later I picked up the phone and it was Maureen. "I feel like a human being again," she said, laughing. "That oestrogen worked like a dream!"

NON-PERIMENOPAUSAL CAUSES OF INSOMNIA

As with hot flushes, it is important to investigate all other possible causes of insomnia before treating it hormonally. I begin by asking my patients a host of questions about their medical history, including what drugs—both prescription and over-the-counter—they are taking. Drugs such as diuretics, medications for Parkinson's disease, some antidepressants, some antihypertensives, steroids, decongestants, and asthma medication should not be taken in the evening, as they may prolong sleep onset and interfere with sleep maintenance. Whereas caffeine and nicotine are stimulants that make it hard to fall asleep, alcohol commonly causes waking episodes in the middle of the night. Panax ginseng is also a mild stimulant, so if you're taking it for overall well-being, consider switching to other herbs.

Chronic medical conditions that can disturb sleep include asthma, angina, congestive heart failure, arthritic pain, migraine headache, urinary tract infection, seizures, and gastroesophageal reflux. As mentioned previously, psychiatric problems such as depression and anxiety can cause disturbed sleep patterns as well. Indeed, at least 90 percent of people hospitalized for depression demonstrate some form of sleep abnormality. Sleep apnoea—disturbed respiration during sleep—is another potential cause. More common in men than women, it is often associated with heavy snoring, which can indicate obstructed airways and cardiac arrhythmias. Leg spasms increase with increasing age in both sexes—one study reported an incidence of 40 percent in perimenopausal women—and are frequently at the root of disturbed sleeping.

Stress can have a big effect on sleep patterns as well. Who hasn't lost a night's sleep because they were nervous or upset over something? Or not fallen asleep until the wee hours of the night before a big exam? One of my patients who was going through a rough divorce woke up every night at 3:00 A.M. in panic and watched the clock until daybreak.

If you have sleep problems, you may be suffering what's known as psychophysiologic insomnia, or learned sleeplessness. Basically, this

TIPS FOR GETTING A GOOD NIGHT'S SLEEP

- Go to sleep and wake up at the same time seven days a week.
- Exercise daily, although not within five hours of bedtime.
- Create a restful environment: dark (install heavy window shades or wear eyeshades); quiet (wear earplugs or create white noise, as with an air conditioner); and a comfortable temperature (on the cool side is best).
- Use a humidifier to keep nasal passages moist and prevent stuffiness and snoring.
- Do not eat a heavy meal before bedtime, although a light carbohydrate snack or warm drink (non-caffeinated) may help you fall asleep.
- Take your calcium supplement at bedtime and/or drink a glass of milk.
- Avoid caffeine, especially after 6:00 P.M.
- Avoid excessive fluid intake before bedtime.
- Avoid excessive alcohol and all alcohol in the evening.
- Stop smoking.
- Avoid excessive napping late in the afternoon or early in the evening. However, a short nap—15 to 30 minutes—in the middle of your day, about eight hours before you go to sleep at night, will improve your performance during the day and may help you fall asleep at night.
- Do not eat, read, or watch television in bed—the bed should only be used for sleep and sex.
- Cover the clock.
- Go to bed only when you're sleepy; if you don't fall asleep within five minutes, get out of bed, go into another room, and read, watch television, or listen to soothing music until you feel sleepy again.

means you have adapted associations and behaviors that prevent you from falling asleep. You become anxious about not sleeping, which in turn makes it even harder to fall asleep. You can break this vicious cycle by adopting sleep-promoting habits such as those described in the preceding box. Practicing relaxation techniques such as yoga, meditation, and deep breathing can also help. In severe cases, a short course of sleeping medication may do the trick. A lot of my patients complain that sleeping pills make them feel hungover the next day, however, and there's always the risk of addiction, so it's best to use them for no more than a month.

TREATMENTS FOR INSOMNIA

Herbs

In addition to behavioral modification, there are several natural remedies you can try to help relieve insomnia before resorting to sleeping pills.

BLACK COHOSH (REMIFEMIN). Black cohosh contains phytoestrogens that can help relieve hot flushes. If your insomnia is being caused by night sweats, this herb can help you get a good night's sleep. Take one Remifemin pill in the morning and one at night.

KAVA KAVA. For thousands of years, the herb kava kava has been used in the South Pacific to induce feelings of relaxation. Kava kava contains kavalactones, natural muscle relaxants that make it an ideal treatment for insomnia caused by anxiety. My patients like kava kava because it is nonaddictive and doesn't leave them feeling drugged. I recommend taking between 60 and 120 mg daily, starting with the lower dose and adding more if you need to. Kava kava should never be taken with alcohol, antidepressants, or benzodiazepines.

SAINT JOHN'S WORT. An excellent alternative to antidepressants such as Prozac, without the side effects or addictive potential, Saint John's wort has been proven to improve depression and therefore help with insomnia. The active ingredient in Saint John's wort is hypericin, which raises serotonin levels. The usual dosage is 300 to 500 mg taken three times a day with meals. Start with one tablet at breakfast and work your way up as needed. But don't expect results overnight—it usually takes about six weeks to kick in. Saint John's wort may cause sensitivity to light and to certain foods such as wine and cheese. It should not be taken if you are on bloodthinners or drugs that cause sun sensitivity, such as Retin-A or tetracycline. If you are on an SSRI antidepressant (Prozac, Lustral) or MAO inhibitor, consult your doctor before taking Saint John's wort.

CHAMOMILE. Among its many medicinal attributes, chamomile contains a gentle sedative called alpha–bisabolol that helps relieve insomnia. Try taking a cup of chamomile tea or between 300 and 400 mg dried chamomile before bedtime.

VALERIAN. A mild natural tranquilizer, valerian has antianxiety and mild hypnotic effects, making it a good treatment for insomnia caused by nerves. You'll fall asleep quicker, sleep better, and be less worried about not sleeping. The usual dose is 150 to 300 mg taken half an hour before bedtime. Do not take valerian with barbiturates or you'll be so tired you can't see straight.

Phytoestrogens

SOY AND FLAXSEED. Foods and herbs containing phytoestrogens such as soy and flaxseed have an oestrogenic effect, so they can help relieve menopausal symptoms including hot flushes and insomnia. Try to incorporate 3 to 5 tablespoons (25 to 50 g) flaxseed and up to 50 mg soy isoflavones into your daily diet from food sources only (see Appendix B).

Hormones

If you've tried lifestyle changes and complementary therapies and still have bags under your eyes, hormone supplements may be a reasonable next step.

OESTROGEN. I've found that patients who report changes in their sleep patterns during perimenopause often find relief with oestrogen supplements, either natural or synthetic. If their sleeping doesn't get better or if it only improves temporarily, I suggest they look elsewhere for the cause of their insomnia.

NATURAL PROGESTERONE. Higher doses of natural progesterone cause drowsiness. Lower doses may help you sleep because progesterone acts as a mild sedative.

HEART PALPITATIONS

"I feel as if I'm jumping out of my skin.""It's like there's a drum beating in my chest.""There's a dance going on in there.""My heart feels like it's going to punch its way out of my body."

Heart palpitations often accompany hot flushes in perimenopausal women and can be a contributing factor to insomnia as well. Palpitations occur when the electrical signals that synchronize the pulsing of the heart muscle cells malfunction, causing the heart to beat abnormally. During palpitations, your heart rate is often accelerated from its normal resting pulse of about 70 beats per minute. Episodes can last anywhere from a few seconds to all day long, and they may wake you up during the night. Irregularities such as skipped beats may cause you to feel a stuttering or fluttering sensation, and a racing heart may pound so hard you can hear it.

While palpitations are common side effects of a host of medical problems, they are also a benign symptom of fluctuating ovarian hormones. You can experience them anytime your hormone levels are changing, whether you're premenstrual, pregnant, perimenopausal, or menopausal. Like hot flushes, they seem to be triggered by decreased oestrogen levels, which cause increased levels of noradrenaline, the stress hormone. Noradrenaline interacts with receptors on the surface of specialized heart cells called pacemaker cells, telling them to speed up the heart rate.

Before prescribing treatment, I always refer patients complaining of palpitations to a cardiologist for a complete exam. I recently saw a perimenopausal patient who told me she was suffering hot flushes and severe palpitations, with episodes lasting for an hour at a time several times a day, scaring her out of her wits. She was not a smoker or drinker, took no caffeine or medications, exercised regularly, and wasn't on birth control pills. We discussed her diet, which was balanced, and her stress level, which was high ("Whose isn't?"). Overall, she seemed in good health, although I checked her thyroid hormone levels just to make sure, as thyroid disease can cause palpitations (see Chapter 12).

I also sent her straight to a cardiologist, who performed an ECG and echocardiogram, which were both normal. The cardiologist then hooked up my patient to a Holter monitor for 24 hours, which confirmed that she had a racing heart. Once she had a clean bill of health from the cardiologist, she returned to me and I prescribed a

HEED YOUR HEART!

Although palpitations are generally harmless, call your doctor if your heart beats more than 120 times per minute, either regularly or irregularly, or if your palpitations last more than a few minutes or are accompanied by nausea, headache, faintness, or dizziness. Palpitations may be a sign of serious heart disease or a side effect of a particular drug, such as a high blood pressure medication or a cold remedy.

combination of natural oestrogen and natural progesterone. Two weeks later she reported relief from both the hot flushes and the palpitations.

Like hot flushes, perimenopausal palpitations are not a serious medical concern but may require treatment if they are causing anxiety, discomfort, or insomnia. Particularly when alternate causes—such as stress, a high-sugar diet, drinking, smoking, or ingesting caffeine—are factors, I suggest lifestyle changes and complementary treatments first. Calcium, magnesium, and coenzyme Q10 supplements can relieve palpitations, as can herbs such as hawthorn and black cohosh (Remifemin), and phytoestrogens such as soy, which raise oestrogen levels and restore the balance of neurotransmitters.

If the complementary approach doesn't work, hormone supplements are the next step. Some of the synthetic progestogens given with oestrogen supplements have been shown to trigger palpitations on their own, however, so I always recommend natural progesterone in combination with natural oestrogen. If hormone replacement doesn't ease palpitations, heart medications such as Inderal, a beta-blocker, may do the trick, although they may cause insomnia, fatigue, and depression.

CHAPTER 4

I'm Losing My Mind!
Oestrogen and the Brain

My patient Sue called to say she thought she was losing her mind. The other night her husband came home from work to find her sitting in the middle of the kitchen floor crying her eyes out. When he asked her what was wrong, she couldn't really think of anything, so she blurted out, "My grandmother will never know Oliver" (Oliver being their 2-year-old son). Sue's grandmother has been dead for years.

"I feel premenstrual all the time, blowing a gasket at the slightest little thing," another patient complained. "My husband called to ask if I'd be home for dinner tonight and I nearly bit his head off."

"I took a taxi all the way down to Macy's and when I got there I had no recollection of why I had come," yet another patient regaled me. "So I spent an hour wandering from department to department, hoping something would trigger my memory. I ended up buying some sheets and towels on sale and a new lipstick. It wasn't until I got all the way home that I remembered what I needed—a new coffeemaker!"

Although accounts of "menopausal madness" may make tabloid headlines, fear not—oestrogen deprivation is not going to transform you overnight into a basket case. Nevertheless, you may find yourself experiencing mood changes, headaches, and loss of concentration and verbal memory beginning in your perimenopausal years. For those of us who are under pressure at home, at work, and everyplace in between and need to be mentally sharp at all times, the cognitive effects of perimenopause may be even more disturbing than the physical ones.

You've probably noticed hormone-related changes in your mood, memory, and thinking at various times in your reproductive life. My patients often tell me they're feeling "the three A's"—angry, anxious, and agitated—up to two weeks before their periods. Some who are artists and writers complain that they become less creative premenstrually as well. While you may not have become clinically depressed postpartum, you may have felt anxious, weepy, strangely detached, or out of control immediately after having a baby. Similarly, in perimenopause the waxing and waning of oestrogen levels can cause you to experience a range of cognitive and emotional effects. All these symptoms seem to occur when the oestrogen levels in your brain fall below a certain minimum set point.

Just because oestrogen levels taper off in perimenopause doesn't mean that you'll necessarily become soft in the head. You may feel cloudy, whereas your best friend may still be sharp as a tack. Symptoms that are related to fluctuations in oestrogen levels, such as headaches and moodiness, rather than overall oestrogen decline, will most likely abate when your hormone levels re-equilibrate after menopause. If you can't wait it out, there are plenty of treatment options to help you maintain peak performance throughout your perimenopausal years.

SEX HORMONES AND THE BRAIN

Oestrogen affects many parts of the brain. In the hypothalamus, it regulates levels of neurotransmitters that affect your thermoregulatory and sleep centers. In addition, oestrogen increases hypothalamic production of serotonin and dopamine, neurotransmitters that affect your mood. Oestrogen receptors are also present in the amygdala and limbic system, an area affiliated with emotions, as well as in the hippocampus, a region associated with learning, memory, and spatial reasoning.

Oestrogen also influences communication among the different parts of the brain by promoting growth and stimulation of neurons, the long nerve cells that connect the various brain centers. It's a myth that your brain is fully hard-wired by the time you reach adulthood. In reality, the architecture of the brain is not static but in constant flux throughout your life, with new connections being made and old ones disassembled all the time. One of the reasons you may experience memory loss and fuzzy thinking during perimenopause is because less oestrogen means fewer neurons. Fewer neurons means fewer messages being relayed from the thinking parts of the brain to the parts of the brain where thoughts may be processed or stored as memories.

Another reason for feeling like you're not playing with a full deck is that your brain may not be getting enough oxygen. Oestrogen increases cerebral blood flow by keeping the muscles surrounding the blood vessels relaxed and reducing inflammation in the brain. The blood vessels of the scalp also respond to oestrogen: when oestrogen levels decline, they constrict, causing migraine headaches, another common symptom of perimenopause. Progesterone has the opposite effect of oestrogen, leading to constricted blood vessels and decreased blood flow to the brain.

I'm always telling my patients that oestrogen and testosterone are mood elevators. What do I mean? Both oestrogen and testosterone decrease levels of monoamine oxidase (MAO), an enzyme that breaks down neurotransmitters such as serotonin, dopamine, noradrenaline, and opiates. When oestrogen levels are high, more of these mood-elevating chemicals are free to circulate. Testosterone is converted to oestrogen by the neurons, so it has the same effect. Low levels of brain neurotransmitters cause depression. Antidepressants such as selective serotonin reuptake inhibitors (SSRIs, e.g., Prozac) and MAO inhibitors work by preventing the breakdown of these neurotransmitters, making more of them available in the brain.

I also tell my patients that progesterone will knock them out. Progesterone competes with testosterone for receptor sites on cell surfaces and prevents testosterone from being converted into oestrogen, thereby inhibiting testosterone's mood-elevating effect. Progesterone also suppresses neurotransmitter production and increases MAO activity, slowing down communication among different parts of the brain. When progesterone breaks down, it binds to the same receptors that are affected by barbiturates and most anaesthetics. When your progesterone level is high, you feel fatigued, sleepy, and sedated, as if you'd actually taken these drugs.

A patient of mine who was afflicted with breast cancer in her perimenopause began to have irregular menstrual cycles. I prescribed a progestogen for her to regulate her periods. She swears that it's the best sleeping pill she's ever taken. She takes her pill at bedtime and within fifteen minutes is fast asleep.

THE DEPRESSION DEBATE

Pat, a 50-year-old patient whom I'd put on hormones to control her perimenopausal symptoms, came in for an appointment. When I asked her how she was feeling, she said, "Really down in the dumps. Everything is an effort." After a full exam, I prescribed a test of her hormone levels, including oestradiol, progesterone, testosterone, and dehydroepiandrosterone (DHEA), another male sex hormone. The results were normal for all but her DHEA, which was low. So I prescribed a 25 mg DHEA supplement, and six weeks later she reported that her moods had greatly improved.

"So was my depressed mood because of my perimenopause?" Pat asked.

"In your case I'm not so sure," I replied. "DHEA levels go down as we grow older, and the fact that your mood did not improve on the oestrogen and progesterone, but did on the DHEA, makes me suspect age more than perimenopause was the determining factor. Then again, the interplay of all these hormones is very complex, so it's impossible to say 100 percent one way or the other."

Is depression a symptom of perimenopause or simply a side effect of aging? This is still a matter of controversy. On the one hand, in both men and women depression has been linked to non-oestrogen age-related changes including alterations in thyroid function, declining levels of androgens such as DHEA, silent strokes, and psychological issues around growing older. With age, both sexes produce less dopamine and serotonin, two important mood-stabilizing neurotransmitters.

On the other hand, women suffer depression twice as frequently as men, especially during their reproductive years, signaling a potential link with the female sex hormones. After puberty, the rate of depression in girls rises more rapidly than in boys; a lot of women feel depressed before they get their periods; and a previous history of depression increases the risk for postpartum depression. Numerous studies have shown that hormone replacement therapy relieves depressive symptoms in postmenopausal women. Nevertheless, it is difficult to prove that fluctuating hormone levels actually *cause* depression.

One of the reasons this is so hard to pin down is that people—even research scientists—are very casual about what they call depression. Studies often do not distinguish between major depression—a definable, diagnosable illness—and minor depression or a wide range of nonclinical mood disorders. Those studies that do distinguish between the two report a significantly greater increase in rates of nonclinical mood disorders than of major depression in perimenopausal women.

When mood changes and depression are considered separately, the consensus seems to be that mood changes do peak between ages 30 and 44. Those who suffer major depression during this time usually have been depressed earlier in their lives. If you have a history of mental illness or have suffered premenstrual dysphoric disorder (PDD)—a form of severe depression associated with PMS—or postpartum depression, you should be aware that perimenopause can trigger a recurrence. If your symptoms begin around the same time as other perimenopausal changes and you have no personal or family history of depression, most likely you are suffering hormone-related mood changes rather than clinical depression.

To further complicate the picture, a number of the symptoms of depression are also symptoms of perimenopause. A woman suffering insomnia, fatigue, weight gain, problems in concentrating, and loss of interest in sex might be diagnosed as mildly depressive whereas actually she's in perimenopause. That's why it's extremely important for your doctor to take the time to talk about the bigger picture with you—what other symptoms you are experiencing, whether your bleeding pattern has changed, and what else is going on in your life that could have put you in a funk. If there's a chance your depressed mood could be related to perimenopause, he or she should test your hormone levels rather than just handing you a prescription for Prozac.

To a certain extent, the difference between depressed mood and clinical depression is one of degree—there is a continuum between minor mood swings and major depression. In either case—whether you're downright depressed or just experiencing a bad case of the blues—there's no reason to suffer. There are numerous routes to relief you can explore. Fewer or less severe symptoms that come and go usually indicate depressed mood rather than full-fledged depression and can often be treated with hormones, psychotherapy, or

SYMPTOMS OF DEPRESSION

If you have been experiencing one or more of the following symptoms for at least two weeks, seek professional help immediately.

- feeling depressed, sad, empty, or tearful most of the day
- loss of interest or pleasure in previously enjoyed activities, including sex
- gain or loss (without dieting) of more than 5 percent of your body weight in a month, or a noticeable increase or decrease in appetite almost every day
- sleep disturbances such as insomnia, early-morning waking, or inability to get out of bed
- restlessness or lethargy
- fatigue or loss of energy
- feeling hopeless, pessimistic, worthless, or guilty for no reason nearly every day
- inability to concentrate or make decisions, decreased attention span, forgetfulness
- recurrent thoughts of death or suicide (in this case, do not wait two weeks)

self-help behavioral changes. When symptoms are severe, persistent, and interfere with day-to-day functioning, you may benefit from anti-depressants.

OVERLOAD SYNDROME

A few months ago Joyce, a longtime patient, came to see me. She's 50 years old, perimenopausal, with two grown daughters who are also in the practice. "Laura, I'm going nuts and my husband is ready for a divorce," she proclaimed when I walked into the room. "My hormones are wacked. I'm flushing all the time and my breasts are killing me. I'm under a ton of stress—I just can't handle it!" It turns out that her father had a stroke and she's been flying back and forth to Florida every two weeks to take care of him, in addition to maintaining a busy corporate consulting practice here in New York.

Because she was still functioning at a high level and not experiencing any changes in her sleeping or eating patterns, I didn't think she needed immediate treatment with antidepressants. Rather, I suggested she try some relaxation techniques such as yoga or biofeedback, as well as taking a multivitamin, natural vitamin E, a calcium/magnesium supplement, evening primrose oil, and Remifemin. I also prescribed a natural progesterone. "You can't always take care of everyone else and ignore yourself; it catches up with you," I counseled, and asked her to come back in two months.

Joyce returned two months later. "How's it going?" I asked.

"The stress is still there, but I feel like I'm managing it so much better now. What you said really struck home—I was trying to be Superwoman and ending up just driving myself and everyone around me crazy. Dad's still sick and work is still insanely busy, but I feel much more in control. And I know my family appreciates that I'm functioning better, too."

Although it's out of vogue to talk about midlife crises these days, the truth is that many of us experience major life changes in our perimenopausal years that can throw us for a loop both emotionally and physically. You may be dealing with teenage children or trying desperately to have children if you've chosen to postpone starting a family in favor of a career. You may be going back to work or attaining new responsibilities at work that create added pressure. You may be taking care of elderly parents or suffering the loss of one or both. You may be going through a rocky patch in your marriage. And certainly divorce, which is extremely common at this time, can send anyone reeling.

It's clear that stress can trigger shifts in your reproductive hormones. Haven't we all skipped a period at one time or another because we were uptight about an upcoming event—an exam, a graduation, a wedding? I've had patients who've been diagnosed with cancer and never gotten their periods again. Another lost her 18-year-old son two years ago and hasn't menstruated since. When perimenopausal symptoms such as mood swings and bleeding changes coincide with major life disruptions, it's oftentimes difficult to figure out which is the cause and which the effect.

A similar chicken-and-egg question arises from a fascinating study of 700 women conducted in the Boston area in the United States that revealed a link between a past history of medically treated depression and early menopause. Does depression or its treatment bring on early menopause, or does early menopause result from prior ovarian dysfunction that also happens to cause depression? In other words, who's to say whether you become depressed because of a particular event in your life and your depression causes you to stop bleeding, or you've stopped menstruating and are suddenly deprived of oestrogen, which has triggered a depression?

In general, perimenopausal symptoms themselves—such as hot flushes, night sweats, insomnia, and menstrual irregularities—are associated with higher rates of depressed mood. A follow-up to the Massachusetts Women's Health Study, a five-year longitudinal study of 2,565 women between the ages of 45 and 55, concluded that women who experienced a long perimenopausal period—more than 27 months—were at increased risk of depression. Again, it is unclear whether this is because they were exposed to fluctuating hormones for a longer period or whether their prolonged symptoms increased their stress and emotional volatility. The good news: by the time they reached menopause, women's rates of depression returned to premenopausal levels.

WHEN ALTERNATIVES ALTER THE MOOD

If you've ever craved chocolate to relieve your PMS blues, you know that what you eat can have a direct effect on how you feel. A high-sugar diet can play havoc with your levels of cortisol and insulin (hormones that have to do with sugar metabolism) and decrease your serotonin, causing mood fluctuations. A low-protein diet can also give you the blahs, as protein is needed to manufacture neurotransmitters. To keep an even keel, eat a diet high in protein with a low level of simple carbohydrates (anything white—refined sugar, bread, rice, pasta, potatoes) and don't skip meals, so your blood sugar remains constant. Also, avoid alcohol and recreational drugs like marijuana and cocaine, which contain depressants.

Certain vitamins, minerals, herbs, and foods, as well as exercise, can boost your mood when you're feeling the perimenopausal blues as well.

Vitamins and Minerals

MAGNESIUM. So why *do* you crave chocolate when you're feeling down? It's because chocolate contains magnesium, which relaxes the blood vessels so that more oxygen can flow to the brain. This improves your general sense of well-being and reduces your fatigue. A daily dose of 600 mg magnesium is optimal.

PHOSPHATIDYL SERINE (PS). A lipid essential to brain cell structure, phosphatidyl serine has been shown to relieve depression and improve mood by increasing neurotransmitter formation. Take 100 to 300 mg daily.

VITAMIN B$_6$. Vitamin B$_6$ helps convert amino acids into the neurotransmitter serotonin. By increasing your serotonin level, it improves your mood. I recommend 50 to 100 mg daily; taking more than 200 mg a day has been shown to cause neurologic problems.

Herbs

EVENING PRIMROSE OIL AND BLACK COHOSH (REMIFEMIN). Herbs such as these can help relieve black moods and anxiety by functioning as oestrogen substitutes. I recommend 1,000 to 3,000 mg a day of evening primrose oil and two capsules of Remifemin, one in the morning and one in the evening.

GINKGO BILOBA. This can also raise your spirits by increasing blood flow to your brain. Take 30 to 40 mg three times a day and wait six weeks for results. But don't take ginkgo if you're on bloodthinners or you risk excessive bleeding.

KAVA KAVA. This herb can also help reduce anxiety, mood swings, irritability, and stress. The suggested dose is 60 to 120 mg daily.

SAINT JOHN'S WORT. This "natural Prozac" has gotten a lot of press over the past few years. Dozens of carefully controlled scientific studies have shown that it is as effective an antidepressant as prescription drugs. Saint John's wort is the leading antidepressant in Germany, where it has been used for decades. I tell patients to start with one 300 to 500 mg tablet with breakfast and see how they feel after a few weeks. If you need to, you can go up to three pills a day with meals; but remember, it takes between 6 and 8 weeks to be effective.

Exercise

Exercise can be a natural high. A recent study comparing women who exercised with women who didn't found that those who exercised reported far fewer perimenopausal symptoms, including hot flushes and mood changes, than those who were sedentary. The fatigue and stress associated with vasomotor symptoms such as hot flushes can understandably cause a woman to feel below par. But there is also evidence that exercise affects mood directly by increasing serotonin levels, thereby acting as a natural antidepressant.

Phytoestrogens

SOY AND FLAXSEED. Both contain plant-based oestrogens that can boost your declining oestrogen level and alleviate your mood swings. Try to incorporate in your daily diet 3 to 5 tablespoons (25 to 50 g) freshly ground flaxseed and up to 50 mg soy isoflavones from food, not supplements (see Appendix B).

Diet

OMEGA-3 FATTY ACIDS. When I was a girl, my mother called fish "brain food." Little did she know how on-the-mark she was! The omega-3 fatty acids found in oily, dark-fleshed fish such as salmon, tuna, mackerel, bluefish, sardines, and pompano, as well as in flaxseed, can actually elevate your mood, according to a recent study from the National Institute on Alcohol Abuse and Alcoholism. Simply put, people who eat more of these fish suffer less depression. Another study from England found that people with clinical depression have notably lower levels of docosahexaenoic acid in their blood cells, a primary component of omega-3 fatty acids. Omega-3 fatty acids act like oil in your car engine, lubricating your brain and making the neurotransmitters flow more smoothly. So if you're feeling blue, go fishin'!

Hormones

I always tailor treatments to meet an individual patient's needs. Those who are experiencing only mild mood swings may find that diet, exercise, and herbs are all they require. Others who are more severely affected may need to go straight to hormones in order to prevent their mood from worsening and becoming full-fledged depression.

LOW-DOSE BIRTH CONTROL PILLS. I don't recommend low-dose birth control pills for treating mood disorders. Why not? Because only one-third of patients on birth control pills will feel better, whereas one-third will feel worse and one-third will remain the same.

OESTROGEN. Whether it be the low-dose natural oestrogen or standard oestrogen replacement therapy (ERT), I have found oestrogen to improve mood remarkably well. For any patient who still has her uterus, I always balance ERT with oral micronized progesterone.

TESTOSTERONE. If patients fail to improve on oestrogen replacement therapy, I add testosterone to their therapy to give them energy and elevate their mood.

PROGESTOGENS. I dislike synthetic progestogens (Provera) because my patients who have taken them become moody and depressed, and they also gain weight. Natural progesterone suppositories, however, only cause mild and transient drowsiness, which can be minimized by taking the drug at bedtime.

DEHYDROEPIANDROSTERONE (DHEA). If you're suffering symptoms of depression and your test has shown low levels of DHEA, you could benefit from a 25 to 50 mg daily supplement. Do not take DHEA unless you have had your levels checked.

WHEN ALL ELSE FAILS

If an oestrogen/progesterone combination or oestrogen replacement with testosterone fails to elevate mood, or if a woman has a past personal history of depression, family history of mental illness, severe depressive symptoms, or contraindications to oestrogen therapy, antidepressants are the treatment of choice. There has been some speculation that oestrogen supplements may enhance the activity of antidepressants, but no formal studies have been published to substantiate this hypothesis.

TOBY—STUBBORN DEPRESSION

About a year ago I saw Toby for the first time. New to me and new to New York, she'd just moved up from Atlanta in an attempt to make a fresh start after a nasty divorce. It seems her husband made a huge success of his business and decided he needed a younger wife. Not that Toby is anything to sneeze at—at age 44 she looks to be in great physical shape with bright blue eyes and a magnificent complexion. Dressed to the nines that day in an apricot silk suit, her blond hair blown into a slightly stiff bob, she could easily have passed for a native of Park Avenue. But as soon as we began to talk, it became obvious she wasn't a local. It wasn't just her accent that gave her away, but a certain softness and vulnerability—she hadn't yet developed the hard shell she'd need to endure life in this tough town.

While taking her medical history, I learned that Toby's former gynaecologist had identified her as perimenopausal and prescribed hormone supplements because she was suffering scanty periods and severe hot flushes. She was taking synthetic oestrogen and progestogen. Her periods were now about 33 days apart and her hot flushes were under control. "But in some ways I feel worse than ever," she sighed.

"Can you be more specific?" I probed.

"Well, I just don't feel like myself. I usually have a lot of energy, but now I can hardly get out of bed in the morning. My whole life I've been known as the soul of patience, but now I'm snapping at everyone. I used to have a whole lot of zest for life; now nothing excites me anymore. I feel like I'm under a black cloud but also in some kind of plastic bubble—cut off from other people and from my own feelings."

"These are all symptoms of depression," I explained. "Do you have a history of mental illness in your family?"

"Eccentrics, yes, but really ill, no."

"Have you ever been treated for depression in the past?" I asked.

"No," she replied.

"And these symptoms have all set in after you've been on hormone supplements?"

"That's right."

"Well, the first thing I'd like to try is switching you from synthetic oestrogen and progestogen to natural oestrogen and progesterone. A lot of my patients have complained that Provera makes them depressed." I explained how progesterone affects the human brain and mentioned that up to 30 percent of women report depressive symptoms when taking oral contraceptives, another combination of oestrogen and synthetic progestogen.

"I'd like to see you again in two weeks," I concluded, "but call me sooner if your symptoms get worse."

I didn't hear from Toby. Two weeks later she reported that her symptoms were the same, although to me she seemed to have taken a turn for the worse. For one thing, she didn't look as well put together—her make-up was a little less carefully applied, her nail polish was chipped, her shoulders drooped. I also noticed that her clothes were a little bit baggy. "Have you lost weight?" I asked.

"I don't know—I guess so. I just haven't had much of an appetite recently," she responded in a monotone. "It's really hard, moving to a new city and all, Dr. Corio. I spend most of my time alone in my apartment thinking about how badly my life turned out. Just a couple of years ago I had everything—a beautiful home, tons of friends, a terrific husband who I *thought* loved me. Now I've got nothing. If only we'd had children, then maybe I wouldn't be so lonely all the time." Tears welled up in her eyes.

I put my arm around her. "I know it's hard to understand, but you have to realize that this is your mood speaking, not the real you. I think it's time you saw a psychiatrist about getting some antidepressants and some psychotherapy. Not all patients respond to natural oestrogen and progesterone. And you could also use some emotional support."

I referred her to an excellent psychiatrist who prescribed Lustral, a selective serotonin reuptake inhibitor (SSRI) that boosts mood by increasing circulating levels of serotonin. Six weeks later Toby called the office.

"How are you feeling?" I asked.

"Well, at least I can get out of bed in the morning." Things were looking up. "But I can't say I'm my old self. I still feel sad a lot of the time, even though I can put a smile on my face and pretend otherwise. Let's face it, the facts haven't changed—I'm a 44-year-old single woman starting life all over again from scratch. That's enough to depress anyone!"

"How's it going with the psychiatrist?" I queried.

"I've been seeing her for about a month and it's going well."

"Good. You didn't become depressed overnight, and it'll take some time to recover. The antidepressant has helped restore your ability to function physically. The talk therapy will help you understand what's causing your depression emotionally. Keep me posted on how things are going, okay?"

"Will do," she promised and hung up the phone.

Four months later Toby called to check in. "The therapist has been such a wonderful support. She's helping me deal with all these issues. I'm beginning to understand all sorts of things about my past and my marriage and gradually accepting them."

"And you're still on the antidepressant?" I asked.

"Yes. My doctor thinks it's important for me to keep my mental strength up while I'm opening all these cans of worms."

"She's right. Keep up the good work and I'll talk with you soon."

MEMORY CHANGES

A friend of my mother's can remember the tiniest details from her childhood in Brooklyn, including her best friend's address and the names of the local butcher and shoemaker. But she hasn't the foggiest idea what she ate for dinner last night. At age 79, she's entitled to forget a few details. A 47-year-old patient of mine began to notice a similar pattern of lapses in her memory. She could recall the names of all of her college roommate's boyfriends—no mean feat, she assured me—but she'd hang up the phone with a client and five minutes later, when her secretary asked for the name to put it in the appointment book, she wouldn't have a clue. She told me she writes everything down on little pieces of paper; the problem is, she can never remember where she put them.

Are these kinds of middle-age memory changes normal, or are they something we should worry about? And why can we remember certain things, often those from our deep dark pasts, and not others? The answers have to do with the nature of memory itself.

Basically, there are three different types of memory. Short-term memory allows you to perform simple tasks such as balancing a checkbook. Working memory is a little more complex. It involves holding information in your mind and carrying out some decision-making activity based on that information. Long-term memory involves recalling material days, weeks, months, or years after it has been presented.

Think of it in terms of clothes, one of my favorite things to think about. Short-term memory is the sweater you take off when you run inside for a minute and don't even bother to put it away. Working memory is the clothes you hang in your closet each night. Long-term memory is the stuff you wouldn't be caught dead in but keep in the attic because you can't bear to throw it away.

Short-term memory does not change substantially with age. Working memory, however, in which new information must be both retained and acted upon, peaks at age 45, but then decreases in both speed and accuracy as we grow older. That's why you may find yourself having to read a recipe several times over before you really grasp it, or keep detailed shopping or "to do" lists. Long-term memory is affected by age, but not consistently. You may not be able to spontaneously recall a certain situation, say your Sweet Sixteen celebration, but if someone prods your memory, it all may come flooding back to you down to the last detail.

One of the reasons you may be remembering less as you grow older is that you're more distracted. When you're being pulled in eighteen different directions it's hard to focus on a new piece of information and deposit it in your memory bank. If you're not paying attention, it's easy to let names, dates, phone numbers, and driving directions float in one ear and out the other. By periodically reminding yourself to slow down and really listen to what people are saying, you'll find you retain these bits of information much better.

Genetics definitely play a role in memory, although no specific "memory gene" has been identified. If you're lucky enough to have been born to parents with impeccable memories, you're likely to stay sharp as you grow older, too. By contrast, if you've been unlucky enough to have been subjected to chronic stress throughout your life, it may have a negative effect on your memory.

Another reason for memory changes is simply that your brain isn't as young as it used to be. Cerebral blood flow and neurotransmitters must be in adequate supply for the different parts of your brain to communicate with each other. When you age, your arteries harden and your neurotransmitter levels decline, so tasks like recall become harder to perform. Even if a memory was stored years ago, when your brain was performing at its optimal level, it may be difficult to retrieve spontaneously if your brain is now a little sluggish. If your brain isn't completely up to speed, it's also more difficult to store newly acquired information for future use, which is why working memory is affected.

WHY WOMEN FORGET

So why does your memory go to pot in perimenopause? Because oestrogen is essential for keeping up the neurotransmitter levels and blood flow to the brain. Specifically, oestrogen affects levels of acetylcholine, a neurotransmitter derived from choline. Acetylcholine helps foster neuron growth, especially in the hippocampus, the area of the brain associated with memory, learning, and spatial reasoning.

Women are particularly susceptible to loss of verbal memory. I wish I had a dime for every time a patient has said to me, "It's so frustrating—the word is on the tip of my tongue!" Or they mean to say one word but something else comes out. The reason for this seems to go back to how female brains are wired in utero.

Numerous studies have shown that men and women differ in specific cognitive abilities. Women excel in verbal abilities, perceptual speed and accuracy, and fine motor skills. Men, by contrast, excel in spatial and quantitative abilities, and gross motor strength. "Aha!" you may be thinking. "That's why he never wants to talk about things as much as I do. I ask him important questions and all I get is 'Yes,' 'No,' or just a grunt for an answer." While it's tempting to use these neurological discrepancies to support the stereotype about men and women being from different planets, the truth is that the amount of divergence between the sexes is extremely slight.

WHEN IT'S NOT ALL HORMONAL

In addition to age and oestrogen deprivation, certain medical conditions and medications can cause memory loss.

MEDICAL CONDITIONS

MEDICATIONS

- cardiovascular disease
- hypothyroidism
- diabetes
- chronic exhaustion
- poor nutrition
- difficulties with vision and hearing

- sleeping pills
- antianxiety and antidepressant drugs

These differences do exist statistically, however. It is currently believed that they result from prenatal influences on brain organization—whether the foetus was exposed to a higher concentration of androgens, the male sex hormones, or oestrogens, the female sex hormones. Women born with a genetic condition causing abnormally high androgen levels in utero later have lower verbal IQ scores, better spatial abilities, and more learning disabilities than average for women.

Back in 1952 a classic controlled study was published in which twenty-eight 75-year-old women living in an old-age home were given weekly injections of either oestradiol (E_2) or a placebo. After one year, the verbal IQ scores of the women treated with oestrogen had increased significantly whereas the scores of those given the placebo had decreased. None of the women's spatial abilities were affected. The women were then taken off their injections, and a year later all of them scored lower than their original baseline two years earlier, indicating that the boost in memory only lasted as long as the oestrogen supplement. More recent controlled studies of women who have undergone surgical menopause and been given either oestrogen or a placebo show the same results.

Keep in mind that these research results are only theoretically significant. In the real world, most women experience memory changes that are only slightly annoying and do not adversely affect their everyday lives. The exception, however, is in cases of Alzheimer's disease, which I'll discuss shortly.

NICOLE—THE CASE OF THE MISSING GLASSES

The mother of two teenage boys, 53-year-old Nicole is a paralegal at a big corporate law firm. Eminently organized, efficient, and level-headed, she keeps her kids and her husband on track just as she does her lawyers. As we began chatting, she told me that her primary focus was making sure her elder son met his college application deadlines and her younger one found a sensible summer internship.

"And how are you doing?" I asked.

"Not great, Laura," she replied matter-of-factly, then proceeded to reel off a list of classic perimenopausal symptoms: hot flushes, decreased libido, insomnia, urinary incontinence. "But by far the worst is that my memory is shot. I forgot to pick up Tom from his soccer practice Monday night. And on Thursday I was supposed to meet Ryan for dinner with clients and at seven o'clock he called and said, 'Where are you?' I had completely forgotten. On top of that, I spend half my day looking for my glasses. I know it sounds stupid, but it's driving me crazy!"

"That's why mine are on a chain," I said. "How about your periods?"

"They've been getting irregular. The last one was about five weeks ago, but sometimes they come as close as 24 or 25 days."

After a full check-up I told her that I thought she was in perimenopause and recommended she start exercising and taking a daily multivitamin, natural vitamin E, a calcium/magnesium supplement with vitamin D, and soy for general well-being and a few special supplements to improve her memory. Specifically, phosphatidyl serine and acetyl-L-carnitine, and B complex vitamins. I didn't feel comfortable giving her oestrogen because she had a history of deep vein thrombophlebitis. "Even though I'm 99 percent sure your memory problem is a symptom of perimenopause, I'd like you to see a neurologist just to make sure it's nothing more serious."

A month later I received the neurologist's report. Her EEG and MRI were negative, confirming that there wasn't a tumor or blood clot impairing her brain functioning.

When I opened the door to the examining room at Nicole's next visit, the first thing I noticed was the chain around her neck holding her glasses. When I pointed it out she laughed. "Great idea, though it's really just insurance. Overall my symptoms are a lot better, but especially my mind. I don't know if it's the vitamins, the soy, or the exercise—or maybe it's just knowing that I'm not losing my mind—but I feel a lot more relaxed and in control. I didn't realize how stressful it was always to be worrying if I was forgetting something important—not just my glasses."

ALZHEIMER'S DISEASE

While most perimenopausal women aren't dealing with Alzheimer's themselves, all too many are dealing with it in their parents and older relatives. It's a devastating disease that takes as much as if not more of a toll on caregivers as it does on those who suffer it.

Bettina, a 46-year-old patient, was telling me about her mother, who is severely affected. "She lives in southern West Virginia, and I visit her every two weeks, not that she recognizes me half the time," she said.

"That's a big trip," I replied. "Why don't you bring her up here to New York? It'd be so much easier for you, and you could see her even more often."

"I can't," she explained. "She's spent her whole life there and has lived in the same house for the past fifty years. She doesn't remember much, but at least she's in familiar surroundings. If I moved her she'd be completely lost."

"And how are you feeling?" I asked.

"Exhausted. Sad. And scared—not for her, but for me. They say Alzheimer's is hereditary, so every time I forget a name or an address I worry that it's the beginning of the end."

"Listen," I tried to reassure her. "Memory changes are normal for women our age, and yours don't sound like anything out of the ordinary. But if you're worried about inheriting the disease, there may be some things you can do now to protect yourself for the future."

Alzheimer's is a form of progressive dementia that affects women up to three times more often than men, and it tends to affect women's verbal memory more severely than men's. The fact that

RISK FACTORS FOR ALZHEIMER'S DISEASE

Although Alzheimer's disease can only be diagnosed through neurological testing, there are certain risk factors that will raise your doctor's antennae that your memory changes may be more than just the effects of aging and fluctuating hormone levels:

- female gender
- family history of dementia
- increasing age
- head trauma
- thyroid disease
- depression
- exposure to aluminum or solvents
- family history of Down syndrome (trisomy 21)

women live longer than men does not entirely account for this gender gap. Other factors seem to contribute to the differences in frequency and course of the disease—including sex hormones. Although Alzheimer's generally doesn't set in until the postmenopausal years, if you are at risk for the disease, oestrogen supplementation during your perimenopausal years may delay its onset and severity.

In addition to the beneficial effects oestrogen has on healthy brains, it has a particular property that protects against Alzheimer's. The disease is characterized by formation of beta-amyloid plaques on the neurons of the central nervous system. In a test tube, oestradiol (E_2) prevents beta-amyloid buildup. Oestrogen also blocks plaque formation because it reduces circulating levels of apolipoprotein E, which is needed to transport beta-amyloid to the brain. Furthermore, oestrogen may control certain inflammatory responses that trigger beta-amyloid accumulation.

The neurotransmitter acetylcholine also responds to oestrogen levels, and low acetylcholine has been associated with Alzheimer's. If your oestrogen level increases, so does your acetylcholine, so oestrogen replacement can add further protection. Taking B complex vitamins, which contain choline, a precursor to acetylcholine, may also help you defend against the disease.

Recent studies in which women suffering from Alzheimer's were given either oestrogen supplements or a placebo have reported improvements in cognitive functioning, especially related to verbal skills, in the oestrogen-treated women. In one, postmenopausal women who took oestrogen were 40 to 60 percent less likely to develop the disease than were their counterparts who didn't take hormone supplements.

In another study that looked at the influence of body weight on Alzheimer's, it was found that women with higher body weight scored better on naming tasks—not surprising, because postmenopausal women's primary source of oestrogen is fat tissue. By contrast, women with a family history of Alzheimer's who undergo an early menopause (before age 47) and are therefore more oestrogen deprived than average women have a significantly increased risk of developing Alzheimer's. Although oestrogen is by no means a cure for this devastating disease, in the future it could be used to mitigate some of its effects.

It is interesting that recent research has shown that tamoxifen, a drug used to treat breast cancer, may also protect against Alzheimer's. A recent survey of 93,031 women over age 65 who lived in nursing homes in New York State in 1993 found the incidence of Alzheimer's to be one-third lower in those who had received tamoxifen.

By contrast, smokers are more than twice as likely as lifetime nonsmokers to develop Alzheimer's and other forms of dementia. Although researchers have not yet pinpointed the mechanism underlying this link, it is probably partly because smoking constricts blood vessels, thereby decreasing oxygen flow to the brain, and partly because smoking lowers oestrogen levels.

FEEDING YOUR BRAIN

Our brains, like the rest of our bodies, benefit from a nutritious diet and regular exercise. Several supplements are proven brain-builders, so don't forget to take your vitamins!

Vitamins and Minerals

B COMPLEX VITAMINS AND FOLIC ACID. Research into the B complex vitamins has shown that several of them have a direct effect on

PREVENTIVE THERAPY FOR ALZHEIMER'S DISEASE

If you are at risk of developing Alzheimer's disease, ask your doctor about nonsteroidal anti-inflammatory drugs (NSAIDs) in addition to oestrogen supplements. Patients with rheumatoid arthritis have a reduced risk of Alzheimer's disease. It turns out that the nonsteroidal anti-inflammatory drugs they take—including aspirin, ibuprofen, and naproxen sodium—have a protective effect because they reduce inflammation that can compromise blood flow to the brain. Cox-2 inhibitors (Celebrex), a new family of anti-inflammatories, provide the same benefits to memory without severe gastrointestinal side effects. NSAIDs also prevent tiny blood clots from forming and cutting off circulation in the brain. Studies are presently under way to see if NSAIDs may be used to treat Alzheimer's in the future.

cognition. People who take vitamin B_6 do better on memory tests than those who don't, and people with low amounts of vitamin B_{12} and folic acid have poorer spatial copying skills than those with normal amounts. Moreover, choline, another B complex vitamin, is needed for the manufacture of acetylcholine, an essential neurotransmitter for a healthy memory. To keep your memory up to par, take 50 to 100 mg vitamin B_6, 50 to 100 mcg vitamin B_{12}, and 400 mcg folic acid daily. In addition take either a 1,250 mg tablet of lecithin (sold with choline and inositol in it) or from one to three 250-mg choline/inositol tablets daily.

ANTIOXIDANTS. Vitamin E, vitamin C, and mixed carotenes are antioxidants that protect neurons from damage by free radicals. In addition, vitamin E slows the progression of Alzheimer's disease. I recommend 400 to 800 IU natural vitamin E, 1,000 mg vitamin C, and 3 to 6 mg mixed carotenes daily.

PHOSPHATIDYL SERINE (PS) AND ACETYL–L–CARNITINE (ALC). The building block of all brain cells, PS is a lipid that is needed to manufacture neurotransmitters. It improves attention, concentration, recall of numbers and words, verbal ability, and both short- and long-term memory. One study concluded that it brought patients in

---

BLUEBERRIES FOR YOUR BRAIN

Of all the antioxidant-rich fruits and vegetables, blueberries have emerged as the leader of the pack in terms of improving short-term memory. Rats that were fed blueberry extract equal to half a cup of blueberries a day for eight weeks outperformed their blueberry-deprived counterparts in negotiating mazes. They also had better balance, coordination, and motor skills.

---

their sixties back twelve years in mental functioning. Taken with PS, ALC improves the supply of acetylcholine and promotes efficient energy use in the brain. It improves mood, memory, and judgment. I prescribe 100 to 300 mg a day of PS and 500 to 2,000 mg a day of ALC.

Herbs

GINKGO BILOBA. This powerful antioxidant enhances memory by improving blood flow to the brain. It is reported to improve short-term memory and concentration in people with early Alzheimer's disease. In Europe, ginkgo is the most commonly prescribed agent for boosting memory. The recommended dose is 120 to 160 mg divided into three doses a day, except if you're on bloodthinners, in which case you shouldn't touch it, as you could bleed excessively.

Phytoestrogens

SOY AND FLAXSEED. As mentioned previously, these products contain phytoestrogens, which are strong antioxidants that can support brain functioning, including memory. Incorporate up to 50 mg soy isoflavones into your daily diet from food products, not supplements or powders (see Appendix B), and sprinkle 3 to 5 tablespoons (25 to 50 g) of freshly ground flaxseed on your food each day.

Exercise

People with chronic high blood pressure perform poorly on visual and verbal memory tests. Aerobic exercise lowers blood pressure and improves circulation, boosting brain function and memory. So get out and move for 30 minutes at least three times a week.

Oestrogen

In addition to protecting against beta-amyloid plaques, boosting acetylcholine, and increasing circulation to the brain, oestrogen—standard as well as low-dose—is a powerful antioxidant and anti-inflammatory, improving memory and concentration. Of the three oestrogens, oestradiol (E_2) has the strongest beneficial effect on cognitive functioning, stimulating regeneration of damaged neurons and production of neurotransmitters.

MIGRAINE HEADACHES

A lot of my patients come to me complaining of headaches. When I ask if they're migraine headaches, I often get a blank look. "What's the difference?" they ask. The difference between migraine headaches and, say, tension headaches is that migraines cause throbbing pain on only one side of the head and are often preceded by an aura such as the smell of ammonia or flashing lights. Ninety percent of sufferers have nausea, 33 percent experience vomiting, and most become highly sensitive to light and noise.

Women are far more susceptible to migraine headaches than men, suffering them an average of three times as often over a lifetime. About one in five adult American women have had at least one debilitating migraine. Prior to the onset of menstruation and after menopause the ratio between the sexes is more equal, but during perimenopause, when the incidence peaks, women are at even greater risk. Because women's suffering increases during the reproductive years, it has long been suspected that there is a connection between migraine headaches and the oestrogen cycle.

Studies of menstrual migraines bear out this theory. One-third of women who suffer migraines have their first headache at menarche; about two-thirds get them on or around the first day of their period, when oestrogen levels are lowest. The prevailing wisdom is that menstrual migraines are caused by the sudden withdrawal of oestrogen during the late luteal phase of the cycle.

THE MIGRAINE CONNECTION
The number of women seeking treatment for migraine peaks at perimenopause

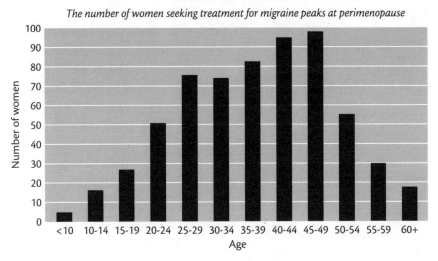

Women who take oral contraceptives frequently suffer migraine headaches during the pill-free week, after experiencing high levels of oestrogen for 21 days. Recently a perimenopausal patient of mine who is on birth control pills began experiencing menstrual migraines. I decided to have her take three months' worth of active pills before withdrawing, so she would have a period only once every three months, which is enough to protect her uterus from cancer. She still gets menstrual headaches, but only four times a year. Women who receive cyclic hormone replacement therapy, which is also administered in a three-week-on, one-week-off pattern, often experience migraine headaches during the off week. I find that using a patch with continuous oestrogen wards off this problem.

One of the most reliable "cures" for migraine headaches is pregnancy, which relieves occurrence in 70 percent of women. During pregnancy, oestrogen levels are maintained at a consistently high level. Postpartum, however, women frequently experience migraine headaches with a vengeance. You'll be happy to know that the incidence of migraine headaches also plummets after menopause, when oestrogen levels are consistently low. The exception is after surgical menopause, when migraine headaches increase, probably because of the sudden cessation of oestrogen production. When women go through natural menopause, oestrogen production decreases more gradually.

In general, for oestrogen withdrawal to trigger migraine headaches, prior oestrogen levels have to have been consistently high for a prolonged period. The peak in migraine headaches between ages 40 and 49 therefore likely reflects the dramatic fluctuations in oestrogen levels characteristic of perimenopause, rather than a gradual decline.

Because oestrogen maintains vascular dilation and flexibility, withdrawal constricts the blood vessels—one explanation for how oestrogen withdrawal may contribute to the onset of headaches. In addition, it is believed that oestrogen withdrawal throws off the balance of neurotransmitters, which may also contribute to migraine headaches.

A colleague of mine who deals with PMS sent me a lovely patient who was experiencing approximately twenty-three migraine headaches a month. He suspected it wasn't PMS but perimenopause and felt that I could help the woman. After reviewing her history, I discovered that not only was she having migraine headaches, which run in her family, but she was also suffering vaginal dryness and decreased libido. But the worst, by far, were the headaches, which were making it nearly impossible for her to function. Her periods were slightly shorter than normal but regular.

I decided to prescribe the continuous low-dose transdermal oestradiol patch because it would keep her oestrogen level consistent. In a month she reported back to me that her headaches had improved significantly—she was down to just seven a month. Eventually, as her perimenopause progressed, I switched her to the standard patch (twice the amount of the low-dose patch) with oral micronized progesterone and oral micronized testosterone, and her symptoms and headaches continued to improve.

TREATMENTS FOR MIGRAINE HEADACHES

Numerous drugs are available to treat migraine headaches. Some drugs are taken consistently as a prophylactic measure, and others are taken at the first twinge. There are also complementary and natural hormonal treatments that are worth investigating.

Vitamins and Minerals

MAGNESIUM. As mentioned previously, magnesium relaxes blood vessels and lowers blood pressure, which makes it an important mineral for preventing migraine headaches. Make sure you get 600 mg a day.

Non-Hormonal Causes of Migraine Headaches

Although hormones play a large role in women's migraine headaches, there are a number of other common causes as well. Different people have different triggers, so if you suffer migraine headaches, try to be aware of what you have recently eaten, done, or been exposed to that might have brought on a particular episode.

- anxiety and insomnia
- becoming overtired
- missing meals and letting your blood sugar fluctuate
- bright lights (resting in a dark room can help alleviate the pain)
- MSG
- chocolate
- red wine and other alcohol
- foods that contain nitrates (bacon, cold cuts)
- moldy cheeses
- birth control pills
- asthma medication
- certain heart and stomach drugs

If you suddenly begin experiencing migraine headaches in perimenopause, don't just assume it's hormonal. See a neurologist to rule out any other causes.

Herbs

FEVERFEW. This herb has been proven to reduce the number and severity of migraine headaches. Its active ingredient is parthenolide, an anticoagulant that also makes the blood vessels less reactive to environmental changes. Like aspirin, it is not recommended for anyone taking bloodthinners such as heparin or Coumadin. Take one 125 mg tablet daily.

BLACK COHOSH (REMIFEMIN). This acts like oestrogen and helps ward off migraine headaches as well. Take one Remifemin pill in the morning and one at night.

Phytoestrogens

SOY, SOY, SOY! If you suffer migraines, you'd better develop a taste for tofu and other soy foods, as genistein, the active phytoestrogen in soy, balances hormone levels and prevents the oestrogen drop that causes migraine headaches. Eat foods containing up to 50 mg soy isoflavones daily (see Appendix B).

Hormones

OESTROGEN. The most important criterion for oestrogen therapy in women with migraine headaches is that it be continuous, as in the patch. Unlike taking oestrogen orally, which causes your levels to go up and down each day, the patch is always on you, giving you a constant dose. I prefer to give the patch with natural progesterone because synthetic progestogens (Provera) are known to cause headaches.

TESTOSTERONE. Adding either synthetic or natural testosterone to your oestrogen replacement therapy can help relieve migraine headaches if oestrogen isn't working on its own.

CHAPTER 5

Not Tonight, Honey: Sexual Changes and Other Embarrassments

One of my grandmother's more outlandish friends was a former actress named Stella. I must have been 16 or 17 when—probably after a couple of vodka tonics—she drew me aside and confided in me about her new boyfriend, Hank. "He's 84, a lawyer, and still goes to the office every day. He loves to play golf on the weekends. And he's terrific in bed!" I remember doing a double take. Bed? As in sex? At that time Stella must have been in her late seventies. I didn't think women that age could still have sex—or were even interested.

Now I know otherwise. In twenty years of practice I've seen numerous women in their sixties, seventies, and eighties who are enjoying rich, satisfying sex lives. Indeed, approximately 70 percent of healthy 70-year-olds continue to have sexual intercourse on a regular basis. And there's absolutely no reason why they shouldn't. Just because a woman is past her childbearing years doesn't mean she has to give up intimate relations.

What's the secret to maintaining a terrific sex life? As a doctor, I've followed numerous patients from one stage of life to another, and one of the things I've noticed is that those who remain sexually active in their perimenopausal years continue to have vibrant sex lives as they grow older. Unfortunately, those who give up on sex in their forties or fifties because of psychological or physical problems find it harder to pick up the ball again later in life.

In perimenopause some women begin experiencing symptoms such as painful intercourse, vaginal itching and dryness, vaginal and urinary tract infections, incontinence, and loss of libido that may not only make sex a turn-off but cause day-to-day life to become uncomfortable and, at times, embarrassing. Fortunately, as the generation that grew up with the Pill and sexual liberation, we're less likely to suffer these complaints in silence, as our mothers might have done. And doctors and scientific researchers are responding to our demands with treatments that can reverse these changes.

The first step toward relief is admitting the problem to your physician. I routinely ask my patients about any changes in their sex lives, but many doctors wait for the patient to take the initiative on this sensitive topic. As intuitive as some of us pride ourselves on being, remember: we are not mind readers. *It is your responsibility to inform your doctor of any changes in your vagina, your sex drive, or your urinary pattern.* Only when the problem is out in the open can it be addressed successfully.

WHEN SOMETHING'S UP DOWN THERE

"Dr. Corio, can I talk with you about something?" the conversation often begins.

"Of course—anything," I respond.

"For the past few months I just haven't been that into sex. My husband wants it and I end up making excuses. Part of the problem is that it just doesn't feel as good anymore."

When I probe further, a typical list of symptoms includes vaginal dryness, burning, and itching that make intercourse uncomfortable or even painful—a condition affecting 40 percent of perimenopausal women. A patient may also report more difficulty becoming aroused and reaching orgasm that, if and when it does occur, is nothing to write home about.

The first thing I do is reassure my patient that these problems are not necessarily a reflection on her relationship and do not indicate that she is "past her prime" or nearing the end of her sexual life span. Rather, they are most likely biological in origin, the result of declining oestrogen levels.

Patients often come to me with these complaints early in perimenopause, when they are just beginning to notice changes in their menstrual cycles. The reason is that vaginal tissue is loaded with oestrogen receptors. Like the canary in the coal mine, the condition of your vagina is an early warning sign that your hormonal balance is beginning to change.

HELEN—DIAGNOSING THE PROBLEM

About fifteen years ago—long before I was familiar with the symptoms of perimenopause—one of my patients, named Helen, reported that she was having sexual problems. A freelance graphic designer, she was 42 years old at the time and had been married to David, an executive chef, for about a decade. They had no kids and lived in a fabulous loft downtown, near David's restaurant.

"Congratulations," I greeted her. "I saw David got three stars!"

"Thanks," Helen replied with a sigh. I was immediately suspicious. Why wasn't she more excited?

"Is there something wrong? Do you want to talk about it?" I asked.

"Ever since *New York* magazine labeled David one of the 'hot' chefs in town, his ego has exploded. He's been impossible to live with—when he's home, that is, which isn't often. I know I should be thrilled for him; it's what he's always wanted and we're certainly enjoying the success financially. It's just that it's all about him these days, and I feel like this shadow lurking in the background."

"That's perfectly understandable," I reassured her. "Don't beat yourself up feeling guilty about it."

"I know I shouldn't, but I can't help myself," she responded. "And to make matters worse, our sex life has gone down the tubes."

"Well, I'd expect it would be a little tough with the hours he works—"

"No, it's not that," she interrupted. "It's me."

I asked her what she meant and she reeled off a list of symptoms: vaginal dryness, burning, irritation, and pain on intercourse.

"How are your periods?" I queried.

"Normal," she shrugged.

"I'm going to do some cultures of your vaginal lining to see whether you've picked up some kind of bacteria, but I have a strong suspicion that it's yeast." I prescribed Canesten vaginal cream and told her to start using it right away. "You may also want to talk with a therapist about the difficulties you're having with David. Sometimes stress in a relationship can actually cause physical problems that affect your sex life."

I didn't see Helen until her next annual exam. She reported that she was still not lubricating during intercourse and that now on top of the vaginal complaints she had burning in her urethra every time she urinated.

"My suspicion is that this is a case of chronic yeast infection," I told her. "It's really hard to get rid of. But I'd like you to see a urologist about the pain when you urinate just to rule out any urinary tract infections. By the way, how are your periods?"

She said that they'd been getting a little farther apart and that occasionally she would skip one. I noted this fact in her chart but, focused on the yeast idea, gave it little attention. "And what about you and David?" I asked casually.

"Not good. We were in couples counseling for about six months and nothing was getting better, so we've decided to try a separation."

"I'm sorry to hear that," I said.

"Yeah, I'm sorry, too," Helen responded.

The urologist gave Helen a clean bill of health, and she continued with a series of yeast treatments. At her next exam she reported the same symptoms inside her vagina as well as irritation outside, and the feeling that she had to urinate all the time. Again, I took cultures for everything I could think of. They all came back negative.

Then it dawned on me. I had her come in on day three of her next period and took a blood sample. Sure enough, her hormones were nearing the menopausal range. "I think I've figured out what the problem is," I told her. "I want you to start using this vaginal oestriol cream daily. After the first two weeks you can go to every other day. If your symptoms improve, taper off to three times a week as maintenance."

Helen called me two months later. "What a relief!" she said. "I can't believe I suffered all those years and this little tube cleared the whole thing up in only a couple of months. You know, I was really getting worried that I'd never be able to have sex again. Since David and I split up, I've been scared to start dating because I knew that if I met someone I wanted to sleep with, I wouldn't be able to stand the pain. Now I feel like I can start living again."

WHY YOU'RE DRY

There are two reasons for vaginal changes during perimenopause. The first is decreased blood flow. As you may recall, oestrogen is a vasodilator that increases the diameter and flexibility of blood vessels. Decreased oestrogen means constricted blood vessels and lowered circulation. Cells that are normally puffed up and plushy become thin and dry; like dry skin anywhere else on your body, they become prone to itchiness and irritation. Vaginal lubrication is also affected by circulation. Unlike, for example, the way your underarms sweat when liquid is secreted from glands under the skin, the vagina is moistened through a process called transudation. Basically this means that liquid seeps from the blood vessels into the spaces between the cells that line the passage, and eventually into the vagina itself. Without adequate blood supply to the area, the tissue does not contain enough fluid to lubricate the vaginal walls, and intercourse becomes much more difficult and uncomfortable.

The second reason for vaginal symptoms has to do with changes in the tissue itself. Like all mucous membranes—in your nose, your eyes, your mouth, your stomach, your urethra—your vagina is lined with epithelial tissue, which is made made up of three types of cells: superficial, intermediate, and parabasal. When we do a smear test, we take a sample of these cells from the upper part of the vagina and cervix. In the absence of adequate oestrogen the protective superficial layer, which is exposed to the outside, thins out or disappears altogether, whereas the internal intermediate and parabasal layers increase. Cigarette smoking has a similar effect. By contrast, when you have too much circulating oestrogen, the superficial layer becomes proliferative and the parabasal layer is lacking.

If you are suffering vaginal symptoms and experiencing pain during intercourse, you may develop a condition called *vaginismus,* or spasming of the vaginal muscles. The origin of this problem is actually in your brain, which after a time becomes wired to associate sex with pain. As a defensive reflex your brain will then, at the first sign of sexual arousal, send messages to your vaginal muscles ordering them to contract so as to prevent penetration. This, of course, makes intercourse even more agonizing, and eventually you may—understandably—lose your desire for sex altogether.

When I asked one perimenopausal patient why she was having sex less frequently, she said, "To be honest, it takes so long to get the juices flowing that half the time I fall asleep. Why bother?" Again, the problem is likely to be declining oestrogen and its effects on blood flow, nerve response, and muscle tone. Just as men with circulatory problems have trouble becoming erect, women with diminished vaginal blood flow do not achieve clitoral erection, making sexual arousal hard to achieve. Decreased oestrogen also leads to decreased responsiveness of the nerve endings in the clitoris and surrounding areas. When you finally do have an orgasm, it may feel weak because oestrogen receptors on the muscle cells supporting your vagina, uterus, and pelvic floor—the muscles that provide the rhythmic contractions felt during climax—are not being stimulated.

A South American patient of mine came in for a routine exam. I asked her if anything was new since we'd last talked. "My husband is the most wonderful Latin lover, but now I can't stand to have him touch me!" she exclaimed. When I probed what she meant by this, she said, "Literally, when he touches me it hurts." It turns out she was also experiencing sensitivity to certain clothing—she could no longer tolerate wool and was wearing mostly cotton—and occasional numbness and itchiness in different parts of her body. Although I'll discuss various skin changes associated with perimenopause in detail in the next chapter, it is important to note here that symptoms such as these, collectively known as *peripheral neuropathy,* can have a negative impact on sexual desire.

TREATMENTS FOR VAGINAL SYMPTOMS

I always feel terrible when patients tell me that they've been suffering vaginal symptoms that have compromised their sexual enjoyment for years but have been too shy to mention them. Speak up! There's nothing to be embarrassed about, and fortunately there are many excellent treatment options available.

WATER–SOLUBLE MOISTURIZERS. If your complaint is mostly dryness, burning, and itchiness of the vulvular and vaginal tissues, you could try one of the many nonprescription vaginal moisturizers that line chemists' shelves, such as Replens and Summer's Eve. A good over-the-counter natural vitamin E compound is Carlson's KEY-E ointment or suppositories, which should be applied once every two or three days.

WATER–SOLUBLE LUBRICANTS. According to Drs. Marcia and Lisa Douglass, authors of *Are We Having Fun Yet? The Intelligent Woman's Guide to Sex*, every woman, no matter what age, should use a lubricant for better sex. And certainly if your perimenopausal vaginal symptoms are making intercourse uncomfortable, run—don't walk—to the nearest chemist. I'm a big believer in water-soluble lubricants—some days I feel like I should just put a fishbowl full of Astroglide samples on the reception desk with a sign: "Take a handful on your way out." K-Y Jelly, K-Y Silk E, Abelene Unscented Cream, Touch, Lubrin, and Moist Again are other brands you might try.

OESTROGEN. Oestrogen improves vaginal moisture, elasticity, and thickness. Because vaginal tissue is so sensitive to oestrogen, a very low dose can reverse perimenopausal discomforts. It is especially effective when applied directly to vaginal tissue as opposed to being taken orally. *Oestriol cream,* for example, works wonders, especially for my perimenopausal patients. Their vaginal tissues bounce back pretty quickly because they haven't been deprived of oestrogen for very long. If you wait a number of years before seeking treatment, however, it may take up to six months to see results. *Oestradiol cream (Orthodinoestrol)* also works well. Note that oestrogen creams should not be used as lubricants.

The *oestradiol ring (Estring)* is just as effective as the cream. Some women prefer it because it only needs to be changed every three months, whereas the cream has to be applied daily in the beginning, followed by a slow tapering down. The oestradiol ring also gives a slow, steady dose, very little of which goes into your bloodstream, making it a good choice for women with or at risk of breast cancer. It looks similar to the ring on a diaphragm and shouldn't affect your partner.

I often prescribe *low-dose oral contraceptives* because they not only improve the dryness and control other perimenopausal symptoms but also provide birth control, which, let's not forget, is still a consideration! *Oral oestrogen replacement therapy* increases blood flow to the vagina and thickens the lining of the vagina. The *transdermal oestradiol patch* also helps. But vaginal oestrogen is superior to oral or transdermal when it comes to treating vaginal symptoms.

PROGESTOGENS. Adding synthetic or natural progesterone to your oestrogen regimen can relieve painful intercourse. The reason is not clear, but one theory is that progesterone reduces pain perception in the central nervous system.

TESTOSTERONE. When applied directly to vaginal tissue, testosterone ointment, cream, or gel thickens the vaginal tissues and increases moisture and sensitivity. Ointments remain local, whereas gels and creams are absorbed into the bloodstream and can lift the libido.

SEX. Last but not least, have sex. If it's too painful, then masturbate. Have you heard the old adage "Use it or lose it"? Well, it's based on fact. There's a proven correlation between frequency of intercourse or self-stimulation and vaginal health. The reasons are not 100 percent clear, but my guess is that both biological and psychological factors are at play. On the one hand, orgasm triggers a flood of neurotransmitters from the brain, which can have physical as well as mental effects. On the other hand, feeling attractive and sexy can also alter your brain chemistry, priming your body to act on those feelings. In general, sex increases blood flow in the vaginal tissue, which can help relieve and even prevent vaginal symptoms on its own or enhance the therapeutic effects of oestrogen supplementation.

WHEN YOU'VE LOST THAT LOVIN' FEELING

One of the biggest secrets I've discovered being a gynaecologist is how many women at midlife are *not* interested in sex. The reasons vary— their busy lives, their partners' busy lives, lack of a partner, or just plain lack of desire. Remarkably often, women have no problem with this, seeing it as a new life stage when they can direct the energies they used to spend on sex toward other things, like their careers, their children, or themselves. If a woman does find loss of libido to be a problem, however, it's important to figure out what may be causing it and try to find a cure.

In many ways, the brain is the ultimate erogenous zone, as sexual responsiveness depends as much on the state of the mind as on that of the body. Mind-body interaction is a two-way street, with physical changes being capable of influencing thought, and thought being capable of influencing physical changes. If vaginal symptoms are making sex a pain, the oestrogen supplements that treat them will also make sex more enjoyable and desirable. Although oestrogen does not have a direct effect on libido, it can help by elevating mood and relieving hot flushes and insomnia. Let's face it—if you're feeling worthless, dropping dead of fatigue, or flushing every hour, you're unlikely to want to get romantic.

Because Saint John's wort and ginkgo biloba elevate your mood, they can also improve your libido.

TESTOSTERONE—A MIRACLE HORMONE?

"My husband's on Viagra and—can I tell you something? I could care less," one of my patients recently confided. A year earlier I'd prescribed the low-dose transdermal oestradiol patch and progesterone to alleviate her many perimenopausal symptoms, which included sleep disturbances, memory loss, hot flushes, decreased energy, fatigue, joint pain, and decreased libido. Even though most of them were improved, she still was dragging and now reported absolutely no interest in sex. I added testosterone to her hormone replacement therapy. Two months later she faxed me: "That testosterone gave me a real zip! And so far no signs of a beard."

There's been a lot of talk recently about using testosterone to boost libido in women. Although testosterone is known as the male sex hormone, women naturally produce testosterone as well, only at much lower levels. In perimenopause your testosterone level may increase, decrease, or stay the same.

The main sign that you may be one of those women whose testosterone level has gone down is an otherwise inexplicable loss of sexual interest and enjoyment. Testosterone influences your sex drive by working on the brain level to increase your sexual fantasies and desire. It also increases your genital sensitivity and the intensity of your orgasms. There is no evidence that it affects performance, however; oestrogen seems to be what's required when physical problems such as vaginal dryness or painful intercourse are causing decreased libido.

Just the other day I was doing a breast exam on a 49-year-old patient whom I'd put on natural oestrogen, progesterone, and testosterone a while back. "Dr. Corio," she said timidly, "I have to tell you something. After you put me on those hormones, my husband and I could not be in the same room together!" She blushed from her head to her chest. "It was like we were two kids again! I even began to have dreams about sex. Isn't that a sin?"

"No way—that's great!" I replied, palpating her left breast.

"Now it's calmed down a bit," she added, "but I'll never forget those few weeks!"

This patient, who had complained of decreased libido, clearly benefited from testosterone in her perimenopause. But there are others who do not require it until several years after menopause.

When I was a resident twenty years ago, I was taught that if a woman had a hysterectomy after age 40, you took the ovaries out with her uterus in order to prevent ovarian cancer. We now know that not only is the risk of ovarian cancer very low, but you can still get it even if you have your ovaries removed. Today we leave the ovaries if at all possible, because they continue to produce testosterone for four or five years after you go through menopause.

Several patients have come to me after other doctors had performed hysterectomies including removal of the ovaries, putting them into surgical menopause. In spite of being placed on all different kinds of oestrogen, they were still feeling terrible. No one had thought to give them testosterone. I added testosterone to their regimen, and to my satisfaction their fatigue, moods, hot flushes, and libido all improved.

To measure testosterone levels in my perimenopausal patients, I use saliva testing. If the level is low, I add testosterone to their oestrogen replacement therapy. Along with testosterone, I always prescribe lots of sex. If you take androgen supplements to boost your libido and engage in frequent sexual activity, you'll find your sexual desire and enjoyment of sex are enhanced.

Combined oestrogen/testosterone pills such as Estratest can be used, but they contain synthetic oestrogen and testosterone and you may need to adjust your dose. You can also get sublingual testosterone lozenges, but my patients who are on the go find them hard to use— they have to be refrigerated at all times. I am eagerly awaiting the approval of a transdermal testosterone patch, because I think it will be more effective than oral testosterone.

Testosterone may decrease your HDL, or "good," cholesterol level, but not to abnormally low levels, and it also may in very rare cases adversely affect your liver. It is therefore important to have your blood tested periodically for cholesterol and lipid levels and liver function if you are taking testosterone.

VIAGRA FOR WOMEN?

Unfortunately, that little blue pill that's getting your husband's train out of the station won't do you any good. One of my patients who was suffering libido problems decided she would give it a try. She took a pill and lay down on the bed. Meanwhile, her husband went into the bathroom and got ready. He showered and shaved, splashed on cologne, brushed his teeth, and put on his black silk robe. He emerged from the bathroom to find her snoring loudly. She was unarousable. They laughed for days.

But there's hope on the horizon. Trials are in the works for a new Viagra cream for women that will work directly on the vaginal tissues. Sounds good to me!

WHEN IT *IS* ALL IN YOUR HEAD

At any age, poor body image, previous sexual abuse, depression, anxiety, sociocultural taboos, and relationship problems can affect a person's sex life. Perimenopause adds several more layers of psychological stress that can damage your sexual self-image. For one thing, you have to deal with all the negative social and cultural images of aging, from the old maid to the old hag. Believing that sexual desire and attractiveness decline with reproductive ability will make such a decline a self-fulfilling prophesy—if you don't feel sexy, you won't act sexy; and if you don't act sexy, you won't feel sexy.

Although I always recommend my patients maintain a regular exercise pattern, doing so can specifically help increase low sex drive. For one thing, exercise improves mood by stimulating the brain to release opiates and neurotransmitters such as serotonin. It also increases circulation and brings more blood to all areas of the body, including tissues that may be suffering from oestrogen deprivation. It helps keep weight gain—which can inhibit desire in you or your partner—under control. But perhaps most important of all, exercise will make you feel better about your body. Poor body image is one of the major reasons women of all ages avoid intimate contact. It's especially prevalent in the perimenopausal years when all the magazine covers, television shows, and movies featuring barely post-adolescent women may be making you feel especially over-the-hill. Now more than ever you should do everything you can to feel good about yourself. Stretch, swim, jog, dance; get a massage, a manicure, a haircut; go to a spa—do whatever makes you feel sensual, sexy, and self-confident about your body.

"Milt and I have had a lovely romantic life for twenty-five years now," a 51-year-old patient told me. "It's never been swing-from-the-chandelier kind of sex, but it's been perfect for us. Now he's beginning to have some difficulties, which I completely understand. The problem is that he's so embarrassed that he won't even come near me, for fear of starting something he can't finish. This makes me feel terribly undesirable. I wish he'd realize that it's not all about intercourse—I love *him*, not his penis!"

When women reach perimenopause, men, who are often older than their partners, may begin experiencing sexual dysfunction, suddenly throwing a wrench into a sexual dynamic that may have been running smoothly for decades. Any unresolved sexual difficulties you may have experienced in the early years of your relationship are likely to resurface during this time. Because it may seem like it's too late to alter the old sexual script, you may accept these changes as inevitable and slide into platonic companionship without making an effort to discuss your feelings with each other or a professional. Embarrassment and inertia are no reasons to deprive yourself of the joys of sexual intimacy, however. If you find yourself in this situation, I urge you to seek the help of a sex therapist or psychologist because it doesn't have to be this way.

Many of my perimenopausal patients who find themselves in new relationships, by contrast, *are* experiencing swing-from-the-chandelier kind of sex. One recently told me that she and her partner were feeding each other samples of Brie at the cheese counter of her local gourmet store when they became so overcome with lust that they dropped their shopping baskets and raced home to bed. Another called her beau at work and he left his desk on Wall Street in the middle of trading hours to run to her apartment for a quickie. (He ended up making several hundred thousand dollars that afternoon anyway.) There's no reason you can't fan the flames of a long-term relationship at this time, either. Try some of the tips on pages 108–109 to refresh your romance.

CHECK YOUR MEDICINE CHEST

All too often, sexual problems are caused by drugs or medical conditions and have nothing whatsoever to do with your age, your attractiveness, or your relationship. Antihistamines dry up mucous membranes, for example, having the same effect on the vaginal lining as oestrogen deprivation does. In fact, any drug with the side effect of dry mouth will dry up your other epithelial tissue, including the vagina. Antidepressants, such as Prozac, Lustral, Seroxat, tricyclics, and MAO inhibitors, act on the neurotransmitters in a way that decreases sexual libido and causes difficulty reaching orgasm. If this is a problem for you, ask your psychiatrist about switching to another antidepressant, such as Wellbutrin, that doesn't have as many sexual side effects. Certain antipsychotics such as Haldol and beta-blockers such as Inderal can have the same effect. Digoxin and Tagamet can also impair sexual function.

Chronic conditions such as diabetes, pulmonary disease, hypertension, thyroid disease, and endometriosis can cause sexual problems, as can any sexually transmitted disease. Even yeast infections can make intercourse painful. Physical ailments such as arthritis and other musculoskeletal conditions may make sex uncomfortable. And the diagnosis and treatment of cancers of the breasts, reproductive organs, or genital region can have a profound effect on sexual function—both physically and psychologically.

Unfortunately, people are often unaware that their physical health may be affecting their sexual desire and mistakenly blame themselves or their partners, causing all kinds of unnecessary psychological and emotional trauma. Before torturing yourself this way, talk to a doctor about the changes in your sexual response. I always ask my patients what medications they are taking—herbs as well as drugs—and what medical conditions they are suffering. If your doctor doesn't ask, volunteer the information: "I'm not sure whether this has anything to do with my symptoms, but I happen to be taking allergy medication." Switching drugs or simply understanding that an underlying medical issue is the cause of your sexual problem can often provide relief, both from the problem itself and also from the stress and damage to your self-esteem that the problem may have caused.

Spicing Up Your Sex Life

If your sex life is getting stale, here are ten simple ideas for adding a little zing:

1. *Flirt.* Cast your mind back to the days when you and your partner were first falling in love, before it all became routine. Resurrect some of the fun, flirty things you used to do, such as calling and leaving sexy messages on his answering machine (or, these days, e-mail), leaving provocative notes in unsuspecting places like his briefcase or toolbox, or dropping the occasional double entendre into your conversation.

2. *Make a date.* Remember dates? The anticipation, the excitement? Why not make one with your partner? Sure, you see him every night, but pick one evening and make it special. Plan in advance what you're going to do—a romantic dinner, a seaside stroll, a night at the opera—get dressed up, spend some extra time on your make-up and hair, try a new perfume. And remember, the date doesn't end when you get back home. Have some candles strategically positioned, dim the lights, play soft music, and let the seduction begin.

3. *Dress sexy.* How many times have you walked by a lingerie shop, or through the lingerie section of a large department store, caught a quick glimpse of some frothy concoction, and quickly turned your head, saying, "Not for me"? Well, why not? Whatever your idea of sexy clothing, be it a lace nightie or a sports bra, indulge yourself.

4. *Break the habit.* If you usually have sex on Saturday nights in bed after the kids have gone to sleep, try Thursday afternoon on the kitchen table while they're out at soccer practice. Or Tuesday morning in the shower. Or lunchtime Friday on the back lawn. If you can swing a weekend getaway, even better; but often changing the routine at home can help bring back that spontaneous, uninhibited honeymoon feeling.

5. *Don't forget foreplay.* Sex isn't just about intercourse. In fact, most women find hugging and cuddling and talking sexier than the act itself. Don't deprive yourself of this part of the experience—and don't let your partner rush you through it either. One great way to keep him at bay and prolong the excitement is massage. Buy some scented massage oil and a book on sensual

massage. If you're having difficulty lubricating, it's especially important to take the time to prepare yourself, body and mind.

6. ***Turn things upside down.*** While you're at it, why not try some new positions? If he's usually on top, flip him over. Use your bedroom furniture creatively—the edge of the bed, the chair, the windowsill, in front of the mirror…

7. ***Tell him what you want.*** Communication is the key to good sex. If you can't bring yourself to verbalize, point and push him in the right direction. If you can talk openly about your desires, don't stop there. Share your fantasies and encourage your partner to do the same. Sexual desire starts in the brain, after all, so acting out some of the scripts you've written in your mind can really jump-start your libido. Plus, talking about sex is incredibly sexy.

8. ***Practice in private.*** All too often women don't even know what makes them feel good because there are such strong societal taboos against exploring our own bodies. But if you don't know, how can you expect him to? Find a time and place where you can have some privacy—the bathtub is a good spot—and let your hands wander. Once you know what turns you on, you can show him. And you may find the act of showing a turn-on in and of itself.

9. ***Exercise.*** Exercise is one of the best libido-boosters around for the reasons I've explained previously. This doesn't mean you have to start training for the marathon. Figure out a realistic program that includes activities you enjoy, not ones you view as torture. If you hate going to a gym, try bicycling, playing tennis, jogging, speedwalking, or doing yoga. If you find it easy to talk yourself out of your intended activity, exercise with a partner or join a class. Peer pressure will help keep you from making excuses.

10. ***Seek inspiration.*** There are lots of good books and videos available to give you ideas on new positions and techniques that can help you help yourself. If you're self-conscious about buying them at your local book or video store, or checking them out of the library, order them by mail, over the phone, or on the Internet.

VAGINAL AND URINARY TRACT INFECTIONS

Perimenopausal women are especially prone to vaginal infection *(vaginitis)* and urinary tract infections, or UTIs *(cystitis)*. Recall the changes in epithelial tissue we discussed earlier? When oestrogen levels are normal, cells of the thick superficial layer contain abundant glycogen. As these cells shed during their normal life cycle, they feed the Döderlein's lactobacilli, an innocuous organism that inhabits the vagina, which then produce lactic acid. One of the reasons our bodies happily host this parasitic organism is that the lactic acid it releases keeps the normal vaginal pH between 3.5 and 4.5, too acidic to support invading infectious agents.

When oestrogen levels decline, the superficial layer of the epithelium thins and there is not enough glycogen available to maintain a healthy colony of Döderlein's lactobacilli. Without the lactic acid they produce, vaginal pH increases to between 6.0 and 8.0. (Your doctor can measure this using a pH indicator strip—a small piece of specially treated paper that is swiped against the inside of the vagina.) In this more neutral environment, women become susceptible to all kinds of contaminating organisms. If you notice the sudden appearance of a thin, grayish vaginal discharge, see your doctor, as this is often a sign of a bacterial infection.

Because the openings to the urethra and vaginal canal are located so close together—they become even closer during perimenopause, as part of the overall thinning of the vaginal tissue—the urinary tract often becomes infected by any opportunistic organisms that may have invaded the vagina. Furthermore, like the vagina, the urethra is lined with epithelial tissue, which, in response to decreased oestrogen, also begins to become thin and dry. Without a thick protective layer of superficial cells and with increased pH, the urinary tract is similarly vulnerable to infection.

WAYS TO PREVENT VAGINITIS AND CYSTITIS

Antibiotics are the standard treatment for both vaginitis and cystitis. If you are prone to these infections during your perimenopausal stage, here are some tips for prevention.

THE BREAKFAST OF UTI CHAMPIONS

"I thought cystitis was a honeymooner's disease," one of my patients wondered. "We've been married twenty-five years and all of a sudden I'm getting these recurring urinary tract infections." I did a full exam and found nothing unusual. As prevention against future infection, I recommended the Breakfast of UTI Champions: organic yogurt with live acidophilus, a blueberry muffin, and artificially sweetened cranberry juice (sugar feeds bacteria). "I thought those were just old wives' remedies," she said, eyeing me a little dubiously. I explained that those old wives knew what they were talking about: blueberries and cranberries contain hippuric acid, which prevents unwanted bacteria from sticking to the bladder lining and initiating an infection. They also increase the acidity of vaginal secretions, while the acidophilus bacilli in the yogurt replace the natural flora that have died off.

Vitamins and Minerals

VITAMIN C. Vitamin C acidifies the urine, making the bladder inhospitable to bacteria. Take 1,000 mg daily.

Herbs

UVA URSI. Also known as *bearberry* or *mountain box*, this herb is used as a urinary antiseptic specifically for UTIs. It has antiviral, antibacterial, and antifungal properties and helps heal damaged tissue. But its active ingredient, arbutin, only works if your urinary tract has a basic pH. If you are already taking vitamin C or drinking a lot of cranberry juice to acidify your urine, uva ursi won't help you. I recommend 250 to 500 mg three times a day; but remember, uva ursi is not a cure. If you do not feel better after a couple of days, consult your physician, as you may need antibiotics.

Oestrogen

Oestrogen restores the pH in the bladder and vagina, making them welcoming to those nice lactobacilli. It also thickens the lining of the urethra and vagina, so that they are less prone to infection. Vaginitis and cystitis respond particularly well to local oestrogen: either *oestrogen cream* applied vaginally or the *vaginal oestrogen ring (Estring)*. You may find that either standard or low-dose oestrogen taken orally or oral contraceptives also provide some relief, but they may not be as effective as oestrogen applied locally.

Other Recommendations

Last but not least, maintain good hygiene, wear cotton underwear, drink at least eight 8-ounce glasses of water daily, and urinate frequently, especially after intercourse. Also, if you are a diaphragm user, you may need to try an alternative form of birth control, as the diaphragm increases the risk of urinary tract and yeast infections. In cases of vaginitis I do *not* recommend douching, as the pressure of the liquid drives bacteria up the vagina, increasing the risk of much more serious pelvic infections.

WHEN YOU JUST CAN'T HOLD IT IN

There's a sneaky little problem that most perimenopausal women are loath to mention: urinary incontinence. But the fact of the matter is that this embarrassing problem is incredibly common. Eleven million American women have difficulty controlling their bladders. One out of four women between the ages of 30 and 59 report occasional incontinence, with the incidence rising to three out of five between ages 45 and 54. Even if you're not wetting your pants, you may feel a frequent urge to urinate that has led you to limit your liquid intake after a certain time of night or refrain from drinking anything within an hour of a long car ride.

During perimenopause, 30 percent of women report incontinence at least once a month. Most of these are instances of stress incontinence: a little squirt when you cough, sneeze, laugh, or exert yourself. (Dribbling tends to be a greater problem postmenopausally.) Urge incontinence, which happens when you just can't wait, also becomes an issue. "It's like this Pavlovian reflex," one patient told me. "The minute I put the key in the lock, I have to go. Even though the bathroom is only ten feet from the front door, I can barely make it in time. And sometimes I'm too late."

The vagina, vulva, urethra, and lower part of the bladder were embryonic neighbors, and all contain large numbers of oestrogen receptors. Just as vaginal tissues respond to lack of oestrogen by drying up and becoming less flexible and responsive, so do the tissues that line the urethra, the blood vessels that feed it, and the muscles that surround it. In particular, these sphincter muscles, which are usually tightened to hold urine but which the brain signals to relax when it's time to go, are weakened by oestrogen deprivation, making it hard to hold back the flow. This loss of muscle tone, combined with the thinning of the urethral tissue due to changes in the epithelium and decreased blood flow, reduces the pressure in the urethral canal that under normal circumstances prevents urine from escaping the bladder.

The first thing I do when a patient comes in complaining about urinary incontinence is run a urine culture to rule out any infection. Vaginal infections and constipation can also cause incontinence. In addition, I ask what medications she is taking, as certain blood pressure medications, antidepressants, antipsychotics, over-the-counter diet medications, cold remedies, sedatives, painkillers, antihistamines, decongestants, nasal sprays, and diuretics can all contribute to the problem. If you're suffering incontinence and you think it may be because of a medication, ask your doctor if there is an alternative drug you can take.

Believe it or not, certain foods and drink can trigger incontinence. Alcohol, caffeine, artificial sweeteners, carbonated beverages, citrus fruits and juices, highly spiced foods, and tomatoes and tomato-based products can all trigger leakage. Smoking can contribute to stress incontinence as well.

METHODS FOR TREATING INCONTINENCE

Pelvic floor exercises (Kegels) and bladder training are extremely effective ways to manage incontinence. But before beginning self-help exercises, see a doctor to make sure there isn't a physical problem underlying your incontinence. There are several drugs and devices he or she can prescribe that may help keep you dry. If all else fails, you may need surgery.

Self-Help Techniques

PELVIC FLOOR EXERCISES. Often called Kegel exercises after the physician who introduced them in the United States, pelvic floor exercises have been known for centuries to be a good general health practice for women. In the hatha yoga tradition, they are referred to as "private meditation" because, if they are done correctly, no one need know but you. Ideally, every young woman should learn them during her teenage years and practice them for the rest of her life, as they are the number-one way to strengthen the muscles that surround the vagina and support the bladder, uterus, and rectum. An added bonus: they can improve your sex life by making your vagina tighter, increasing stimulation for both you and your partner.

Many women are taught pelvic floor exercises for the first time during childbirth classes, as they prepare the muscles used to push out a baby. Most women do not continue these exercises after their babies are born, however, which is a particular shame, as vaginal birth increases the risk of incontinence later in life. Those who do continue have much less chance of developing incontinence as well as prolapse of the uterus, bladder, and/or rectum when they reach perimenopause. The good news is that up to 80 percent of women who suffer incontinence may be cured by regularly doing these exercises.

Kegel exercises are extremely easy to do once you figure out the right muscles to contract. At first it takes a lot of concentration, but after doing them for several weeks you'll find it much easier and be able to do them in a variety of positions. To start, lie on your back with your knees bent and your feet flat on the floor. Imagine that you're in the middle of urinating and the doorbell rings. The muscles you use to stop the flow of urine are the ones you want to isolate. Start by constricting those muscles; then slowly work your way up the vagina, imagining ring upon ring of muscles going all the way up into your pelvis. It's like riding an elevator, constricting at each floor until you reach the top. Once you do reach the top, hold the contraction as hard as you can—at first you may only be able to do so for two or three seconds; eventually you should work up to ten. Then slowly ride the elevator down, releasing each ring until you reach the bottom. Take a deep breath and relax completely before repeating the exercise.

Begin by doing at least ten repetitions twice a day. Work up to as many as you can, but at least fifty daily. You'll notice improvement within a few weeks. You may find that a few Kegels performed right before doing something that usually causes you to leak, such as heavy lifting, or when you feel an urge to urinate coming on, can prevent an episode of incontinence.

The hardest part about this exercise is isolating the right muscles— your thigh and gluteal muscles should not be involved. Also, beware of the tendency to bear down, as if you were making a bowel movement, as this is the opposite of what you want to do. Rather, think about pulling the anus upward and inward along with the vagina. Once you become proficient, you'll find you can do these exercises anywhere—standing on the checkout line at the supermarket, talking on the phone, sitting in traffic, riding the bus. The more the merrier!

BLADDER TRAINING. If you suffer incontinence, you can train yourself to avoid urinating at inopportune moments. Much the way you would toilet-train a toddler by putting her on the toilet at specific times whether or not she has to go, such as before bedtime or before leaving the house, bladder training involves making yourself urinate at specific intervals. Gradually stretching out those intervals trains the bladder to accommodate more fluid. Although tedious, bladder training is extremely effective, curing incontinence in more than half the women who maintain the program for a minimum of six weeks.

The first step is to keep a voiding diary for at least three days in which you record every time you urinate, voluntarily or involuntarily, day or night. A typical example looks like this:

SAMPLE VOIDING DIARY

Patient ___Lorraine___

Address ___Feb 12, 2000___

INSTRUCTIONS: Place a check in the appropriate column next to the time you urinated in the toilet or when an incontinence episode occurred. Note the reason for the incontinence and describe your liquid intake (for example, coffee, water) and estimate the amount (for example, one cup).

Time interval	Urinated in toilet	Had a small incontinence episode	Had a large incontinence episode	Reason for incontinence episode	Type/amount of liquid intake
6-8 a.m.	6:30 ✓ 7:30 7:45	✓ 7:00		sneeze	coffee 2 cups
8-10 a.m.	✓ 8:10 8:40		✓ 9:00	exercise class	2 cups coffee
10- noon	10:15 ✓ 10:30	✓ 11:15		laughing	1 bottle water (16 oz)
Noon-2 p.m.	noon ✓ 12:25 1:30	✓ 1:00			½ bottle water (8 oz)
2-4 p.m.	2:10 ✓ 2:40 3:10	✓ 3:45		cough	1 cup coffee
4-6 p.m.	4:15 ✓ 4:50 5:40	✓ 5:00		running for the phone	½ bottle water 8 oz. lemonade
6-8 p.m.	6:00 ✓ 6:30 7:30				8 oz. OJ
8-10 p.m.	8:00 ✓ 8:45 10:00	✓ 9:15		lifting kids into bed	
10-midnight	11:15 ✓ 11:45				
Overnight	3:00 4:15 ✓ 4:30				

No. of pads used today: ___8___   No. of episodes ___7___

Comments: ___miserable day   Exhausted.___

Based on your diary entries, figure out the average time between voidings during your waking hours. In the sample case presented here, the average time is 30 minutes. It may be 15 minutes; it may be an hour. Your initial voiding interval will be your average rounded down to the nearest 15-minute increment. If your average is every 40 minutes, for example, your initial interval will be every 30 minutes. This means that you must urinate every half hour from the time you wake up in the morning to the time you go to bed at night. It's okay to push it five or ten minutes in either direction, but just make sure that you get back on schedule the next time.

Once you can comfortably maintain this routine without any accidents between voidings, increase the interval by 30 minutes. If you find that too big a leap, scale back by 15 minutes. It will probably take at least a week to become relaxed and confident with each new interval. Your ultimate goal is to achieve two- to four-hour intervals.

When you feel the need to go but it's not yet time, there are several strategies you can try to forestall the urge. The first is to distract yourself. Pick up a book, do a crossword puzzle, make a phone call, knit, pay some bills—anything to keep your mind occupied. "It's mind over bladder," I tell my patients. The second is to practice relaxation techniques such as deep breathing. If the urge to urinate makes you feel anxious, you may need to relax before you can begin to distract yourself. The third is to tighten the pelvic floor muscles a few times, an exercise that can reverse incontinence in and of itself.

Urethral Devices

PROSTHESES. You may have heard about plastic or silicone pads, caps, or patches used to cover the urethra. These prescription prostheses work by changing the angle between your urethra and your bladder so you don't leak urine. The latest breakthrough is a device called Introl Bladder Neck Support Prosthesis. It has to be fitted by your doctor, but then you can insert it, remove it, wash it, and lubricate it daily.

CAPS. FemAssist is a prescription soft rubber cap that you put over the opening of your urethra. It is held in place by suction. You need to take it off every time you urinate.

PATCHES. A new prescription product, the Impress Softpatch, is a small disposable foam pad, like a mini sanitary napkin, that you place over the opening to your urethra. You change it every two to three hours during the day and can wear it all night except when you're having sex.

Oestrogen

Perimenopausal incontinence may be successfully treated with oestrogen in either cream or pill form. *Before prescribing oestrogen to treat incontinence, however, I always recommend that my patient see a urologist to rule out any other non-hormonal causes.*

Drugs

Ditropan and Detrusitol are commonly prescribed for treatment of an overactive bladder with symptoms of urinary incontinence, urgency, and frequency.

Surgery

There are several different surgical techniques for treating urinary incontinence. All of them are based on the same principle. Basically, we want to make it harder for the urine to flow down the urethra, normally a straight shot. Using slings or suspensions, we lift the urethra, so the urine has to go uphill first, making it harder for urine to leak out involuntarily. Collagen or silicone injections can bulk up the tissue surrounding the urethra, tightening the sphincter and making it harder for urine to pass through.

DENISE—PROLAPSED EVERYTHING

"It's totally mortifying," Denise confided, looking me straight in the eye. "Every time I have sex, I pee."

Denise was a new patient, a 47-year-old advertising executive who had been raising three teenage children on her own since her husband was killed in a rock-climbing accident two years earlier. She was smartly dressed in a revealing black jumpsuit I recalled seeing recently in *Vogue*. Her dead-straight henna-red hair was cut in a dramatic, asymmetrical do. Brusque and self-confident, she exuded command as well as creativity.

"How long has this been going on?" I asked.

"Ever since I started having sex again, about two months ago. Before that, with Bob's death and all, I'd gone through a long dry spell, so I wouldn't have noticed any problem. Now that I'm back in the swing there have been several men in my life, but this peeing problem is really putting a damper on things."

I asked her about the deliveries of her three children, and she told me they'd each been nearly 10 pounds, delivered vaginally. Two years after having her third, she had surgery to repair her prolapsed bladder *(cystocele)* and confessed that she'd been living in fear of a repeat occurrence ever since. "I'm the Queen of Kegels," she told me. When I asked if anything other than sex set off spontaneous urination, she mentioned high-impact aerobic exercise. "I used to jog six miles a day but haven't been able to do that for seven or eight years. Now I ride a stationary bike for about forty-five minutes each day and do a lot of free weights."

"How are your periods?" I queried.

"Getting a little further apart, now about thirty-five days. They used to be twenty-eight, twenty-nine."

"And what are you using for birth control?"

"Condoms—I'm not taking any chances!" she replied, raising her carefully tweezed eyebrows.

When I performed an internal exam, I was confronted with not only a prolapsed bladder but a prolapsed cervix, uterus, and rectum as well. Everything had fallen down.

"While the Kegels may have prevented this from happening earlier, it looks as if those three deliveries really damaged the muscles in your vagina that support all these organs," I explained. "There's only one option at this point."

"And that is?"

"Surgery," I replied. "Providing you don't want to have any more children—"

"You've *got* to be kidding!"

"—I'd like to remove your uterus and cervix, and repair your bladder and rectum."

"That sounds pretty major," she commented.

"It is, but the muscles are shot; no amount of oestrogen or exercise will help at this point."

"Will I have to go on hormones afterward?" Denise asked.

"No, because I'll be leaving your ovaries, so you won't go through surgical menopause. But two weeks after the surgery I will start you on some vaginal oestriol cream to help build up the tissues."

"Then let's do it as soon as possible," she said decisively. "I'll call you to schedule an appointment as soon as I get back to the office and check my book. It's taken me a few years to get my life back together, and now I don't want anything to stand in the way of my happiness."

"Good for you," I said. "I'll see you soon."

THE COLLAGEN CONNECTION

Even though vaginal delivery can definitely weaken the muscles of the pelvic floor, I don't usually see prolapse of the organs of the lower abdomen until perimenopause—often years or even decades after the initial damage was done. I also see prolapse in women who have never had children. Part of the reason is that declining oestrogen leads to loss of urogenital muscle tone. But even more important, scientists are just discovering, are oestrogen-related changes in collagen.

You've probably seen ads for face creams that claim to be "fortified" with collagen, or heard of people having collagen injections to get rid of wrinkles. As I'll explain in the following chapter, collagen does play a crucial role in keeping your skin looking younger. It also is a major factor in maintaining bone density, which we'll discuss in Chapter 8. Indeed, collagen is in many ways a miracle molecule, performing a wide range of important tasks throughout the body. Because it is oestrogen-sensitive, however, all of those tasks are affected during the perimenopausal years.

Among its many functions, collagen is the major constituent of connective tissue. A flexible but non-elastic protein, it is found outside the actual cells, providing the scaffolding that holds the tissue together. Less collagen means less support for organs that the connective tissue is supposed to hold in place, such as the bladder, uterus, and rectum. Women with genital prolapse have decreased Type I collagen, and women with stress incontinence produce 30 percent less collagen than do those with normal urination. In the case of incontinence, reduced collagen may be affecting the urinary tract at two levels. On the one hand, the bladder itself may be prolapsed. On the other, connective tissue that surrounds the urethra may be weakened, decreasing the pressure that holds urine in.

Although oestrogen therapy cannot reverse organ prolapse, it can relieve stress incontinence by contributing to the buildup of collagen in the urethral sphincter.

PROLAPSE—SYMPTOMS AND RELIEF

Most of my patients don't come to me saying, "Dr. Corio, I think I have a prolapsed uterus." Rather, they complain that their diaphragm doesn't fit anymore or that they're having trouble using a tampon—they put it in, but it pops right out. Some find intercourse uncomfortable, as if there's not enough room for the penis. Others notice "pressure" or "feel like something's falling out." Women with prolapsed bladders may notice that they have to adjust their position to get just the right angle in order to urinate. Women with prolapsed rectums may find they have to insert a finger into their vagina to assist with bowel movements.

Once we've discussed their symptoms, I perform a vaginal exam. Sometimes I can see right away that an organ is protruding into the vaginal canal. Other times, I ask the patient to cough or bear down as if she is making a bowel movement. The pressure will force any prolapsed organs to pop out. Alternatively, I may perform a manual exam while my patient stands, using gravity to help show me what's what.

Once a prolapsed organ has been diagnosed, the only treatment is surgery or a vaginal pessary (which is left in all the time and is changed every three months by your doctor). I generally don't recommend pessaries in perimenopause because they make it impossible to have intercourse. Rather, for a prolapsed bladder or rectum, I repair the damaged connective tissue surgically. In addition, if the uterus is prolapsed, I recommend a vaginal hysterectomy if the patient is through with childbearing. If she still wants children, I tell her to conceive as quickly as possible, but I warn her that she may need a pessary in her first trimester.

Of course, an ounce of prevention is worth a pound of cure. Even though there's nothing you can do to repair connective tissue that is already damaged through difficult vaginal deliveries, you can strengthen the muscles of the vaginal walls to help compensate for this weakness and keep the organs in place. Kegel, Kegel, Kegel! Do up to 100 repetitions a day. Pelvic floor exercises are discreet, so you can do them anytime, anywhere. Who knows—that woman sitting next to you at the beauty salon may be doing her Kegels, too.

CHAPTER 6

Mirror, Mirror, On the Wall: Visible Signs of Perimenopause

This past summer my close friend Michelle called me, very upset. "I don't know what to do, Laura, I feel like my body is falling apart. I've gained twelve pounds in the past year, which means I now have to lose nearly thirty to get back to where I want to be. And when I look in the mirror I see a St. Bernard—I've got *jowls!* The wrinkles are so bad I'm considering having plastic surgery. What do you think?"

"If it'll make you feel better about yourself, go for it," I responded. Michelle had been a heavy smoker since we were teenagers, so her skin had aged prematurely. She'd tried every skin product on the market, but to no avail.

After discussing the pros and cons with her for a while, I suggested she make an appointment with a plastic surgeon I know. They met, and in the early fall she had her face lifted and her eyes done.

For the week following surgery, Michelle was forbidden to smoke. When the time was up, she decided to take the opportunity to kick the habit altogether. "That first week was so hard, I figured I may as well continue—it couldn't get any worse," she told me when I stopped by to see how she was doing. "Besides, smoking is what made me look like such a hag in the first place. If I want this lift to last, I'd better start taking better care of my skin."

"Yes," I agreed. "It's major surgery, not something you want to have to go through every five years."

"And as long as I'm on this self-improvement kick," Michelle continued, "I'm going to tackle my weight. You're a doctor—what really works?"

"Diet and exercise are the only way to take it off and keep it off," I responded. "And I don't mean just calorie-counting. You've got to really rethink the way you and Dan eat." Michelle and her husband would typically split a pound of pasta and half a loaf of Italian bread for dinner. "Some fat is okay, but you have to radically cut the simple carbohydrates, add fruits and vegetables, and load up on protein. I guarantee you'll see results."

Following my advice, Michelle went on a high-protein, moderate-carbohydrate, lower-fat diet. She refused to give up the heavy cream in her morning coffee but switched from cereal or a brioche to eggs and lean cold cuts for breakfast. For lunch she'd have tuna salad or a chef's salad with oil and vinegar dressing. For dinner she ate a much smaller portion of pasta, but with two or three huge meatballs. And throughout the day she snacked on fruits and nuts. Because she had a bum knee, she didn't exercise at all. Nevertheless, in six weeks she'd dropped 25 pounds.

"I feel incredible!" she said to me over coffee, her new face glowing. "Guys are looking at me in a way they haven't for years. If Dan weren't so proud of me I'd worry about him being jealous."

"You really do look fabulous," I said in awe. While I knew her new diet would work, her weight loss had surpassed even my expectations. "Now it's time to go shopping—doctor's orders!"

Like Michelle, most women in their perimenopausal years notice changes in their appearance and worry that they're beginning to look like their mothers. The timing is not a coincidence: even though environmental and genetic factors determine a good deal of how we look as we grow older, hormones also play an influential role. Oestrogen affects hair, skin, and nails in much the same way it does urogenital tissue, which we discussed in the previous chapter. Perimenopausal women may notice more wrinkles as the collagen supporting the skin becomes less elastic, and skin itself may become dry, itchy, and tingly. Nails and hair also become thin and dry, and hair loses its shine because reduced oestrogen contributes less to oil production in the scalp.

Adding insult to injury, many women also find that they are gaining weight even though they haven't increased the amount they eat or decreased their exercise. "I just can't seem to lose these extra ten pounds, and they all seem to be in my middle," a patient moaned one afternoon, not unlike half a dozen others I'd seen that day. "I went to

Saks to try on pants this morning and couldn't close the waist on any of them. It was so depressing!"

Although there may not be a way to maintain the hourglass shape you've come to know and love without resorting to architectural lingerie or plastic surgery, you definitely can take off the extra weight or—better yet—prevent it from accumulating in the first place. Ideally, we would still weigh what we did when we were 20 years old. But it's especially important not to let weight gain get out of control at this stage of life. Increased fat, particularly in the abdominal area, can put you at risk for a host of illnesses, including breast, uterine, and colon cancer, heart disease, diabetes, and stroke. Now is the time to commit to a healthy diet and exercise plan if you haven't done so already. In addition to improving your physical health, you'll find it rejuvenates your mind and your body image as well.

OESTROGEN AND YOUR SKIN

Skin is an amazing organ. Not only is it our first line of defense, protecting us from all kinds of environmental assaults such as pollution, infection, and radiation, but it also helps regulate our temperature, release toxins, and communicate with the outside world. The skin is also the mirror of a woman's health. In that split second when I walk into an examining room and get a first impression of a patient, I gather a great deal of information from the state of her skin. The skin reveals all your secrets: whether you smoke or drink or sit in the sun, whether you're stressed out or relaxed, whether you're exercising and eating a healthy diet or munching crisps on the couch. It can also indicate, in a non-scientific way, the state of your hormones.

In perimenopause, women notice that their skin begins to lose the bloom of youth. Declining oestrogen causes a reduction in skin's elasticity, thickness, moisture, and shine and contributes to the development of fine lines and wrinkles. This is because many of the most important components of skin—capillaries, connective tissue, fat cells, hair follicles, and oil glands—have oestrogen receptors, making them responsive to changes in hormone levels as we age. To understand how oestrogen's effect on each of these elements changes the appearance of your skin, we need to take a closer look at the structure of skin itself.

THE LAYERS OF THE SKIN

Skin is by far the largest organ of the body, accounting for 10 percent of the weight of the average woman's body. It is made up of three distinct layers, the *epidermis,* the *dermis*, and the *hypodermis*.

The epidermis, or outermost layer, is primarily composed of two types of cells: *basal cells* and *squamous cells*. Their job is to protect the skin against the outside world. Both produce *keratin,* a dense protein that gives skin a waterproof surface and is the first defense against environmental skin damage. This layer also produces *melanin,* the pigment that gives skin its color and provides resistance to ultraviolet rays.

Basal cells originate in the bottom layer of the epidermis. As they mature, they rise to the top and flatten out, becoming squamous cells. Squamous cells are constantly dying and flaking off, making room for new skin cells to emerge. In our youth, we lose and replace a layer of skin cells each day; by the time we reach our postmenopausal years, that rate has halved. Old skin cells make our skin look old. That's why products and treatments such as loofah sponges, scrubs, alpha hydroxy acids, Retin-A, chemical peels, and dermabrasion, which remove the top layer to reveal the healthier skin beneath, can help us look younger.

The middle layer, or dermis, is mostly made up of fibroblasts, connective tissue cells that have oestrogen receptors on their surfaces. When these receptors are stimulated, the water content of the cells increases; in the absence of oestrogen, the cells become thin and dry. The dermis also houses blood and lymph vessels, sebaceous and sweat glands, sensory and motor neurons, hair follicles, muscles, elastic fibers, and, of course, collagen—a number of which also respond directly to oestrogen stimulation.

Adequate blood flow is critical to maintaining healthy skin, and oestrogen plays a key role in maintaining vascular dilation and flexibility. Smokers and people with heart disease, both conditions that constrict blood vessels, are often notable for the yellowish tinge of their skin, a sign that it is not receiving enough circulation. At the opposite end of the spectrum, pregnant women, whose blood volume nearly doubles and who are full of oestrogen, often have magnificent thick, glowing skin.

One of oestrogen's main roles in skin is to stimulate the fibroblasts to produce collagen and elastic fibers. As you'll recall from the previous chapter, collagen keeps your gynaecologic tissues strong. Declining oestrogen, sun exposure, and aging in general cause reduction and atrophy of collagen, resulting in skin that sags and fails to snap back after a pinch. Oestrogen also maintains the water-binding capacity of collagen, so when your oestrogen levels decrease, your skin becomes thin and dry like parchment. Because 70 percent of the dermis is Type I collagen, this layer is especially vulnerable to declining oestrogen levels.

Sebaceous glands produce *sebum,* an oily substance that keeps skin supple and moist. Sebum production peaks in adolescence, and overproduction can be a problem at that time of life, contributing to acne. With age, sebum production naturally declines, causing our skin to become drier and rougher and to develop fine lines. Sebaceous glands also appear to be responsive to oestrogen, hence the common perimenopausal complaint of scaly skin that has lost its luster.

Between the epidermis and the dermis is a thin layer of connective tissue called the *basement membrane.* Made up of collagen fibers, blood vessels, and nerve endings, the basement membrane is the glue that holds the top and middle layers of skin together. As oestrogen levels decline and collagen content decreases, the basement membrane loses its stickiness. When the dermis and epidermis no longer fit together tightly, deep wrinkles begin to appear.

The innermost layer of skin, or hypodermis, contains sensory and motor nerves but is mostly made up of fat. Babies have an incredibly thick hypodermis, which accounts for their deliciously velvety skin. In evolutionary terms it makes sense for women of childbearing years to have more of this subcutaneous fat than men because it insulates the body, which could at any time be harboring a foetus. Oestrogen stimulates cells in the hypodermis to retain fat; when oestrogen levels decrease as the childbearing years draw to a close, the fat is broken down and the skin thins and loses its plushness, becoming more like men's.

SO, WILL OESTROGEN MAKE MY SKIN LOOK YOUNGER?

In a word, yes. One of the wonderful side effects of oestrogen replacement therapy is more youthful looking skin. My patients often request oestrogen supplements expressly to treat aging skin. I have no problem prescribing for this reason, not only because I believe that feeling younger helps people act younger, but also because signs of oestrogen depletion in the skin are an excellent indicator of the state of other oestrogen-dependent parts of the body—most important, the bones.

Like skin, bones contain a large amount of oestrogen-responsive Type I collagen. When collagen levels decline during perimenopause, the connective tissue that holds bones together weakens, leading to loss of bone mass and, in the worst-case scenario, osteoporosis (see Chapter 8). In a fascinating study done at the University of Barcelona, researchers showed an absolutely parallel trajectory between skin collagen and bone density. Both peak between ages 35 and 40, then precipitously decline. The exciting news that skin and bone respond to oestrogen decline in perfect sync means that in the near future it may be possible to determine bone loss through a simple skin thickness test, rather than via the costly bone densitometry scan we use today.

THE COLLAGEN/BONE CONNECTION
Skin collagen and bone density change in sync as we age.

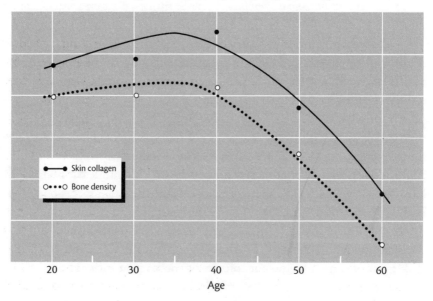

Restoring collagen quality and quantity is key to improving skin appearance. Lots of skin creams tout their collagen content, but the fact of the matter is that collagen is too large a molecule to be absorbed through the dermis. The only way to increase collagen and prevent its future loss is to elevate declining oestrogen levels. Numerous studies have shown increased skin thickness and hydration in women taking oestrogen supplements compared with those who do not. Oestrogen therapy also helps maintain the health of the elastic fibers that keep skin taut and the subcutaneous fat cells that keep skin cushy and soft.

CREEPY CRAWLY SKIN

Does your skin feel dry and itchy, like little creatures are crawling all over you? You're not alone—this is a common side effect of perimenopause. As your skin becomes drier and thinner because of oestrogen depletion, you are more susceptible to itches and rashes. Oestrogen supplements will increase the moisture content of your skin, making it less crusty and irritable.

One of my perimenopausal patients who alternates between a standard dose of oestrogen one day and low-dose the next (so as not to aggravate her fibroids) says that when she goes to the lower dose, she feels like scratching her skin off. Another patient who has suffered severe psoriasis all over her body for her whole life noted a marked improvement in her skin within 48 hours of going on oestrogen replacement therapy.

When skin becomes dry, not only do fine lines appear but the incidence of skin conditions such as psoriasis, eczema, and rosacea increase. If you're predisposed to any of these ailments, likely as not you'll notice more frequent outbreaks as you enter your perimenopausal years. A patient of mine came in for her regular check-up not too long ago complaining of ugly red, dry, itchy blotches on her cheeks. She also suffered vaginal dryness and hot flushes. I prescribed a transdermal oestrogen patch and suggested she see a dermatologist about her face. Lo and behold, she called me six weeks later to say that before she'd had a chance to see the dermatologist, her skin had cleared up. It seems the oestrogen patch increased the water-holding capacity of the fibroblasts in the skin cells throughout her body, helping repair the damage to her face and prevent future irritation.

In an intriguing study, two groups of women were given oestradiol (E_2) and oestriol (E_3) creams, respectively, to apply directly to their skin. Within six to eight weeks of treatment, women in both groups were found to have improved skin moisture and vascularization, and more and thicker elastic fibers that made their skin firmer. Wrinkles actually flattened within 16 weeks for 80 percent of the women using the oestradiol cream and within 15 weeks for 90 percent of the women using the oestriol cream. In both groups, pore size was reduced in 90 percent of the cases around 13 weeks after treatment had begun.

What excites me most about these findings is the evidence that direct application of oestrogen to the skin can have such dramatic effects.

In the not-too-distant future I foresee a whole new line of cosmetic products containing oestriol compounds. The reason I say oestriol rather than oestradiol is that although both were shown to have beneficial effects, oestriol worked slightly better, just as it is the preferred oestrogen for treating vaginal symptoms. (I wouldn't recommend rubbing your vaginal oestriol cream on your face, however, as we have no idea what dose is safe for cosmetic use.) In addition, oestriol is generally safer than oestradiol, as it does not affect uterine tissue. Oestradiol can cause abnormal bleeding in women who still have a uterus.

Another way oestrogen supplementation improves skin appearance is by stimulating the sebaceous glands to produce sebum, the body's natural moisturizer. For women whose perimenopausal symptoms include dry skin, this is a great relief. But how about women who experience the opposite?

Unfortunately, some women find their skin begins to look a bit *too* young during perimenopause—they break out with acne as if they were reliving their teenage years. The reason for this is that decreased oestrogen levels lead to proportionately greater circulating testosterone. Women prone to acne have sebaceous glands that are extremely sensitive to testosterone and overproduce sebum in response to this hormonal imbalance. In their case, oestrogen treatment can restore a normal level of sebum production by decreasing the relative amount of circulating testosterone, therefore reducing the incidence of acne. Certain birth control pills can also relieve acne by regulating the hormone levels.

NINE WAYS TO PRESERVE YOUR SKIN

In addition to oestrogen decline and sun exposure, age itself is a factor in skin deterioration. Simply put, as we grow older our bodies repair themselves less efficiently, so as collagen and elastic fibers break down, our skin gradually loses its resilience. Although there's nothing you can do to stop this process, there are a number of lifestyle modifications that can slow it down.

1. STOP SMOKING. Smoking makes signs of skin aging exponentially worse—I can usually pick out a smoker from twenty yards away just on the basis of her skin. Nicotine accelerates collagen loss and constricts blood vessels, reducing blood flow especially to extremities such

THE SUN AND YOUR SKIN

At the age of 74, my mother looks amazing—she doesn't have a line on her face. My sisters and I, while by no means prunes, definitely don't look as remarkable for our ages. We've all got similar genes, so what's the difference?

The answer is photoaging, the number-one cause of skin deterioration. Most of our mothers came of age in an era when a pale complexion was considered beautiful. They never sat out in the sun. Our generation, by contrast, was raised to believe that tanning was healthy, even sexy. I shudder to think back on how, as a teenager, I used to slather myself in baby oil and lie on the beach frying day after day. And do you remember those aluminum reflectors some of us held under our chins?

I remember pooh-poohing my mother when she'd say, "If you sit out in the sun that way, your skin is going to look like shoe leather by the time you're 50." Sadly, her dire predictions were true. Sunlight not only breaks down the collagen and elastic fibers that give our skin structure and resilience but is the leading cause of skin cancer as well.

"But I use moisturizer with SPF 30 every day," you may respond. That's great, but be aware that not all products with a high sun protection factor protect you from wrinkles or age spots. There are actually two different kinds of ultraviolet rays in sunlight, UVA and UVB. UVB rays, commonly known as "burning rays," are the demons that can lead to skin cancer. UVA rays are called "tanning rays" because they take longer to produce a sunburn than UVB rays. The problem is that UVA rays penetrate the skin more deeply than UVB rays, breaking down the support system of collagen and elastin beneath the skin's surface. Because they reach the lower layers of the skin, they may also prove to be a risk factor in melanoma, the most dangerous form of skin cancer. So make sure to read the fine print on your sunscreen and moisturizer: it should say that you are getting *both* UVA *and* UVB protection.

as the hands, feet, and skin. Without adequate nutrition, skin health declines and the face takes on a sallow tinge. Nicotine also distorts the surface cells of the skin so that they no longer fit neatly together, causing wrinkles to appear.

2. DRINK IN MODERATION. Excessive alcohol intake can have just as bad an effect on skin as smoking, but for the opposite reason.

Alcohol dilates blood vessels, causing that telltale "one too many" flush. Regular consumption of more than a couple of drinks a day can cause the flush to become a chronic condition. In this case, the tiny blood vessels under the skin lose the ability to constrict and may appear as a network of spider veins on the nose, cheeks, and upper chest that can eventually become swollen and disfiguring.

3. EAT ENOUGH FAT AND PROTEIN. Protein is necessary for tissue growth and repair. Without adequate protein in your daily diet you won't have enough raw material to replace lost hair and skin cells. You need 0.8 grams for every 2.2 pounds of body weight. That's 47 grams a day for a 130-pound woman. Fat is also a key ingredient for healthier-looking skin. People on low-fat diets have dry skin, a pasty complexion, and deep lines, especially around the nose and mouth. Eating adequate fat (30 percent of your daily calories) will give you better skin tone and a smoother, rosier complexion. (See Chapter 13 for more on diet.)

4. RELAX. A patient named Sabine told me that she used to have deep grooves between her eyebrows and lines in her forehead. One day she was in yoga class and the teacher instructed the students to relax the bridge of the nose. "I never realized I was tensing the bridge of my nose—I never realized I *could* tense the bridge of my nose—but the moment she said, 'Relax,' I felt my whole forehead opening up. I tried it in front of the mirror when I got home, and sure enough, my face smoothed out. So I began practicing, reminding myself to relax the bridge of my nose several times a day. Now I've trained myself not to store tension there, and the creases are virtually gone."

Many of us hold tension in the muscles of our face. Under stressful or painful circumstances we scrunch these muscles up, causing tiny lines and eventually deep creases to appear. When the pain or stress is relieved, these wrinkles disappear spontaneously. More often than not, however, tensing the facial muscles has become a subconscious habit and we have to make a conscious effort to relax them.

5. GIVE YOUR SKIN—AND YOURSELF—A WORKOUT. If you've ever had a good facial, you know that massage can also loosen muscles under the skin. In addition, facial massage stimulates blood flow, restoring skin health and complexion. Exercise benefits the skin for the same reason—when your skin flushes, it's a sign that oxygen-rich blood is pumping vigorously through all those capillaries close to the surface.

6. REST. As we all know, a good night's sleep can do wonders for the skin (once the designs from the pillow have worn off). Sleep affects your metabolic functions, and not getting enough can cause premature aging throughout your body.

7. KEEP HYDRATED. One of the best prescriptions for maintaining healthy-looking skin—and your health in general—is to drink at least two quarts of water a day. That's eight 8-ounce glasses. Fruit juice counts; coffee, tea, and soda do not. The reason as far as skin is concerned is that as we age our sweat glands shrink and work less effectively. Our skin, therefore, receives less hydration, which contributes to its thinning, dryness, and loss of sheen. Drinking lots of water forces those glands to keep active, pumping sweat through the layers of the skin and lubricating the surface.

8. LUBRICATE YOUR SKIN. Make moisturizing a part of your daily routine. Wash with a moisturizing soap, add moisturizing gel to your bath water, and apply moisturizer liberally to your skin immediately after bathing or showering, when your pores are open. Moisturize your face both in the morning and before bed. Your daytime cream or lotion should contain sunscreen; for nighttime, you may consider one of the many "replenishing" creams, as they tend to provide heavier moisturizing. Just as eating fat is good for your skin, putting fat directly on your skin is also beneficial. So look for products that say they contain essential fatty acids. And don't feel you have to go for the most expensive product on the market, particularly if the high cost will induce you to skimp.

9. TAKE YOUR VITAMINS. *Vitamin C* stimulates the growth of new collagen, so it is one of the most important vitamins you can take for your skin. Be sure to get at least 1,000 mg daily. Both vitamin C and *vitamin E* are antioxidants, which pick up free radicals that can damage your skin cells. Vitamin E seems to help prevent wrinkles and smooth fine lines. Take 400 to 800 IU natural vitamin E a day.

> ### CHEW ON THIS
>
> A patient recently called me to ask whether the fact that she had lost four teeth in the last two years could be related to her perimenopause. It seems so. Your gums are skin, after all, and there are lots of oestrogen receptors in the gingiva. As your oestrogen levels wax and wane, your oral tissues will thin, making you susceptible to receding gums and infection. *If your gums are sore or bleeding more than usual, or your mouth is dry, consult a periodontist immediately.* Studies have shown that perimenopausal gum disease will resolve after three weeks on hormone replacement therapy.

HAIR AND NAILS

Like skin, hair and nails tend to become drier and more brittle as oestrogen levels decline during perimenopause. Oestrogen therapy, either synthetic or natural, can reverse these changes. Sabine, my yoga-practicing patient, decided to take phytoestrogens including soy and black cohosh (Remifemin) to treat her perimenopausal symptoms, which included hot flushes and mood swings. "It's amazing," she reported back to me. "My nails are gorgeous! They used to be ridged and break all the time. Now they're growing like crazy. Even my manicurist noticed the difference."

As with sebum glands in the skin, sebum glands in the scalp produce less oil when oestrogen levels wane. The result is dry, dull, brittle hair. Oestrogen can remedy this; alternatively, a moisturizing shampoo with vitamin E can help restore hair's shine.

As oestrogen levels wane and proportionately more testosterone flows through the system, women often experience *hirsutism*—hair growth in awkward places, such as the face, chest, lower abdomen, and thighs. Even though tweezing, waxing, or electrolysis can remove unwanted hair, to prevent growth from recurring it is necessary to restore the hormone balance by taking an oestrogen supplement. Unwanted hair growth can also result from the use of drugs associated with androgen excess such as phenytoin, anabolic steroids, danazol, and minoxidil, or from an adrenal disorder such as Cushing's syndrome or hormone-secreting ovarian tumors (polycystic ovaries). It is

CAUTION: DON'T BORROW HIS HAIR RESTORER

If you're suffering hair loss, you may have heard mention of a "wonder drug" called Proscar. Although Proscar has been approved for men, it is not recommended for women because it is such a powerful cause of birth defects that just a drop on a woman's skin can damage a foetus. While it looks as if Proscar may be given the nod for postmenopausal women, the jury is still out as to whether it may ever be okay to use during perimenopause.

important, therefore, to report this symptom to your doctor and not shy away from admitting it out of embarrassment.

The opposite problem—hair loss from the scalp—affects some 20 million American women, about one in four, usually beginning in their thirties. Most of these cases are caused by a hereditary condition called *androgenic alopecia,* or female-pattern baldness. Women with this genetic predisposition have hair follicles that are extremely sensitive to testosterone, which causes the follicles to shrink and produce shorter and finer hairs or none at all. When these women enter perimenopause and experience an imbalance of oestrogen and testosterone, their hair thins all over their scalp. The only approved treatment is a 2 percent solution of Loniten (minoxidil), which has positive effects in 44 to 63 percent of women who try it. Unfortunately, it is somewhat pricey (around $30 per month) and must be continued indefinitely.

The second most common cause of hair loss in women is an autoimmune condition called *alopecia areata,* in which hair falls out in bunches leaving perfectly circular bald patches. There is no treatment for this problem; the hair usually grows back in six months to two years.

Hair loss in women can also be a side effect of certain medical conditions, the most common being anaemia and thyroid problems. For this reason, I always test a patient's blood for its red cell count, ferritin, TSH (thyroid-stimulating hormone), and free T_4 levels when she complains of losing hair. I then send her to a dermatologist to rule out any skin condition of the scalp that may be affecting the hair follicles, such as psoriasis. If there is no skin disorder, I suggest she see an endocrinologist to rule out any hormone imbalances.

Once the cause of the hair loss is determined, treatment of the underlying condition should solve the problem. I once had a

OTHER RISK FACTORS FOR HAIR LOSS

Stress. In general, stress can cause hair loss. In particular, it is one of the triggers for alopecia areata. If your hair is thinning and there is no medical or hereditary explanation, take a step back and assess the stress level in your life. Try to slow down a bit and incorporate a few moments of relaxation into your routine, be it through meditation, yoga, or a nightly hot bubble bath. Also, relax your scalp and increase blood flow to the hair follicles by massaging your head when you give yourself a shampoo.

Childbirth. "After giving birth my hair has been falling out all over the place," complained one of my patients. "Between me and the cats, our bathroom is a mess!" On average, adults lose about 100 hairs a day as part of the natural cycle of hair growth and loss. The high levels of oestrogen experienced during pregnancy prevent hair from falling out, causing most women to enjoy a head of lush, thick hair. After the baby is born the cycle kicks in again, and all those hairs that should have fallen out over the past nine months do so, in addition to the normal 100 a day. In most cases this is a temporary condition and the hair will return to its normal thickness in about six months or, if you breastfeed for longer than that, after you wean the baby. In the meantime, treat your hair gently, using conditioner, towel drying, and avoiding harsh treatments such as permanents, coloring, and hair relaxers.

Too little protein. As with skin, hair health reflects your diet—a telltale sign of anorexia nervosa is dry, brittle, thin hair. If you don't consume enough protein, your body won't have the resources to maintain good hair quality and quantity.

perimenopausal patient who suffered a massive haemorrhage as part of a wildly fluctuating menstrual pattern. Her red blood cell count dropped acutely, and at the same time her hair fell out in clumps. As soon as I put her on iron supplements and corrected the bleeding problem, her hair stopped falling out.

In addition, there are more than 290 medications known to cause hair loss in women. Some of the more common ones include oral contraceptives; beta-blockers such as Inderal; lithium and other antidepressants; bloodthinners such as Warfarin; and amphetamines. Sometimes simply changing medication can solve the problem. Certain other medical conditions such as high fever or severe infection, flu, kidney disease, leukaemia, lupus (SLE), and cancer can also cause hair loss. In general, if you are suffering hair loss, it is imperative to give your doctor a full description of any other symptoms or health problems you may be suffering, or drugs—prescription, over-the-counter, or complementary—you may be taking.

WHY WEIGHT?

No, there's nothing wrong with your scale—the two, five, seven, ten, or twelve pounds you've gained over the past year or so are real. "But how could that be?" you may ask. "I'm not eating more than usual, yet the dial keeps going up." If it makes you feel better, you're not alone. Between ages 35 and 44, more women tend to become overweight than at any other time in their adult lives. Indeed, 52.7 percent of women in the United States between ages 40 and 49 are overweight or obese. The sad fact is that perimenopause is associated with a slowing down of the metabolism, so that even the most careful eaters find themselves putting on the pounds.

The most basic reason why your metabolism downshifts during perimenopause is a loss of lean body tissue. As we grow older we tend to move more slowly and exercise less than we did in our youth. Whereas adults on average lose 0.5 pound of muscle mass each year after age 20, in women over 35 the rate accelerates to 1 pound a year. With each lost pound of muscle mass you burn 50 fewer calories per day, a decrease in basal metabolism that can lead to 5 extra pounds of fat per year. By menopause women need only two-thirds the calories they needed at age 20 to maintain a constant weight.

Another 5 pounds can come simply from not ovulating. Progesterone, which is released upon ovulation, signals the hypothalamus to increase the core body temperature, thereby increasing the resting metabolism rate. That's why pregnant women, who have very high circulating levels of progesterone, feel hot all the time. Anovulation reduces energy expenditure by 15,000 to 20,000 calories per year. This explains not only the weight increase experienced by perimenopausal women but also that of women with conditions such as polycystic ovaries who fail to ovulate regularly.

Decreased oestrogen can also lead to increased weight. Oestrogen stimulates production of a protein called sex hormone binding globulin (SHBG), which binds circulating androgens, decreasing androgen

BELLY BASICS

Even if you haven't been gaining weight in perimenopause, you may have developed a bit of a belly. "I look like I'm four months pregnant!" one patient cried. If you're suffering bloating and fluid retention, here are some tips:

- Limit your salt intake.
- Try natural diuretics such as tea, strawberries, grapefruits, and grapefruit juice.
- Ask your doctor about prescribing a potassium-sparing diuretic such as spironolactone (Aldactone). I find it works beautifully for my patients with PMS or perimenopausal fluid buildup.

availability. When oestrogen levels decrease, so do levels of SHBG, thereby freeing up more androgens to affect the system. Among other things such as hirsutism and sebum production, androgens stimulate production of insulin, which stores fat. Overproduction of insulin, in turn, can lead to insulin resistance, which, as I'll explain shortly, is a syndrome that makes it even harder to control your weight.

There is some interesting evidence from animal studies that oestrogen may have an effect on appetite as well. Rats that had their ovaries removed and therefore produced very little oestrogen exhibited an increased desire to eat and drink. Their appetite went back to normal, however, when they received oestradiol (E_2) supplements. Similarly, ovariectomized baboons, monkeys, and guinea pigs all demonstrated decreased appetite when given oestradiol. While it has not been shown that anovulation causes increased appetite in human females, there is a chance that perimenopausal women may actually be eating more than they think.

Is oestrogen going to be the next miracle diet pill? Maybe yes, maybe no. When postmenopausal women have been given high doses of oestrogen, they've experienced an increase of lean body mass without gaining any extra weight. Whether the same effect can be enjoyed by perimenopausal women on lower doses of oestrogen remains to be seen.

Of course, all this being said, there are always those disgustingly lucky women who sail through perimenopause without gaining an ounce. Factors such as genes, race, lifestyle, diet, libido, and mood may influence body composition in such a way as to affect whether a particular individual is liable to increase or maintain her weight during this

PILLS THAT CAN PACK ON THE POUNDS

Certain drugs can cause weight gain. If you are taking any of the following medications and packing on the pounds, ask your doctor about ways to control your weight.

- Provera (medroxyprogesterone acetate)
- antihistamines
- beta-blockers
- steroids
- insulin
- lithium
- tricyclic antidepressants
- neuroleptics (epilepsy drugs)

time of life. Even if you're not blessed with the right combination of fat-resistant variables, however, there are still steps you can take, such as diet and exercise, to keep your body within bounds (see Chapter 13).

SHAPESHIFTING

"I'm in better shape now than I've ever been in my life!" cried a fortysomething patient. "I do two hundred crunches every morning and take an aerobics class four times a week, but my waistline keeps getting bigger."

"I know, it's really a drag. It must be very frustrating to be working so hard and still feel like your waistline isn't under control. Unfortunately, as your hormones change, so does your body. It's all part of perimenopause."

Even those lucky women who don't gain weight during perimenopause will find that their shape shifts from the more feminine gynoid or pear shape to a more masculine android or apple shape. Fat melts away from the hips and thighs and magically materializes in the belly and breasts. Whereas 80 percent of premenopausal women have a gynoid shape, less than 50 percent do in perimenopause; and after menopause only 40 percent retain their waistline. This metamorphosis is independent of any change in the lean-to-fat mass ratio.

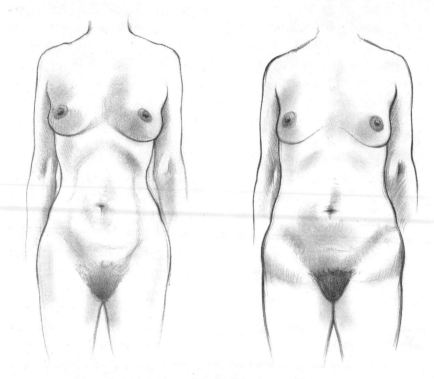

"Pears" often become "apples" during perimenopause.

Contrary to popular belief, the greatest change in body fat distribution takes place *before* menopause, not after. This is because oestrogen is responsible for maintaining our curvaceous silhouettes. It keeps our waists small by stimulating what are called *lipolytic enzymes* to break down fat in the abdominal region. At the same time, oestrogen stimulates an enzyme called *lipoprotein lipase* to store fat in the lower body. When oestrogen levels begin to wane, these oestrogen-dependent enzymes slow down, so fat begins to build up in the waist and disappear from the hips.

Another reason why women put on weight around the middle at this stage of life is that abdominal adipose tissue has more receptors for androgens and other steroid hormones such as cortisol than other fat tissue does. During perimenopause, when androgenic activity increases in proportion to oestrogenic activity, the abdominal region becomes more susceptible to cortisol-stimulated fat accumulation than other parts of the body. For the same reason, women who take steroid medication, such as hydrocortisone to treat lupus, put on weight around the middle, as do women with polycystic ovaries, who produce an excess of male sex hormones.

A higher waist-hip ratio is not merely a cosmetic issue but a serious health concern as well. It's a major risk factor for cardiovascular disease, diabetes, stroke, and cancer, especially of the breast, uterus, ovary, and colon. Elevated levels of androgens cause increased blood pressure, low-density lipoprotein ("bad") cholesterol, and oestrone (E_1). They also raise blood levels of insulin, a hormone produced in the pancreas that is responsible for energy storage, spurring the vicious cycle known as insulin resistance.

Whereas we've traditionally thought that increased waist-hip ratio was an inevitable side effect of aging in women, it's beginning to look as if it ain't necessarily so. Oestrogen replacement therapy has been shown to decrease the waist-hip ratio of postmenopausal women. So there's a possibility that at the lower doses taken perimenopausally, oestrogen may prevent the increase in waist-hip ratio altogether, not only helping us maintain our girlish figures but also decreasing our risk for these major medical problems later in life.

One thing to be aware of, however, is that taking a synthetic progestogen (Provera) may negate the positive effects of oestrogen on your figure and metabolism. Studies of monkeys have shown that when oestrogen is taken with synthetic progestogen, the monkeys' weight, waist-hip ratio, and insulin resistance all increased. This was not the case when the monkeys were given oestrogen with natural progesterone.

INSULIN RESISTANCE

Whenever I see a perimenopausal patient, the conversation invariably drifts toward weight. "So what are you eating?" I ask. "Bread, potatoes, pasta, rice, bagels—is that your diet?"

"That's me!" they respond. "Everything white."

"That's the problem!" I answer.

Most of these women believe that they are actually watching their weight: they are eating the high-carbohydrate, low-protein, low-fat diet that they have been told for years is the miracle way to shed pounds. If this is indeed such a miracle, then why are the populations of many Western countries today fatter than ever before, and not experiencing good health? The answer to this question lies in insulin resistance, or Syndrome X.

The symptoms of insulin resistance are all too familiar. You gain weight—as many as 20 pounds since you were 20 years old—and have a tough time taking it off. You eat sporadically, skipping meals and then chowing down. You experience problems concentrating, lack energy, crave sugar, feel fatigued and bloated, and have aging skin, hair, and nails. In addition, you notice your blood pressure and cholesterol levels beginning to creep up when you go for your annual physical. Long-term high insulin levels can also contribute to depression and mood swings, fertility problems, and migraine headaches.

So how do we become insulin resistant? Basically, by eating too many of the wrong type of carbs (see Chapter 13). Carbohydrates are broken down into glucose (sugar) in the body. So when we pig out on potatoes, for example, our blood sugar goes up. The pancreas then releases insulin, which lowers our blood sugar by helping transport that sugar to cells where it is stored to fuel normal cellular functions.

If you keep eating carbohydrates day in and day out, your insulin levels remain high. Eventually, when insulin escorts the sugar molecules to the various cells of the body, they shut their doors. They are full up and have become resistant to insulin. At that point, glucose is instead transported to the liver, where it is converted into glycogen and triglycerides—fat. In other words, *it's not fat that makes you fat, it's carbohydrates!*

If insulin resistance goes unchecked, fat cells eventually become so full that they, too, will hang out the "No vacancy" sign. At this point there is no place for excess dietary sugar to be stored, so it remains in the bloodstream and is excreted in urine. Ultimately, the pancreas becomes exhausted and ceases to produce insulin. The result is Type II, or non–insulin-dependent, adult-onset diabetes, which is a severe risk factor for coronary artery disease, the leading cause of death in women.

The best way to ward off diabetes is to avoid insulin resistance by keeping your weight and blood sugar under control. How you do that most effectively depends on your genes. Twenty-five percent of the population can handle carbohydrates and lose weight without any difficulty by eating bagels and pasta and just counting calories. At the opposite end of the spectrum are the 25 percent who have an elevated insulin response to carbohydrates (like my friend Michelle) and do magnificently on a moderate-carb, high-protein diet. The rest of the population responds normally to carbohydrates; they can eat a moderate amount, but if they gorge they'll put on weight and court insulin resistance.

If you have been trying to lose weight by eating a high-carbohydrate, low-protein, low-fat diet and not succeeding, it's not your fault; indeed, for 75 percent of the population that's not the ideal diet. Try increasing

PERIMENOPAUSE AND DIABETES

The two greatest risk factors for Type II diabetes, a disorder that affects women above all, are obesity and age. (One in four women over the age of 85 suffers the disease.) As we become fatter and fatter as a population, however, insulin resistance and Type II diabetes are manifesting themselves in people at younger and younger ages.

Half of the women who develop Type II diabetes do so during perimenopause because oestrogen-related changes in body composition contribute to the development of insulin resistance, the precursor to this disease. Women at particular risk of developing non–insulin-dependent diabetes at this time of life include those with a history of gestational (pregnancy) diabetes, those with a family history of diabetes, and those who are obese and/or suffer high blood pressure. In addition, black people tend to have much higher rates of diabetes than do members of the general population.

Complications of the disease include high blood pressure and high cholesterol, which can lead to severe cardiovascular disease. In addition, diabetics may suffer kidney failure, deterioration of the retina, and peripheral neuropathy (in which nerves to the hands and feet are damaged). Because of these associated problems, diabetics should be under close medical supervision and follow the recommendations of the British Diabetic Association regarding diet and self-care.

your protein and scaling down your carbs to six to seven servings a day of low-glycemic carbohydrates such as fruits and vegetables (see pages 338–339). And add back some polyunsaturated fats such as nuts and olive oil—after all, fat is what fills us up and helps keep our skin looking young. Don't be fooled by foods labeled "fat free"—they're often full of sugar and surprisingly high in calories.

In the end, calorie counting is still important, as is regular exercise—both aerobic and weight-bearing. Aerobic exercise will help you to maintain your cardiovascular fitness and control your weight, and weight-bearing exercise will build up your bones and muscle—an extremely insulin-friendly type of tissue—and keep your metabolism running efficiently. For more details on the optimal perimenopausal diet and exercise plan, see Chapter 13.

My Biological Clock Is Ticking: Changes in Fertility

Thanks to the women's movement, most women are no longer slaves to their reproductive organs. Unlike our foremothers who had to marry young for security reasons and were kept barefoot and pregnant—metaphorically speaking, at least—for most of their adult lives, we have the freedom to educate and support ourselves. Homemaking and childrearing are only two of a myriad of life options. And with the availability of convenient, affordable birth control, we can control our fertility and "have it all" exactly when we want it.

Up to a certain point. Eventually, most of us will come face to face with biological reality. Whether it's when your birth control fails or when you wake up to the fact that you may have missed the baby boat, each of us confronts the limits imposed by our reproductive life at some time or another. And as an Ob/Gyn at the turn of the millennium, I'm finding more and more women wanting to push those limits.

Why? Because women today are starting families at a much later age than their mothers did, sometimes having their first child in their late thirties or early forties. During the 1990s there was a 22 percent decrease in the number of women who said they wanted to conceive before age 35, and since 1970 there has been a 50 percent increase in the number of women who have had their first child after age 40. While there are many good reasons for delaying childbirth, including increased maturity and financial security on the part of the parent, older mothers run the risk of decreased fertility that is a direct result of perimenopausal changes.

As we age, our eggs are of poorer quality and much less readily fertilized, often requiring drugs and/or surgery to stimulate conception. Older eggs are also associated with more chromosomal abnormalities in the foetus, which leads to a higher miscarriage rate. Pregnancy becomes riskier, with a significant increase in pregnancy-induced hypertension and gestational diabetes. And delivery complications such as failure to dilate are also more common, yielding a higher rate of cesarean sections in older mothers.

At the opposite end of the spectrum, unwanted pregnancy is an issue for many perimenopausal women. Over age 40, women become extremely lax about birth control, resulting in a high rate of abortion and increased risk of sexually transmitted diseases. But 50 percent of women over age 40 are still potentially fertile, and even after age 50 there is a chance of conceiving. For this reason, I always ask my patients about birth control and thoroughly discuss the options, which include barrier methods, IUDs, oral contraceptives (which have the added benefits of reducing other perimenopausal symptoms), progestogens, and sterilization.

ANNETTE—THE RACE AGAINST THE CLOCK

"She's 41 but she doesn't look a day over 35," said Halley, my nurse/technician, describing the new patient she had shown into Room 3. And she was right. I opened the door to greet an attractive woman with elbow-length auburn hair, glowing pale skin, and lively green eyes. I noted an athlete's body under her slim gray pantsuit.

"Don't tell me—Armani, right?" I asked.

"Absolutely!" Annette responded with a smile. "Nice to meet you, Dr. Corio," she said, extending a smooth hand with trim coral nails.

"Likewise," I replied.

Over the next few minutes I learned that Annette, an entertainment lawyer, and her husband, Stan, a theater director, had just moved to New York from Los Angeles. Married for eleven years, they only began trying to have children eighteen months ago, during which time Annette had suffered three miscarriages.

"The first was so early that we couldn't recover any foetal tissue. The pathologist said the second foetus had a genetic abnormality known as Turner's syndrome. The third had another genetic problem,

Down's syndrome. Stan and I are in great shape—we swim, ski, bike, jog; don't smoke, drink, or do drugs—and there are no genetic abnormalities in either of our families. My periods have always been perfectly normal. So why is this happening?"

"There may be no one specific cause," I explained. "It could simply be a factor of age. You may look great, take care of your body, and feel as energetic as you did at 30, but inside the clock is still ticking. Your ovaries are aging, and age is the number-one contributor to infertility."

"But my mother didn't go through menopause until she was 50, and I don't have any symptoms yet," she protested.

"That doesn't matter," I said. "Our fertility starts declining at least ten years before we enter menopause, even before we notice any signs of *peri*menopause. It doesn't sound like you're having any trouble getting pregnant—"

"Stan just has to look at me!"

"—so the problem isn't that you're not ovulating, but that the eggs you're producing are genetically abnormal. I'm going to do a complete exam and infertility workup. First I'll take blood to check your hormone levels and your thyroid function. I'll also have immunology studies done on your blood to make sure that your body isn't fighting off the pregnancies. Then I'll do vaginal and cervical cultures to rule out any infection. You and your husband should both have a blood test to check your genetics. I also recommend a hysterosalpingogram, transvaginal sonogram, and a biopsy of your uterus. If everything comes back okay, you can keep trying or use donor eggs."

"So you think if I get pregnant with a good egg that will solve the problem?"

"It would help, but it's no guarantee. The fact that you've had three miscarriages already means that you have what we call recurrent miscarriage. Normally, it's like throwing dice at the craps table—each time you get pregnant you have a certain percentage chance of miscarrying. Once you have three, however, your chances increase."

"All this just because I chose to put off having a child," Annette moaned. "I feel like going outside and shouting at all the twentysomethings I meet, 'Go forth and multiply!' "

"Yes, it's a nasty joke Mother Nature plays—when we're young and foolish we're most likely to have a child; when we're older and wiser we run into trouble. But just think of how much more you have to offer that child when it finally comes," I suggested.

"You're right. Five years ago I was so wrapped up in my career I wasn't the least bit ready to be a mom. Now I'm in a place where I can give it my all. Plus, Stan and I are rock-solid emotionally and financially. I'm not sorry I waited, though I sure wish I didn't have to go through all these disappointments."

"Fortunately, there are a lot of options these days," I said. "Let's not waste any more time!"

WHAT CAUSES GENETIC PROBLEMS?

I didn't want to discourage Annette by mentioning it, but in fact our fertility peaks at age 24; from then on it's downhill. Our ovaries have a finite number of eggs, which are dying off all the time. The healthiest ones develop earlier in our reproductive life; by the time we're in our mid to late thirties we start releasing ones that are less responsive to hormonal stimulation, causing irregular and anovulatory cycles.

Those that do get released have a greater chance of containing genetic abnormalities. A 24-year-old, for example, has a 10 percent chance of experiencing a miscarriage due to a foetus with an extra copy of chromosome number 21 (trisomy 21), which causes Down syndrome. A 45-year-old woman, by contrast, has a 53 percent chance of miscarriage due to Down syndrome. In general, genetic abnormalities are seen in the foetuses of 26 percent of women under age 35 and 78 percent of women over age 35.

Even though women over age 40 have a higher rate of miscarriage than younger women, they still have a good chance of having a healthy baby. Miscarriage is nature's way of eliminating unhealthy foetuses so the ones that do come to term are less likely to have genetic abnormalities.

We are just now beginning to understand what might cause these chromosomal abnormalities in the eggs of older women. There seems to be a problem with the mitochondria—small bodies that float around in the cytoplasm of the cell that play an instrumental role in dividing up the chromosomes to make germ cells (eggs and sperm). Right now exciting research is being done to determine if inserting the cytoplasm from a donor egg into the egg of an older woman can avert chromosomal mutations. If this technique works, it could be an excellent option for older women who up to now have had to rely on egg donation—an effective technique, but one that results in children who are not genetically related to their mothers.

OTHER EFFECTS OF AGE

If you put off childbearing, you face a greater risk of having physical problems with your reproductive tract that can cause infertility. In comparison with younger women, you have likely had more sexual partners by the time you try to conceive, so you've had more opportunity to become infected with sexually transmitted diseases such as gonorrhoea or chlamydia that cause pelvic inflammatory disease (PID). Even after these infections are cured, they may leave scar tissue in the Fallopian tubes. This can inhibit conception by preventing sperm from swimming up the tubes and preventing eggs from floating down. Even in the absence of PID, the motility of your Fallopian tubes decreases with age, making it harder for them to grab ripened eggs as they are released from the ovaries.

Nowadays, having blocked Fallopian tubes is not as dismal a prognosis as it was years ago. With the advent of in vitro fertilization, which I'll discuss shortly, we can bypass the tubes and you can still get pregnant with your own eggs.

Age also increases your risk for endometriosis, a condition present in at least 25 percent of infertile women. This is a common disorder in which the endometrial tissue that lines the uterus migrates to other parts of the pelvis (and on rare occasions to other parts of the body), where it continues to grow and bleed on a monthly cycle. It can cause infertility by latching on to the inner surface of your Fallopian tubes or the outer surface of your ovaries, causing scarring or blood-filled cysts. Endometriosis tissue anywhere in your pelvic cavity releases prostaglandins, hormones that affect ovulation and both sperm and tubal motility. Women with endometriosis also have an increased risk of miscarriage. In Chapter 11 I'll explain more about this condition.

Not all women with endometriosis have fertility problems, however. I once did a cesarean section on a full-term woman and was stunned to find endometriosis all over her pelvis just as I was delivering her healthy 8-pound son.

Fibroids, which I'll also cover in greater detail in Chapter 11, are benign growths in the uterus. At least 20 percent of women over age 35 have them (even more in those of African origin) and for the most

HIS CLOCK'S TICKING, TOO

Although it is generally accepted that male fertility does not significantly decline until age 64, the chance of a man impregnating a woman does decrease with age. One study reported that only one-third of men over age 40 impregnated their partners within six months of trying, compared with three-quarters of men under age 25. A small part of this difference may be chalked up to "male menopause": men's testosterone levels go down about 1 percent a year beginning at age 40, resulting in diminished sperm production and quality. Men's libido also wanes with age, leading them to have sex less often and therefore be less likely to impregnate their partners. Mostly, however, the decline is the result of sexual dysfunction (impotence), which affects 50 percent of men over age 40.

part find them innocuous. Problems arise when fibroids begin to bleed or get so big that they deform the uterus. Large fibroids inside the uterus (submucosal fibroids) can prevent implantation of the embryo or miscarriage. They can also cause premature labor (see Chapter 11).

Surgery to remove fibroids that are causing infertility problems is usually successful. A perfect example is a 40-year-old patient of mine who was having trouble conceiving her second child. After a full workup I sent her to an infertility specialist who did a pelvic sonogram, which revealed a large submucosal fibroid blocking the entrance to the uterine cavity and the Fallopian tubes. He removed it vaginally with a resectoscope, and she got pregnant shortly thereafter.

INFERTILITY—THE BASICS

The party line is that a couple is considered infertile if they have been trying to conceive for at least a year without success. That's all very well and good if you're 25 years old; if you're 40, you don't have a year to fool around. If a woman is between 35 and 40 years old, I begin investigating the problem after six months. In women who are 40 and over or who have irregular periods, I check their FSH level immediately, because if it's high, they may wish to begin fertility treatments right away.

Now, when I say trying, I mean really trying. When I see a couple who are concerned about their fertility, I first take a detailed sexual history. "We haven't been using birth control for nine months, and nothing's happened," a typical patient tells me.

"Are you tracking your ovulation?" I ask.

"Oh, yes," she responds. "I take my temperature every morning before I get out of bed."

"And are you having sex in the days leading up to ovulation?"

"Well, most of the time. This past month didn't work out because Hugh was out of town on business, and the month before I was working late those nights and was just too exhausted . . ."

It turns out that in the past nine months this couple may only have had unprotected sex at the right time of the month about half the time. That's not really trying for nine months.

If a couple has been diligent, however, and still has had no success, we begin an infertility workup in which we systematically examine all the possible causes of the problem in the hope of zeroing in on and treating exactly what's wrong.

To begin, I ask the woman the following questions:

Did your mother take DES? (Diethylstilbestrol was a hormone given to many women in the 1950s and 1960s to prevent miscarriage that ended up causing reproductive problems in their daughters.)

Did you ever use an IUD (intrauterine device)?

Did you ever have pelvic inflammatory disease (PID)?

Did you ever have a sexually transmitted disease?

Did you ever have abdominal surgery?

Do you smoke?

Do you drink?

Did you ever use drugs?

Are you taking any medications or herbal products?

Does your partner suffer impotence?

Have you noticed any changes in your periods recently?

DR. CORIO'S PREGNANCY PRESCRIPTION

What do I tell women without any obvious fertility problems who want to conceive?

- Approach your ideal body weight, eat a balanced diet, and don't skip meals (especially breakfast!).
- Reduce your alcohol intake—and your partner's—to one drink a week or fewer.
- Stop smoking.
- Cut down the caffeine to one cup a day.
- Don't use any lubricants or jellies such as K-Y Jelly—they kill sperm.
- Have sex every other day beginning four days before ovulation and up to four days after (every day will decrease your partner's sperm count).
- Start taking folic acid or prenatal vitamins and calcium supplements as long as possible before you begin trying to conceive.
- Keep exercise in moderation.
- Have your partner wear boxers (see page 155).
- Relax, have fun, give it six months, and enjoy the fact that for the first time in your life you don't have to feel guilty about not using birth control.

If she answers "yes" to any of these questions, it gives me a good idea of what might be the source of the problem.

In general, 40 percent of infertility can be traced to the man, and the remaining 60 percent can be traced to the woman. Twenty-five percent of all cases (40 percent of those in which the problem lies with the woman) are caused by hormonal imbalances that affect ovulation. These could result from perimenopause, but they could also be due to excessive weight gain or loss, overexercise, stress, and conditions such as polycystic ovaries, pituitary adenomas, and thyroid disease.

Another 25 percent are caused by peritoneal problems such as PID, endometriosis, or adhesions from prior abdominal surgery. Five percent result from uterine factors such as fibroids, polyps, a previous history of abortion, dilation and curettage (D&C), or exposure to DES

CAUTION! HERB AND DRUG ALERT

Some popular herbs have recently been shown to affect fertility in both men and women. Saint John's wort and echinacea purpurea damage sperm and inhibit their motility, and ginkgo biloba prevents sperm from penetrating the egg.

I also tell my patients that herbs are off-limits if they're pregnant. Many herbs, including black cohosh, chasteberry, feverfew, ginseng, goldenseal, Saint John's wort, and ginkgo, can cause bleeding, contractions, and—potentially—miscarriage.

Certain prescription medications may affect fertility as well. High doses of steroids such as hydrocortisone and prednisolone can prevent the pituitary gland from producing adequate levels of FSH and LH. Tranquilizers and some older antihypertensives can raise prolactin levels, interfering with ovulation.

(one of the effects of being exposed in utero is an abnormal, T-shaped uterus). And the remaining 5 percent result from cervical factors such as surgery (biopsy, D&C, abortion, LLETZ [large loop excision of the transformation zone]) infection, or exposure to DES, which can affect the quality or quantity of cervical mucus.

CAUSES OF INFERTILITY

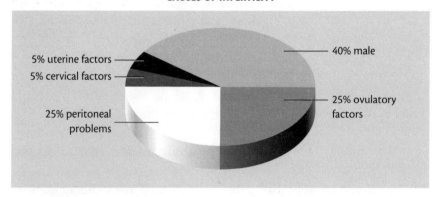

5% uterine factors
5% cervical factors
40% male
25% peritoneal problems
25% ovulatory factors

FAT AND FERTILITY

Fully 12 percent of all infertility cases can be traced to weight problems. If a patient is less than 95 percent or more than 120 percent of her ideal body weight (see Chapter 12), my first recommendation is that she gain or lose accordingly. More than 70 percent of over- or underweight women experiencing fertility problems who correct their weight disorder conceive spontaneously. Take the following two cases, for example.

Ursula, now age 35, has been a patient of mine for seven years. During that entire time she has been trying to get pregnant. She came in last autumn for a check-up, and when I weighed her she was 270 pounds. "You've got to lose some weight," I told her. "Your excess fat is producing androgens that are throwing off the hormonal balance needed for ovulation." I told her that one study showed that the chance of a woman becoming pregnant decreased from 63 to 32 percent with increasing waist-hip ratio. I put her on a low-fat, moderate-carbohydrate, high-protein diet. Two months later she had lost 20 pounds and conceived. I sent her directly to a nutritionist because her challenge now is to not gain any weight during her pregnancy.

Ava, on the other hand, is a stick—five-foot-four and 108 pounds. She exercises fanatically and has less than 10 percent body fat. In her late twenties she had one child; five years later she wanted another but couldn't conceive. She tracked her basal body temperature for three months, and it showed that she was not ovulating. I took her bloods and found her oestradiol to be 20 pg/ml—far below normal. "You must gain weight," I counseled. "With so little body fat you aren't producing enough oestrogen to ovulate. Increase your calories, especially complex carbohydrates and fats, and we'll see what happens." Sure enough, she put on 7 pounds, her oestradiol rose to 76 pg/ml, and with a cycle of Clomid she got pregnant.

THE PROBLEM: HIS OR HERS?

If a patient answers "no" to all the questions on page 150, we have to begin at ground zero.

First I send both my patient and her partner for complete physicals to rule out any health problems that may be affecting their fertility. If everything looks good, I send the partner for a sperm analysis. The reason I do this right away is that infertility is much easier to diagnose in men—all it takes is ten minutes and a magazine with pictures of scantily clad women! Secret catalog. Analyzing semen under a microscope immediately reveals whether low sperm count (less than 20 million sperm per cubic centimeter), abnormally shaped sperm (morphology), or poor sperm movement (motility) is a problem, or whether there is an infection present in the seminal fluid. If the sperm analysis comes back abnormal, I repeat it; if it again comes back abnormal, I refer the partner to a male infertility specialist.

In the case of Annette and Stan, in addition to sending them both for genetic counseling, I recommended he have his sperm analyzed. Even though I was especially concerned about the quality of Annette's eggs, I wanted to make sure nothing was wrong on his end as well. His results were normal, allowing us to focus our efforts exclusively on her.

If the semen analysis comes back fine, the next step is to look at the woman. The first thing I do before I begin the complete workup is to check her hormone levels on day 3 of her cycle. Why? Because if her FSH and oestradiol are in the perimenopausal range, her ovaries may be resistant to any kind of help. At the same time I like to check the woman's TSH and free T_4 blood levels to make sure there is no thyroid disorder, and her prolactin level to see if a pituitary adenoma may be affecting her fertility. Medication to treat these conditions will restore fertility if they are the only problems.

Of course, perimenopause is by definition a time of flux. Because your FSH is going up and down from month to month like a yo-yo, it's perfectly possible to have an FSH of 25 mlU/ml one month and conceive the next. As a case in point, consider Julie, a former lawyer turned full-time mom. At age 35, two years after having her second baby, she started having irregular periods and began experiencing hot flushes. I did her bloods and found her TSH and prolactin to be normal, but her FSH and oestradiol were very high—74 mlU/ml and 63 pg/ml, respectively. Three months later when I checked her bloods again her FSH was 22 mlU/ml and her oestradiol was 126 pg/ml.

"You're definitely in perimenopause," I told her.

"But I want to have another child," she responded. "Does this mean I can't?"

"No," I answered. "Keep trying. During some cycles your FSH will be high, and during some cycles it will be lower. When it's down, you can still get pregnant." Sure enough, four months later she missed her period and a pregnancy test came back positive.

One complication of Julie's case was that because of her perimenopausal state she needed progesterone supplements for the first

BUY HIM BOXERS

When the husband of one of my patients went for a sperm analysis and the results were terrible, she confided in me that he wears nylon bike shorts all the time. "And I mean all the time, Dr. Corio—not only at home and at the gym, but under his suit at work."

"There's your problem," I said. "Sperm need to be kept slightly cooler than body temperature to stay healthy. Bike shorts and bikini briefs smush up the testicles into the body so the sperm overheat. Buy your husband some boxers and give it a couple more months." She did, and they conceived two months later.

trimester. She menstruated once after giving birth to her third son, then didn't see another period and began getting hot flushes again and suffering terrible insomnia. She decided to try alternative treatment, so she started eating soy and taking black cohosh (Remifemin). But three months later she said her libido was nonexistent and she wanted to try hormones, so I put her on natural oestrogen, progesterone, and testosterone. She was in menopause at age 37 and today is still on hormone replacement therapy, enjoying her three sons.

TRACKING YOUR OWN OVULATION

The minute they decide to begin trying to get pregnant, many of my patients tell me their cycles become totally irregular. The stress of taking this major life step is certainly enough to throw your hormones off kilter. If you are in perimenopause, of course, your hormones are already unpredictable; they could be in the perimenopausal range one month and completely normal the next. You could have anovulatory cycles mixed in with ones in which you do ovulate, making the conceiving of a baby a bit like playing a slot machine. While performing blood tests every month is theoretically an option, it's less costly and invasive to monitor your own ovulation by using an ovulation kit, a basal body thermometer, or both.

Ovulation kits are easier to use, though more of an investment, than basal body thermometers. The kits are available at the chemist

CONTROL THE CONTROLLED SUBSTANCES

Smoking and drinking have adverse effects on both male and female fertility. Women who smoke experience infertility 46 percent more often than those who don't. Light smokers (up to 20 cigarettes a day) are 75 percent as fertile as nonsmokers, whereas heavy smokers (more than 20 cigarettes a day) are only 57 percent as fertile as nonsmokers. Smoking also increases your chance of having an ectopic pregnancy (a dangerous condition in which the fertilized egg implants in the Fallopian tube) because smoking inhibits the motility of the Fallopian tubes. In men, smoking reduces the concentration of sperm as well as their vigor.

Even a moderate amount of alcohol can impair fertility. A recent study showed that just one drink per week can significantly reduce the rate of conception. Whereas women who abstained from alcohol entirely had a 24.5 percent rate of conception, those who consumed *less than* one drink a week had only a 17.3 percent rate. Those who had between one and seven drinks per week had a rate of 11.9 percent.

Men are equally affected. One of my patients had been trying to get pregnant for several years. She'd been to several infertility specialists; none of them had been able to help her. In conversation one day it came out that her husband consumed between four and five drinks every night. I had her bring him in, then read him the riot act. He cut down to one drink a night and she was pregnant in two months.

The same study charted caffeine intake and found that women who abstained from alcohol but drank more than 100 mg caffeine a day (one cup of coffee or two colas) had a conception rate of 18 percent. By contrast, women who drank no alcohol and kept their caffeine intake down to less than one cup of coffee a day had a conception rate of 26.9 percent.

and run about £20 a month. Starting four days before you expect to ovulate, you stick a piece of paper treated with a chemical that detects LH in your first urine of the day. When the paper changes color, it indicates that you are experiencing an LH surge and will ovulate twelve to twenty-four hours later. No LH surge, no ovulation that month.

Using a basal body thermometer takes more diligence than an ovulation kit but provides useful information that a kit does not. The thermometer itself—specially calibrated to the tenth of a degree—

only costs about £10 at the chemist. The trick is that you have to take your temperature for five minutes every day at the same time, before you get out of bed, shower, or have a cup of coffee. (Patients of mine who frequently travel to different time zones often find it difficult to keep track.)

Starting on day 1 of your cycle (the first day of your period), plot your temperature on a graph. In the first half of the cycle it should be in the 97° range. It will drop down by a few tenths of a degree for a couple of days just prior to ovulation. Once ovulation has occurred, it will slowly rise above 98° and stay there until the day before you menstruate, when it will drop down again. (If you're pregnant, it will remain above 98°.) At the end of a cycle, you will have a biphasic curve (two plateaus) if you ovulated and a monophasic curve (a flat line) if you didn't.

Recently a patient came to me and said, "Dr. Corio, I'm not ovulating. My temperature never goes above 97°." Upon further inquiry, I found that when she starts her cycle her temperature is in the 95° range—she just happens to have a low basal body temperature. She's having a perfectly normal biphasic cycle, just lower than other people.

In addition to indicating whether or not you ovulated, a basal body thermometer reveals information about the timing and quality of your ovulation. One of the things I look for is whether the second half of

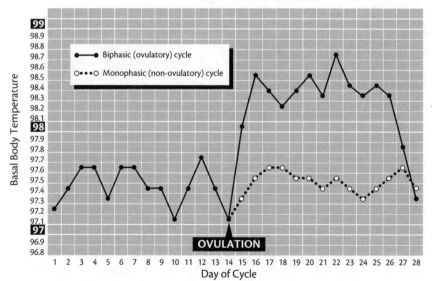

BASAL BODY TEMPERATURE CHART

the biphasic curve rises above 98° and remains at that level for at least twelve to fifteen days. If not, it signals to me that we're dealing with a luteal phase deficiency due to inadequate oestrogen and progesterone production—a cause for infertility that requires treatment such as Clomid.

The ovulation kit can be difficult to analyze—many of my patients tell me either that the color change is so subtle that they can't tell for sure if it's real, or that their urine shows a color change for days. Therefore, I like my patients to combine it with the basal body thermometer so that we know exactly when they ovulated and can accurately gauge the temperature change and the length of the second half of the cycle. After three or four months of tracking her ovulation, a patient will come in and we'll analyze the graphs together.

ENDOMETRIAL BIOPSY

Even if the basal body thermometer and/or ovulation kit indicate that a patient has ovulated, I still do an endometrial biopsy ten days after ovulation just to make sure. This entails scraping a tiny bit of tissue from the uterine lining—a very simple procedure that should not cause a problem even if you're pregnant. In fact, I've done numerous endometrial biopsies on women early in their pregnancies and ended up delivering their babies.

Because endometrial development in the second half of the cycle is extremely predictable, by analyzing the sample a pathologist can tell exactly how many days the tissue has matured since ovulation. If there is more than two days' discrepancy between the dating of the uterine tissue and the date you were in your cycle on the day of the biopsy— for example, the pathologist says your uterus is only as thick as it should be on day 16 and the biopsy was done on day 24—you have a shortened luteal phase.

At the same time as the biopsy, I check blood levels of progesterone. If ovulation has occurred, the progesterone level should be greater than or equal to 4 ng/ml. Lower than this indicates that you have not ovulated.

SO WHAT'S THE MAGIC DAY?

My patients often tell me that they've been tracking their ovulation for months but still are not having any success getting pregnant. I ask them when they're having sex, and they say, "The day I ovulate." I tell them that's too late. You want to have sperm already hanging around by the time the egg comes down the Fallopian tube. If you wait until you've ovulated, it could be too late. To get pregnant, I recommend having sex on days 10, 12, 14, 16, and 18 of a 28-day cycle. Earlier is always better than later—most sperm live 2 to 3 days, but some can last as long as 7.

IF YOU'RE OVULATING BUT STILL NOT PREGNANT . . .

. . . and your hormone levels are normal, we move on to another series of tests to determine whether the problem is in the cervix, the abdominal cavity, or the uterus.

THE POSTCOITAL TEST. Remember back in puberty when you first began to notice discharge in your underwear? It was around the time you began menstruating, right? That's no coincidence. The cervix, a knob-like muscle that protrudes into the top of the vagina, keeps the bottom of the uterus shut tight, protecting the pelvic cavity from infection. When your reproductive hormones kick in at puberty, they cause the tissue of the cervix to begin producing mucus, which plays a critical role in conception.

The consistency and amount of mucus you make varies in sync with the menstrual cycle. During infertile times of the month, the cervical opening is plugged with a thick, cheesy mucus that is chemically hostile to sperm; during the fertile time, the opening is lubricated with a thinner, more chemically welcoming mucus that sucks sperm up into the uterus through long thin channels. You've probably noticed these different consistencies when you've wiped yourself after urinating.

In a postcoital test, we examine the quality of your cervical mucus and how it interacts with your partner's sperm. You need to have sex the morning that your temperature drops, usually fourteen days before your period, and come in for an exam within twelve hours. "I woke my husband up at five this morning," a patient recently told me. " 'Today's the day!' I said to him. 'Get to work!' " I then take a sample of mucus from your cervix and look at it under a microscope.

Ideally, there should be plenty of sperm swimming around. If the sperm are shaking but not swimming, if there aren't any sperm, or if they're all dead, then we have a problem. Providing that semen analysis has shown that your partner has an adequate sperm count and that his sperm are healthy, the problem could be that your mucus is toxic to your partner's sperm—you are producing antibodies that are killing them. These antibodies can be detected by a blood test. If you have them, your best bet is IUI (intrauterine insemination, also known as TIH, therapeutic insemination with husband's sperm), a relatively simple procedure. First your partner's sperm are extracted from his semen. Then they are washed and treated with a special activating solution. Finally, they are inserted directly into your uterus via a thin tube through the cervix so they never come in contact with your mucus.

As part of the postcoital test I also check the condition of the mucus. Oestrogen causes it to soften, so that at ovulation it should be the consistency of egg whites. It ought to be clear and also have good spinnbarkeit, or elasticity—I should be able to stretch it about 2 to 3 inches (if you like, you can try this at home). If your mucus is of poor quality, it signals an oestrogen deficiency (which can be treated with oestradiol supplements), cervical stenosis (scarring due to prior surgery or infection), or exposure to DES.

HYSTEROSALPINGOGRAPHY (HSG). HSG, or the dye test, tells us about the shape of your uterus and the condition of your Fallopian tubes. In the first half of the cycle—after bleeding and before ovulation—a radiologist injects dye into the uterus through the cervix, then takes an x-ray of the reproductive organs that highlights the dye. The dye should flow out the Fallopian tubes at the top of the uterus; but if there is a blockage, there won't be any dye spilling into the abdominal cavity. This test also illuminates any abnormality in the shape of the uterus, such as the T-shaped uterus typical of women who have been exposed to DES, or any organic growth such as polyps, scar tissue, or fibroids. At the same time I like the radiologist to do a transvaginal pelvic sonogram to look at your uterus and ovaries. When Annette had this procedure, her uterus showed no scar tissue or abnormalities and her Fallopian tubes were open.

If the Fallopian tubes look clear, I suggest holding off on further treatment, as there is a 30 percent chance of getting pregnant naturally in the next three to six months. This is because the dye itself can force out blood or mucus that may have been blocking the tubes.

LAPAROSCOPY/HYSTEROSCOPY. Even if your infertility workup is completely normal, there is a 68 percent chance that you could have a physical problem that can be detected only by laparoscopy/hysteroscopy. Also, if your tubes are blocked or if you have a normal HSG and don't get pregnant within three months of the test, we need to investigate further by doing a diagnostic laparoscopy/hysteroscopy. Using a small telescope called a *hysteroscope* that is inserted into the uterus through the cervix, I check out the lining of the uterus and the openings to both Fallopian tubes. This tells me whether polyps or fibroids that could be preventing successful pregnancy are blocking the ends of the tubes. If so, they can be removed surgically.

At the same time I like to perform *laparoscopy,* a more invasive but more direct way of checking the status of the Fallopian tubes. Under general anaesthesia, I insert a scope through a small incision under the navel. This gives me a great view of all the pelvic organs. In addition to spotting blocked Fallopian tubes, I can see if adhesions or endometriosis in the abdominal cavity are inhibiting conception. If so, I can laser the scar tissue or endometriosis then and there.

If you have blocked Fallopian tubes, your best option for pregnancy is in vitro fertilization (IVF), in which conception takes place in a Petri dish, bypassing the Fallopian tubes altogether. If your tubes are severely blocked, I can remove them during the laparoscopy/hysteroscopy, as one study shows that doing so in these cases raises the rate of embryo implant with IVF.

IF YOU'RE NOT OVULATING...

. . . and your hormones are still in the premenopausal range, your best bet is fertility drugs. There is a growing number available from which to choose. Usually we start out with Clomid, the mildest, and if that doesn't work we move on to Pergonal or one of the other follicle stimulants.

CLOMID. Patients who aren't ovulating but have some oestrogen, such as those with polycystic ovaries or luteal phase defects, are good candidates for the ovulation-stimulating drug Clomid (clomiphene citrate). Clomid is what's known as an antioestrogen—an oestrogen mimic that outcompetes naturally occurring oestrogen for the oestrogen receptor sites. This fools the body into thinking there isn't enough oestrogen, and when this message gets to the brain the pituitary pumps out extra FSH. If all goes well, this high level of FSH should jump-start the ovaries into ovulating.

I start out my patients on Clomid by prescribing 50 mg a day on days 5 through 9 of their cycle and instruct them to have intercourse every other day after day 9. If they don't ovulate by day 30, we try 100 mg a day on days 5 through 9 the next month, ultimately going as high as 150 mg a day if necessary. Eighty percent of patients on Clomid ovulate, usually between days 14 and 18. After three ovulatory cycles, the chance of conception on Clomid is 55 percent—the same as in the general population.

When a patient reaches the 100 mg level, I administer what's called the Clomiphene Citrate Challenge Test (CCCT). On both day 3 and day 10 of that cycle, I check her FSH. If it's greater than 10 mlU/ml on day 10 after five days on Clomid, she has a poor ovarian reserve and only a 9 percent chance of conceiving during that cycle. By contrast, a woman with a normal CCCT, in which the day 10 FSH level is below 10 mlU/ml, has a 43 percent chance of conceiving during that cycle. The exception is the woman over age 40: even if she has a normal CCCT and day 3 FSH level, she could still have fertility problems simply because of her age.

As I increase the dosage of Clomid, I always do postcoitals at ovulation because Clomid can affect the quality of the cervical mucus. I also do endometrial biopsies each month for patients who have a shortened luteal phase to see if it is being corrected by the drug. Generally I recommend a maximum of three cycles of Clomid.

The advantages of Clomid are that it is safe, effective, and reasonably inexpensive. Side effects are minimal; they may include abdominal swelling, breast tenderness, nausea, headaches, hot flushes, and visual symptoms such as blurring, spots, or flushes. The rate of multiple births, mostly twins, is increased to between 6 and 12 percent.

Because age affects the responsiveness of the pituitary gland, Clomid may not be the best option for women over age 40, who may do better going straight to Pergonal or one of the other FSH-based drugs. These would be administered by an infertility specialist.

PERGONAL, HUMEGON, REPRONEX. For women who don't ovulate with 150 mg of Clomid or do not conceive despite ovulation with Clomid after three months, the next step is to try a class of drugs called gonadotrophins, which include Menogon and Menopur. A combination of FSH and LH made from the urine of postmenopausal women, gonadotrophins are more expensive than Clomid and must be given by injection in the buttock.

The dose is typically one to two ampules (70 to 150 IU) per day; the couple should have intercourse or IUI every day. If the oestrogen level does not rise within five days of beginning the shots, the dose is increased by half again. Four to six days later the doctor checks the oestrogen level and if it still hasn't risen, the dose is increased once more. Each time the doctor checks the oestrogen, he or she will also do a transvaginal pelvic sonogram to look at the uterus and ovaries. When the oestrogen level has risen, the lining of the uterus is plush, and the ovaries are sufficiently large, the doctor gives a shot of HCG, which prompts ovulation.

The conception rate with gonadotrophins is between 50 and 75 percent. They also carry some risks, however. The most serious is ovarian hyperstimulation, in which the ovaries produce too many eggs and become enlarged. Mild cases occur about half the time, whereas severe cases that can result in the ovary rupturing occur less than 2 percent of the time. To avert ovarian hyperstimulation, the doctor must be vigilant about doing transvaginal pelvic sonograms and both doctor and patient must be ready to abandon the treatment if growth gets out of control. Other possible side effects of gonadotrophins include abdominal discomfort, nausea, and headaches.

Women on gonadotrophins have a 26 percent chance of conceiving multiples. Seventy-four percent of those are twins; the remaining 26 percent are higher order multiples. Before embarking on this treatment it is important to think about how you would deal with multiples—if you would go through a pregnancy with any number of foetuses or selectively reduce down to one or two. Because of the ethical issues involved in bringing higher order multiples into the world, many doctors are now counseling patients to abandon cycles in which a large number of follicles mature.

Because the effects of gonadotrophins are long lasting, it is not usually recommended to do cycle after cycle. Rather, do one and then wait a few months before trying again.

METRODIN. This drug, which is also known as a urofollitropin, is simply a FSH preparation without LH. Given exactly the same way as gonadotrophins, it has similar rates of conception and similar potential side effects. It has an advantage over the gonadotrophins in that it can be given in lower doses, carries less risk of ovarian hyperstimulation, and yields fewer multiples—only 10 to 20 percent.

GONAL-F. The most recent addition to the fertility market, this drug, known as a follitropin, is basically synthetic FSH. The advantage is that it is more stable than the gonadotrophins and urofollitropins, which are extracted from human urine. It is administered the same way as the other two types of drugs, has similar side effects, and carries a slightly lower conception rate. The risk of multiples ranges from 15 to 20 percent.

ASSISTED REPRODUCTIVE TECHNOLOGY (ART)

If your tubes are blocked or fertility drugs aren't working, the next option is assisted reproductive technology. This is an umbrella term that includes an ever-increasing number of techniques for joining sperm and egg artificially. Here's a rundown on the four most common, all of which have a success rate of approximately 27 percent.

IN VITRO FERTILIZATION (IVF). This is the oldest and most popular technique, accounting for 70 percent of all ART cycles. First you take fertility drugs to stimulate your ovaries to produce several eggs. The eggs are then harvested through laparoscopic surgery and combined with sperm in a Petri dish (not a test tube). The fertilized eggs are allowed to progress to the embryo stage, then are transferred to your uterus. An interesting study recently reported that waiting two extra days before implantation—five days instead of three, so that the embryos have reached the blastocyte stage (a ball of more than one hundred cells)—can as much as quadruple your chance of getting

FERTILITY DRUGS AND CANCER

Many women worry that taking fertility drugs will increase their risk of ovarian cancer. It is true that women undergoing infertility treatment have a higher incidence of ovarian cancer than women in the general population, but it appears that the cause is not the drugs. Rather, it seems to be years of living with hormonal imbalances—the kinds that lead to fertility problems—that cause cancerous growth of ovarian tissue.

pregnant and reduce your risk of multiples. IVF is the treatment of choice for women with blocked Fallopian tubes and for women who choose to use donor eggs.

GAMETE INTRAFALLOPIAN TUBE TRANSFER (GIFT). In this technique, three to five eggs are removed from your stimulated ovaries and combined with sperm in a laboratory dish. The mixture is immediately inserted into your Fallopian tube, where fertilization occurs.

ZYGOTE INTRAFALLOPIAN TUBE TRANSFER (ZIFT). The only difference between ZIFT and GIFT is that with ZIFT the mixture of eggs and sperm is kept overnight in the laboratory. The next day the doctor can check to make sure the eggs have been fertilized before placing them in your Fallopian tube.

INTRACYTOPLASMIC SPERM INJECTION (ICSI). This technique is used in cases of low sperm count or when the sperm are too weak to penetrate the outer membrane of the egg. Once again, eggs are retrieved from your stimulated ovaries. This time, however, only a single sperm is injected into each egg. The resulting embryos are transferred to the uterus.

USING DONOR EGGS

If your FSH is consistently over 20 mIU/ml and your oestradiol is over 75 pg/ml, or if you're over age 40 and have been unable to conceive either spontaneously or with assisted reproductive technology, it's time to talk about donor eggs. While the ovaries age, mercifully the uterus does not, so perimenopausal—and even menopausal—women still have the option of carrying and delivering a child through egg donation. Whereas the conception rate for women over age 40 trying to get pregnant naturally is 20 percent at best, it is close to 50 percent when they use donor eggs—as good as it is for much younger women. That is because conception rates correlate with the age of the egg. The technique is the same as that for IVF; except instead of having your own ovaries stimulated and eggs harvested, a donor undergoes that part of the procedure. Her eggs are then combined with your partner's sperm and transferred to your uterus.

Something to think about before embarking on this procedure is that the child you will bear will not be related to you genetically. For most women this is a small price to pay for the joy of becoming pregnant and having a child. After all, the baby will at least be related to your partner—50 percent more connection than if you adopted. And because egg banks provide background on the egg donors, you can choose a woman who shares your physical characteristics so that your child may resemble you, too.

PERIMENOPAUSAL PREGNANCY

When a perimenopausal woman does conceive, she has a higher risk of complications in pregnancy and delivery regardless of whether she used her own egg or that of a donor. Incidence of miscarriage, gestational diabetes, hypertension, intrauterine growth retardation (IUGR), preterm labor, and cesarean section all increase with age, especially for women having their first baby over age 40.

MISCARRIAGE. The risk of spontaneous miscarriage rises to 50 percent in women over age 40, as compared with between 15 and 20 percent in the general population. The major cause is chromosomal abnormalities in the foetus, which account for 70 percent of all miscarriages. As we discussed, older women's eggs are far more likely to contain genetic abnormalities than those of younger women, therefore their pregnancies will be more likely to abort spontaneously.

In cases where a woman suffers more than three miscarriages, the problem could be chromosomal, as it was in Annette's case, or it could be something else. (Incidentally, Annette conceived for the fourth time and her CVS [chorionic villus sampling] showed that she's carrying a normal baby girl.) Fifty percent of recurrent miscarriages have no obvious explanation. Some doctors are beginning to think the cause may be immunologic—the woman's white blood cells are attacking the embryo as if it were a foreign object—and are claiming success treating patients with immunoglobulin, a blood product that regulates immune response. To my mind, the jury's still out on this one.

Even if she holds on to the foetus, an older woman has a 35 percent greater chance of experiencing bleeding during pregnancy than a younger woman. Bed rest is the usual recommendation; depending on the cause of the bleeding, medication may also be necessary.

GESTATIONAL DIABETES. A temporary form of diabetes that is the most common of all pregnancy complications, gestational diabetes is far more prevalent among older women than younger ones. One study found the rate to be 7 percent in women over age 40 as compared with 1.7 percent in women in their twenties. It is normal in pregnancy for the placenta to produce hormones that cause insulin resistance; this ensures that you have adequate sugar in your blood to feed both you and the developing foetus. But in older women, aging and weight gain may already have caused insulin resistance. The combination triggers diabetes.

I give all patients a glucose screen for gestational diabetes at 28 weeks, but I screen perimenopausal or obese patients earlier, at their first or second prenatal visit, then later on at 28 weeks as well.

It is important to control gestational diabetes through diet and, if necessary, insulin, because the effect of prolonged high blood sugar on mother and foetus can be serious. In the mother, it can cause full-blown insulin-dependent diabetes, with all its risks and complications (see page 143). High blood sugar can cause a foetus to become too large, requiring early and/or cesarean delivery. It can also cause problems in the infant after delivery, such as the inability to regulate temperature and electrolyte imbalance, and failure to thrive. Basically, the child's system goes into shock—it's been used to a high-sugar environment that has suddenly disappeared. Once the baby is delivered, diabetic symptoms in the mother disappear 98 percent of the time.

HYPERTENSION. If a woman has chronic high blood pressure or shows symptoms of hypertension early in her pregnancy (blood pressure of greater than 140/90), it is important to treat it aggressively so that it doesn't develop into preeclampsia/toxemia. Standard medications for hypertension are not usually used, and common treatments include methyl-dopa and labetalol. Untreated high blood pressure can cause problems in the foetus such as growth retardation or even stillbirth. Hypertension is vastly more common in older women— from five to nine times the rate of younger women—and can occur whether it's your first baby or your ninth.

Preeclampsia, by contrast, more often occurs with first pregnancies and in women who are older or in their teens. It shows up after 24 weeks of pregnancy. Its initial symptoms are elevated blood pressure (140/90 or higher), swelling of the hands, feet, and face, sudden weight gain above and beyond what's normal for pregnancy, and spilling of protein in the urine. Strict bed rest is the order of the day, because if the preeclampsia gets worse, the baby may need to be delivered prematurely.

When women who are close to full term show signs of pre-eclampsia, the best treatment is often early delivery, through either induction or cesarean section. If a woman is not as far along and her doctor feels her blood pressure can be kept under control, she and her baby will be closely monitored with a variety of tests. In 97 percent of preeclampsia cases, the mother's blood pressure returns to normal shortly after delivery. Chronic hypertension, however, remains after the baby is born and requires long-term treatment through medication and/or lifestyle change.

INTRAUTERINE GROWTH RETARDATION (IUGR). As part of your prenatal visits, your obstetrician will measure your abdomen to get an idea of whether your baby is growing at a normal rate. Any suspicion that the foetus is failing to thrive can be confirmed by using ultrasound. In addition to smoking, drinking, and eating poorly, risk factors for growth retardation (low birthweight) include preeclampsia and chronic hypertension. Even taking these medical conditions into account, a woman having her first baby at over age 40 has an increased risk for IUGR and prematurity, suggesting that maternal age itself is a factor.

The statistics on IUGR associated with older mothers also reflect

THE MORE THE MERRIER

Older women are more likely than younger women to carry multiple foetuses, especially fraternal twins, with the incidence peaking between ages 35 and 39. Indeed, over the last twenty years the twin birth rate has risen 63 percent for women ages 40 to 44 and nearly 1,000 percent for women ages 45 to 49. Birth rates for triplets or more have increased nearly 400 percent for women in their thirties and 1,000 percent for women in their forties. This multiple baby boom is primarily a result of increased use of fertility drugs or ART. Twins occur more often naturally at a later age as well, because the increased FSH associated with perimenopause sometimes overstimulates the ovaries so that more than one egg is released in a given month.

the increase in multiple births to women in their perimenopausal years. "The more, the smaller" is generally the rule; moreover, multiples are more likely to be premature and therefore of lower-than-average weight.

PRETERM LABOR AND CESAREAN SECTION. Because gestational diabetes, hypertension, and multiple foetuses are all more prevalent in older mothers, women in their perimenopausal years have a higher risk of preterm labor and cesarean section than do their younger counterparts. Indeed, a recent study found women over age 40 having their first child to have cesarean births 47 percent of the time, more than twice as often as women in their twenties. Including deliveries requiring forceps or vacuum extraction, the rate of operative deliveries for older women rises to 61 percent as compared with 35 percent in younger women.

Even if a perimenopausal woman carries to term, she still has a higher risk of cesarean birth. One reason is that the foetuses of older women are twice as likely to be in the wrong position—breech (head up, tush down) or horizontal—than those of younger women (11 percent versus 6 percent), perhaps because the aging muscles of the uterus are not efficient at turning the baby. Another reason is that older women's cervixes tend not to dilate as successfully. Placenta previa, another risk for preterm labor and cesarean section, increases with women who already have several children and with older women having their first babies.

OBESITY—A BIG RISK FACTOR

Even though pregnancy complications increase with age, they are not inevitable. When the statistics are corrected for weight, it turns out that older women have no greater chance of hypertension, foetal death, and foetal distress than younger women. For these conditions, it seems that weight, not age, is the determining factor—one more reason to keep weight gain under control at this time of life.

In my own practice I find that whereas younger women endure more prolonged, difficult labor in order to have their babies vaginally, older first-time mothers, especially those who have had difficulty getting pregnant, are much more willing to accept the need for a cesarean—after all they've been through, they just want the baby out quickly and safely. Regardless of age, however, when labor fails to progress, it is usually in the best interest of both the mother and child to undertake an operative delivery rather than risk the mother's uterus rupturing or the foetus going into distress.

WHEN INFERTILITY IS *NOT* A PROBLEM

I can't tell you how many patients in their forties tell me that their periods are so irregular that they figure they can't get pregnant and so have stopped using birth control. It makes my hair stand on end! In spite of having irregular cycles and poorer quality eggs, *perimenopausal women are still fertile.* Eighty percent of women between ages 40 and 44 can conceive, although one-third of all pregnancies in this age group end in spontaneous miscarriage. Seventy-five percent of pregnancies in women over age 40 are unintended; as many as half are terminated by elective abortion—only teenagers have a higher rate. The rule of thumb is that you must use contraception for a full year after your last period.

But what kind? At this time of life it often makes sense to reevaluate your contraception choice. Perhaps you've been on the Pill for ten years but, recently divorced, you are now concerned about protecting yourself against sexually transmitted diseases (STDs). Or maybe you've been using the diaphragm while you had your kids but now you're

BIRTH CONTROL OPTIONS AT A GLANCE

TYPE	EFFECTIVENESS
Male Condoms	80–90% (greater with spermicide)
Diaphragm/Cervical Cap	85% (greater with conscientious use)
IUD	Copper 99%
	Progesterone 97%
Norplant	99%
Mini-Pill	96%
Depo-Provera	99%
Sterilization	99%
Oral Contraceptives	99%
Natural Family Planning	65–95%

sure you're finished with childbearing and you no longer want to deal with the nightly ritual. If you are experiencing any perimenopausal symptoms, such as irregular bleeding or vaginal dryness, they, too, may influence your decision. To help evaluate your options, here is a listing of what's out there with particular attention to each method's pros and cons for the perimenopausal woman.

Barrier Methods

CONDOMS. Male condoms (female ones have not been a success) are great for women who are playing the field and concerned about STDs, including AIDS. Because so many midlife women find themselves suddenly single, either because of divorce or widowhood, condoms should not be written off as something only college kids use.

Because of the increased sensitivity of their vaginal tissue, many perimenopausal women experience an allergy to latex, becoming itchy and red after intercourse with a condom. My standard response is to have him wear two—a latex one next to his skin and a lambskin one next to yours (lambskin alone does not protect against HIV, the virus that causes AIDS). When I told this to one patient recently she said, "Are you crazy? I can hardly get him to wear one!" Alas, she's right. But if you don't want to suffer, you'll have to be firm. It's your life; it's your health.

Vaginal dryness can make condom use uncomfortable and also increase the chance of a condom breaking. The solution is to use plenty of spermicidal jelly or water-based lubricant (oil-based lubricants may break or tear the condom)—it'll be more comfortable and provide extra protection.

DIAPHRAGM AND CERVICAL CAP WITH SPERMICIDE. As long as you use them religiously, the diaphragm and cervical cap provide excellent protection against pregnancy. They do not protect you completely against STDs, however, so if you're not monogamous, use a condom as well.

Because the spermicide used with diaphragms kills some of the beneficial vaginal flora as well, it puts women at risk for an increase in yeast and urinary tract infections. Perimenopausal women, who already have decreased vaginal flora and increased incidence of urinary tract infections (UTIs), may find that they're getting infections especially often and opt for another form of birth control.

If you've been using the diaphragm for years, aren't suffering too many UTIs, and don't mind the somewhat messy routine and lack of spontaneity, there's no reason to change now. But do remember to have your doctor check the size periodically—you may need to be refitted if you have gained or lost ten or more pounds or had a child.

Anyone using the cervical cap should go for frequent smear tests because it may cause changes in the cells of the cervix.

THE SPONGE. It's back! Women are celebrating the return of the vaginal sponge because it is an inexpensive, effective, comfortable, and disposable method of birth control.

IUDs

Two types of IUDs are available: a progesterone-impregnated one that needs to be replaced every five years (Mirena), and a copper T-shaped one that can be left in for up to twelve years. IUDs are an excellent contraceptive choice for perimenopausal women. Because there is a slight chance of damage to the Fallopian tubes, I recommend that my patients be absolutely sure they don't want any more children before I insert an IUD, just in case. I also tell them they must be monogamous, monogamous, monogamous! IUDs increase your risk for STDs because the string that dangles down through the cervix into the top of the vagina can be a pathway for pathogens to enter the uterus and cause pelvic inflammatory disease (PID).

One disadvantage of the copper IUD for perimenopausal women is that it can cause heavy periods and spotting, which, if your bleeding pattern is already all over the place, can be intolerable. In fact, I recently had to remove an IUD from a patient of mine who had had it in for four years. Over the past two years her bleeding got heavier and longer until she was bleeding two weeks out of every month. I did a transvaginal sonogram and endometrial biopsy; both were normal. After a long discussion we decided to remove the IUD. She and her husband are now using condoms, and her periods are back to normal—only three to four days, not two weeks.

Combined Hormones

ORAL CONTRACEPTIVES. In the good old days we never prescribed oral contraceptives to women over age 35 because of fear of increasing their risk of cardiovascular disease. Now I'm doing it all the time. Low-dose pills (35 mcg or less of oestrogen) provide great birth control and simultaneously treat a host of perimenopausal symptoms, including hot flushes, memory problems, mood swings, irregular bleeding, and vaginal dryness. While cyclic oral contraceptives may cause menstrual migraines, I've actually prescribed noncyclic ones to treat migraines. What I'm not keen on, however, are the high-progestogen (second generation) formulations because they tend to exacerbate perimenopausal symptoms such as acne, bloating, weight gain, breast soreness, and mood swings. Now a third generation of oral contraceptives are available that are less like male hormones and have fewer androgenic side effects.

The benefits of oral contraceptives go far beyond treating perimenopausal symptoms. Not only do the new low-dose pills *not* increase your risk of breast cancer, but they can actually reduce your risk of ovarian, uterine, and colon cancer. They can build bones and also pose much less cardiovascular risk than their predecessors. Indeed, they may even lower your risk of cardiovascular disease (see Chapter 9). In addition, oral contraceptives reduce your risk of PID, ectopic pregnancies, functional ovarian cysts, chronic cystic breast disease, painful periods, anaemia, and acne.

If you're considering going on the Pill at all, now is the time to do it—if you take the Pill for five years at this time of your life you'll reap the benefits for years to come. I would not recommend oral contraceptives to smokers; women with liver disease or with a history of thrombophlebitis (blood clots); women with breast, uterine, or colon cancer; women who've had a stroke or heart attack; women who've had gallbladder disease during a previous pregnancy; and women with undiagnosed abnormal vaginal bleeding.

Progestogens

These options are particularly useful for women who cannot take oestrogen.

NORPLANT. These days I'm taking out more Norplant implants than I'm putting in. Even though Norplant seems like the ideal contraceptive in theory—insert a half-dozen matchstick-size rods that slowly release progestogen under the skin and you're worry-free for up to five years—it's not all it's cracked up to be. The side effects, which include bloating, weight gain, acne, headaches, and irregular bleeding, only exacerbate perimenopausal symptoms. Roughly half of all women with Norplant have the implants removed before the third year.

PROGESTOGEN-ONLY PILL (MINI-PILL). As with Norplant, the side effects of the mini-pill make it an unpopular choice for perimenopausal women. At this time of life you need an oestrogen boost; by taking progestogen you only increase the hormonal imbalance that's causing all your discomfort. It can cause irregular periods and amenorrhoea. Also, if you miss two pills you must use a barrier method for the rest of the month, because you can become pregnant.

DEPO-PROVERA (DMPA, OR "THE SHOT"). Again, like Norplant, this seems ideal—one injection every three months and no birth control worries. But Depo-Provera is worse. In addition to causing the same unpleasant side effects, it lowers your oestrogen, causing significant loss of bone density, something no woman, and especially no perimenopausal woman, can afford. I also don't recommend Depo-Provera if a perimenopausal woman is thinking about conceiving because it can take up to 18 months for fertility to return after she stops taking DMPA.

Sterilization

Each year 640,000 women undergo surgical sterilization in the United States; nearly 70 percent of American women have undergone surgical sterilization by age 45, making it by far the most popular form of birth control for midlife women. Often it's performed immediately after a cesarean delivery; otherwise, it can be done laparoscopically at any time. The Fallopian tubes are cut, cauterized, or clamped shut (not tied). On rare occasions a cut tube may reattach and a woman can get pregnant. In this case, the fertilized egg is much more likely to implant in the Fallopian tube—an ectopic pregnancy—which is extremely dangerous.

Bilateral tubal ligation (BTL) is essentially an irreversible form of birth control. For that reason I have a hard time recommending it, even though most women in their perimenopausal years have a good idea of whether or not they want any more children. My feeling is that you just never know where life may take you—you may find yourself with a new partner for whatever reason and, even though you may have children from a prior relationship, you may decide you want to have a baby with this new man. Studies show that one in three women who are sterilized regret their decision at some point in their lives.

Back when I first started in practice, I tried to talk a 35-year-old patient without children out of having a tubal ligation. She swore she never wanted children. Three years after I performed the operation she came to me, fiancé in tow, asking whether she could have the procedure reversed. Because I had used clips to close her tubes rather than cauterizing them, there was a slim chance she could regain her fertility if she wanted to undergo several hours of microsurgery under general anaesthesia. She ultimately decided to live with her earlier decision and not have any children (at that time in vitro fertilization was not yet an option).

Nevertheless, the majority of women who undergo sterilization are happy with their decision and enjoy worry-free intercourse with minimal side effects. There may even be benefits: it seems that tubal ligation decreases the risk of ovarian cancer by two-thirds.

Natural Family Planning

Unless you combine it with scrupulous tracking of your basal body temperature and your cervical mucus changes, the rhythm method is not a great idea during perimenopause. Even then, I wouldn't recommend it unless you have no alternative for religious reasons. Think about it: this is a time when your body loses its rhythm—your periods can become wildly erratic—so how can you ever be certain when you're going to ovulate?

If You Do Become Pregnant . . .

THE MORNING-AFTER PILL. The morning-after pill has been around for a long time. There are two types on the market now: PC4 is a megadose of birth control (200 mcg) taken half within 72 hours of unprotected sex, then half 12 hours later. It's extremely effective, but not something you should get in the habit of using. In perimenopause it's especially unwise to subject yourself to such extreme hormonal ups and downs. Side effects include nausea and vomiting, which can last up to one or two days. Women at risk for blood clots or who smoke should not use PC4. The other type is Levonelle 2, which is slightly more effective and associated with fewer side effects.

ABORTION. Whether surgical or chemical, abortion is not to be taken lightly. Unfortunately, all too many perimenopausal women find themselves facing the decision of whether or not to go through with an unwanted pregnancy because after age 40 we tend to become dangerously lax about birth control.

If you choose an abortion, I recommend surgical over chemical. Mifepristone, the "French abortion pill," is the pill version, but I do not recommend it. Do you really want to be expelling the products of conception, an extremely bloody affair, all alone at home? You'll feel nauseous and experience severe cramps, and you may even end up having to undergo a D&C anyway if the abortion is incomplete. Surgical abortion is much faster, less complicated, and less traumatic.

PERIMENOPAUSAL PARENTHOOD

My patients who have become mothers in their perimenopausal years tell me they feel especially lucky. Also especially exhausted. "I never dreamed I'd be 45 and chasing a 2-year-old around the playground. At least it's a good workout!" one mused. Another, who had been a powerful litigator prior to having her first child at age 41, said, "It's definitely easier to work—even the 100-hour weeks I was putting in—than to stay home full-time."

In spite of the sleepless nights and sore backs, however, they all appreciate how wonderful it is to be a mother at this stage of life, when they have so much wisdom and self-assurance. "I can't imagine having a kid in my twenties—*I* was still a kid in my twenties. I had no idea who I was or what my values were. Now, even though I'm a novice at childrearing, I feel I have some solid life experience to offer my son."

The joy is especially poignant for women who have overcome fertility problems in order to have babies during perimenopause. As one patient put it, "I just stand by the bassinet and stare at my beautiful baby and count my blessings."

Part Two

STAYING HEALTHY

CHAPTER 8

Don't Cry Over Spilled Milk: Your Bones

As I began writing this chapter, I happened to receive in the mail the National Osteoporosis Foundation's recommendations for treating osteoporosis. "What luck!" I thought. But when I began to read the pamphlet, I almost threw it out the window. They generously recommend bone densitometry scans—the standard test for measuring bone health—for all women age 65 and older. *Sixty-five?* By that time you might very well have lost half your bone mass and be on your way to spending your golden years bent over like a paperclip!

Osteoporosis is a major public health concern. Eighty percent of its victims are women, for whom it is the fourth leading cause of death after cardiovascular disease, lung cancer, and stroke. A woman is more likely to die of complications from a hip fracture than of breast, uterine, and ovarian cancer combined. In the United States, progressive bone loss affects more than 25 million women, causing 1.5 million fractures a year and costing an estimated $13.8 billion annually in medical bills and lost productivity. One out of every two women over age 50 is at risk for a fracture. One in six will suffer a hip fracture, which can have dire consequences: of those who survive, 20 percent will die from complications within a year, and half will be unable to walk independently again.

The good news is that osteoporosis is a preventable disease, *but only if we catch it early*, when bone loss is just beginning—that is, in perimenopause. I begin talking about bone loss with patients from the very first time they see me, even if they're only in their teens or twenties, as those are the optimal years for building up our bones. Then, at age 45 or at their first hot flush, whichever comes first, I recommend my patients have a baseline bone densitometry scan. Perimenopause is also the time to make sure you are taking a multivitamin with vitamin D and a calcium/magnesium supplement daily and to incorporate other bone-building lifestyle changes if you haven't already. And if your bone density is already poor, now is the time to start treatment, not twenty years from now when the loss will be irretrievable.

THE STORY OF BONE

We begin building strong bones in utero. Pregnant women need to consume 1,500 mg of calcium a day—300 mg more than nonpregnant women of childbearing years—in order to have enough raw material to build their babies' bones and simultaneously maintain their own. Nature gives the foetus priority; it takes whatever it needs. So if a pregnant woman doesn't get enough calcium, it's *her* bones that will suffer and *she* who will be at risk for osteoporosis later in life. If there is a real shortage, of course, the baby can suffer, too.

Babies live on milk for the first year of their lives. The problem starts when they begin drinking juice instead. Children require a lot of calcium to ensure adequate bone growth—from 600 mg per day for toddlers to 1,550 mg per day for teens. In fact, poor childhood nutrition is so closely linked to osteoporosis in adulthood that some doctors now consider osteoporosis a paediatric disease with geriatric manifestations.

When my children were young, it wasn't too hard to get them to drink enough milk and eat enough cheese to meet their daily requirement (broccoli was more of a challenge). Neither of my children consumed huge amounts of juice, but as soon as they discovered soda, we had a problem. Not only does soda lower children's intake of calcium by replacing milk in their diet, but it also contains phosphorus, which inhibits the absorption of any other calcium they may be ingesting.

A full 60 percent of final bone mass is accumulated during puberty, when children go through their big growth spurt. This makes adolescence the most critical time for healthy eating. After reading about several compelling studies showing that girls who drink an extra glass of milk a day have significantly greater bone density than their peers, I had a talk with my 15-year-old daughter. "Marisa," I told her, "I want you to drink a glass of milk with every meal."

"But Mom, milk will make me fat," she protested. I explained that skim milk would not make her fat and she eventually conceded. Now Marisa and I have a new nightly ritual: we sit at the kitchen table together and each drink a glass of milk before bedtime.

Our twenties may be when we do the most damage to our bones. Obsessed with thinness, young women often restrict their intake of cheese and other calcium-rich foods. In an effort to lose weight, they also may exercise excessively and even take up smoking—both risk factors for osteoporosis later in life. "Please, eat yogurt!" I beg my twentysomething patients. "If you don't build up your bones now, you're going to pay for it big-time when you're my age."

Our twenties and early thirties are our last chance for bone building—between ages 28 and 35 we reach our maximum bone density. From there on, it's downhill. "But wait," you may say. "Oestrogen doesn't start declining until perimenopause. Why would I start losing bone in my thirties?" The reason is that bone density is affected by a number of factors other than oestrogen, which I'll discuss shortly. Several of them, including growth hormone and DHEA, begin declining long before perimenopause sets in.

Unless you actively support your bones with exercise and calcium and keep your body mass index (BMI) between 22 and 25 (see page 350 to learn how to calculate your BMI), you can expect to lose between 0.1 and 1 percent of bone density each year from the time you reach your peak until menopause. (A subset of women who are rapid losers may lose as much as 5 percent a year premenopausally.) In the first seven to ten years after menopause, you can lose 3 percent or more a year. These numbers add up: a woman who reaches her peak at age 35 and menopause at age 50 can lose 45 percent of her bone density by age 60. And for every 1 percent of bone you lose, you increase your risk of fracture by 8 percent. In fact, the average white woman will lose 2½ inches in height due to fractures and deterioration of the spinal column unless she takes steps to protect her bones.

We're now beginning to think that accelerated bone loss—loss of more than 1 percent a year—may actually precede menopause by several years, beginning as soon as oestrogen levels start to decline. That's all the more reason to have your bone density checked and begin taking preventive measures in your perimenopausal years.

TOOTH LOSS—A TIP-OFF

Believe it or not, 32 percent of women in the United States have lost all their teeth by age 65. While periodontal disease is the major culprit—brushing and flossing regularly is the best way to maintain dental health—a certain amount of tooth decay may result from osteoporitic bone loss. Basically, when the jawbone begins to shrink, the gums retract and weaken their grip on the teeth.

If you find yourself looking a bit "long in the tooth," mention it to your doctor and ask whether he or she thinks a bone densitometry scan is in order. Although oestrogen therapy has been associated with decreased risk of tooth loss, good dental hygiene and a glass of milk a day are a simpler way to help keep your pearly whites.

WHAT IS BONE AND WHY DOES IT DISAPPEAR?

Most people are under the mistaken impression that bones are a solid, stable, and static part of our bodily architecture. While they do provide the scaffolding that supports our more malleable parts, they are by no means immutable. Bones are constantly being broken down and rebuilt in an endless remodeling process that keeps bone dynamic and elastic. As we grow, bone building outpaces destruction, or resorption. As we pass our peak, however, resorption begins to exceed formation and we begin to lose bone density.

Another popular misconception is that a bone is a bone is a bone. The truth is that there are two different kinds of bone. Cortical bone makes up 80 percent of the skeleton, including the long bones of the arms and legs. Trabecular bone, the bone of the spinal column, wrists, and ankles, makes up the rest. Cortical bone gives you strength, whereas trabecular bone gives you flexibility. The hip bone is a mixture of the two kinds. Trabecular bone has a honeycomb-type structure and, because of its greater surface area, turns over (that is, is broken down and rebuilt) four to eight times as fast as cortical bone, which is more solid. This makes trabecular bone much more vulnerable to osteoporotic deterioration; in fact, the most common fractures—of the spine—occur in trabecular bone.

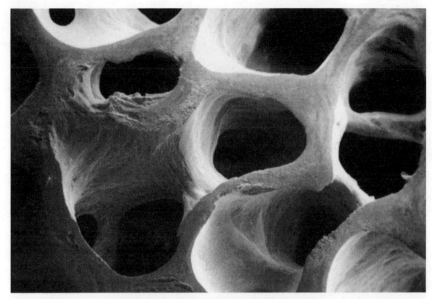

Healthy bone in a 75-year-old woman

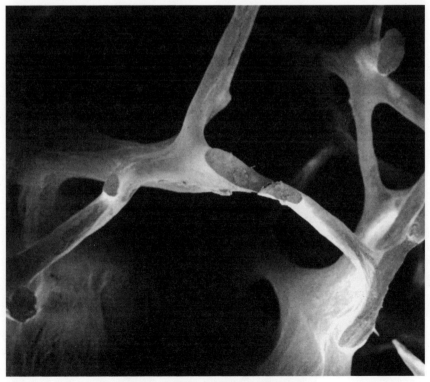

Osteoporosis in a 47-year-old woman
Osteoporosis is not inevitable

Bone turnover involves two types of cells: *osteoclasts*, which eat little pits or "remodeling spaces" into the surface of the bones, and *osteoblasts,* which fill in the pits with calcium phosphate crystals and Type I collagen fibers. This sequence of events is called a bone metabolic unit. An average bone remodeling cycle takes 60 to 100 days; 5 to 10 percent of the skeleton is created and destroyed each year.

Both osteoclasts and osteoblasts have receptors for a variety of hormones that regulate their activity. Oestrogen, for example, inhibits osteoclast activity and stimulates osteoblast activity. Therefore, when oestrogen levels decline, osteoclasts begin to work overtime destroying bone and osteoblasts begin to slack off on rebuilding bone, creating an imbalance that leads to progressive bone loss. Testosterone and progesterone are bone builders, enhancing osteoblast activity. Calcitonin, a hormone produced by the thyroid gland, also builds bone, but by means of a different mechanism: it interferes with osteoclast activity, therefore tipping the balance in the osteoblasts' favor.

The body also makes hormones that promote bone destruction. Why? Because bones are our major storage facility for calcium. Calcium is needed for a number of cellular activities, so our bodies are designed to keep a constant level in the bloodstream at all times. If we don't get enough calcium from our diet and the level begins to drop, we replenish it by raiding our calcium supply—our bones. In fact, 98 percent of the 1 to 2 kilograms of calcium in the body is stored in our bones.

Parathyroid hormone, secreted from the parathyroid glands (which sit right next to the thyroid gland in the neck), is the hormone responsible for regulating blood levels of calcium. If calcium levels decline, we release more parathyroid hormone, which stimulates osteoclasts to break down bone and release calcium into the bloodsteam. Loss of oestrogen makes bone especially sensitive to parathyroid hormone activity—one of the reasons it's more important than ever to maintain your calcium levels during perimenopause. Magnesium deficiency and thyroid disease are two other factors that can impair the function of your parathyroid gland.

Vitamin D plays an important role in maintaining our calcium supply by helping the intestines absorb calcium from the food we eat. When calcium levels in the blood are low, parathyroid hormone tells the kidneys to make a more active form of vitamin D so that the intestines can absorb calcium as efficiently as possible. Normally, the

WILL DHEA HELP MY BONES?

There's a lot of hoopla about DHEA (dehydroepiandrosterone) at health food stores these days, and for good reason. DHEA, a hormone naturally secreted by the adrenal glands, is converted to androgens and oestrogens in fat tissue. As we age, we produce less DHEA, just as we produce less oestrogen. But blood or saliva levels of DHEA correlate even more closely with bone mineral density than do oestrogen levels. In fact, DHEA levels may be an accurate predictor of later development of osteoporosis, so have yours checked.

Taking DHEA supplements will boost your oestrogen and testosterone levels, consequently improving your bone density. I recommend 25 to 50 mg a day. Be careful, however: DHEA may cause irregular bleeding. Also, because it is mostly converted into the male sex hormone, it may have side effects that include acne, hair growth, a negative effect on blood lipids, and liver toxicity. Make sure you have your blood or saliva levels of DHEA checked before you take supplements.

body makes vitamin D in response to sunlight. You only need about 15 minutes of direct sun exposure a day to make enough vitamin D to fulfill all your bodily needs. The problem is that nowadays many of us don't get even that small amount of sunlight. Our lives are spent mostly indoors or in cars; we slather on the sunblock, either straight up or in our moisturizers and make-up; and many of us live in places that just aren't sunny at certain times of the year. For this reason, I prescribe vitamin D supplements to my patients along with their multivitamin and daily dose of calcium and magnesium.

There is anecdotal evidence that women who grow up in the north have a higher incidence of osteoporosis than those who grow up in the south, suggesting that childhood vitamin D levels may affect bone density in adulthood. It remains a question whether this discrepancy will diminish in the future, now that children throughout the West routinely consume foods fortified with vitamin D and calcium.

MAJOR BONE BUILDERS AT A GLANCE

OESTROGEN—Inhibits osteoclast activity; stimulates osteoblast activity

PROGESTERONE—Enhances osteoblast activity

TESTOSTERONE—Enhances osteoblast activity

CALCITONIN—Inhibits osteoclast activity

VITAMIN D—Enhances calcium absorption in the intestine; activates osteoblasts

CALCIUM—Provides raw material for new bone formation

MAGNESIUM—Provides raw material for new bone formation

MIRANDA—CHAMPION BONE BUILDER

Right about the time I was writing this chapter, Miranda came in for her annual exam. I love the fact that although she's a senior vice president of one of the big cosmetics firms, she never wears a drop of make-up. Then again, she doesn't have to—she has a peaches-and-cream complexion framed by a bob of naturally blond hair. At five-foot-ten and about 160 pounds—"I come from a long line of Amazons," she once told me—she's a tall, strong, healthy-looking woman.

Two years ago, when she was 47, Miranda came in complaining of hot flushes, insomnia, palpitations, and irregular periods. I prescribed multivitamins and a calcium/magnesium supplement, and suggested she try taking Remifemin (black cohosh) and evening primrose oil for her symptoms. The herbs kept her symptoms in check for eight months but then they gradually worsened again. "I think I'm ready for the real stuff now," she said.

A week earlier Miranda had had a routine bone densitometry scan. I opened her chart and looked at the results:

Hip:	103 % compared to a young adult
Spine:	115 % compared to a young adult
Wrist:	95 % compared to a young adult

"Miranda, I want to know what it feels like to shake the hand of someone with bones that are a hundred and fifteen percent," I said, holding out my hand.

"Sure, Dr. Corio," she replied, laughing.

We shook hands and then I said, "Seriously, I'm in awe of you. Tell me a little bit about your background."

It turns out that Miranda was born and raised on a farm in Wisconsin—"the land o' cheese." "We didn't drink milk straight from the cow, but we did drink a lot of it. And we worked hard on the farm growing up."

"That is so very interesting." I went on to explain that even though her oestrogen levels were waxing and waning, her bones were in great shape because a high-calcium diet, exercise, good genes, and not being too thin are the most important factors in preventing osteoporosis.

"Looks like I hit the jackpot, especially the not being too thin part!" she joked.

"Hey—would you rather be a twig that snaps in two?" I asked. "Whatever you've been doing, you've been doing right. It just goes to show that if you build enough bone during childhood, you can have perfect bone density right up through menopause."

RISK FACTORS FOR OSTEOPOROSIS

Understanding the risk factors for osteoporosis is an important prelude to making conscious choices that will help you prevent the development and progress of this disease. Unfortunately, some of these conditions you can do nothing about; others, however, are under your control. In addition to having a bone densitometry scan, make sure to discuss with your doctor where you stand in relation to the following risk factors. Then together you can formulate a plan to keep your bones as healthy as possible.

AGE. It's a numbers game: you lose a certain amount of bone mass each year beginning in your late thirties, so the older you are, the greater your chance of brittle bones and fracture.

SEX. The simple fact of being a woman puts you at risk for osteoporosis. Whereas men's bone cells are under the influence of bone-building testosterone for their entire lives, ours begin to be deprived of the stimulating effect of oestrogen in perimenopause. Men eat more than women, therefore getting more calcium into their bodies, and they tend to be more active, which, as you'll see shortly, improves bone health. In addition, we women are generally smaller and lighter than men. Our bones are therefore not as big or as strong to begin with; moreover, they have not been carting around as much weight as men's. As I'll explain shortly, weight-bearing exercise improves bone density.

GENETICS. For a general idea of whether or not you are susceptible to osteoporosis, take a look at your family, especially the women. Did your grandmother shrink a lot and/or have a hump? Has your father suffered a number of fractures? If your mother broke her hip, your own chance of fracturing your hip doubles. Have you yourself had a number of fractures in your adult life? Family and twin studies have shown a strong genetic basis for osteoporosis; the question now is which genes are the culprits.

Genes controlling receptors for hormones and molecules that affect bone remodeling are the logical suspects, and genes for collagen, vitamin D, oestrogen, parathyroid hormone, and various cytokines and growth factors have been examined. Thus far, the gene for the vitamin D receptor, which allows vitamin D to transport calcium into cells, has been most closely studied and has exhibited a strong influence on the disease: it is responsible for 75 percent of the genetic variation in bone mineral density. Women with defective Type I collagen genes have also shown a strong predisposition for osteoporosis. Genetics may also determine whether a woman has a high rate of bone turnover and is a particularly fast loser.

Once we identify the genes that may lead to osteoporosis, we will be able to treat women who carry those genes much more aggressively. In addition to lifestyle changes and supplements, we may be able to prescribe drugs designed specifically to compensate for these genetic flaws. With the incredible advances being made in gene therapy, we may ultimately even be able to treat the problem at its source.

RACE. Women of European and Asian ancestry are far more susceptible to osteoporosis than are women of African, Hispanic, or Polynesian heritage. Osteoporosis occurs in 18.7 percent of non-Hispanic white women as compared with 11.6 percent of all other women. The rule

---

THE COLLAGEN QUESTION

The notion that osteoporosis may actually be a collagen disorder has been gaining currency in the scientific community. We know that collagen levels decline significantly after age 40, leading to loss of thickness and elasticity in skin. Collagen, a connective tissue, also helps hold bones together. As I mentioned in Chapter 6, changes in bone mass closely parallel changes in skin collagen, and both decline with age. In years to come, a skin collagen test may be able to predict bone loss as accurately as a bone densitometry scan can.

---

of thumb is that the lighter your skin and hair, the greater your risk. The reason is that darker people have a lower rate of bone resorption than lighter people.

WEIGHT. Although the Duchess of Windsor may have been right on one count—you can never be too rich—she was dead wrong on the other. You *can* be too thin, and one of the results is osteoporosis. Women weighing less than 127 pounds are at increased risk for the disease, as are women with a history of eating disorders and athletes who have very little body fat.

While I'm not advocating a diet of cookies and cream, a certain amount of fat is beneficial to your bones. For one thing, fat helps the body absorb certain nutrients that are fat-soluble, including vitamin D. For another, bone marrow, where osteoclasts reside when they're not breaking down bone, also contains fat cells. As I explained previously, fat cells convert androgens to oestrogens. Therefore, when women have a little fat on—and in—their bones, the oestrogenic environment will inhibit their osteoclasts from digesting their bone.

SEDENTARY LIFESTYLE. By studying the bones of our foremothers, archaeologists have discovered that osteoporosis was virtually nonexistent 200 years ago. Part of the reason, of course, is that women died a lot younger, and osteoporosis develops with age. But the major factor seems to be that before the invention of modern conveniences such as cars and washing machines and vacuum cleaners, women were on the go morning, noon, and night.

Physical activity—especially weight-bearing exercise such as jogging, playing tennis, dancing, or walking—increases bone mineral density by stimulating new bone growth. Exercise also builds muscle, which pulls and pushes on bone, keeping it elastic. In a study comparing women who exercised three times a week with women who were sedentary over a two-year period, the exercisers increased their bone density by 5.2 percent whereas the non-exercisers lost 1.2 percent of their bone density. (See Chapter 13 for my complete exercise prescription.)

EARLY MENOPAUSE/LONG PERIMENOPAUSE. In the absence of oestrogen, osteoclast activity outpaces osteoblast activity and the resulting imbalance, or "uncoupling," of the bone metabolic unit leads to bone loss. For this reason, women who undergo menopause before age 45 are at increased risk of osteoporosis. In addition, the longer you are in perimenopause, with declining oestrogen levels, the more bone you risk losing. There is a strong correlation between increased hot flushes and decreased bone mineral density, which is why I recommend a bone densitometry scan at the first flush.

SKIPPED PERIODS. At any time of your life, not just in perimenopause, anovulation causes a decline in oestrogen that can put your bones in peril. Premenopausal women who've skipped more than half their periods have been found to have bone mineral density 69 percent lower than women who menstruate normally. It is estimated that just one year of missed periods can cost you 4.2 percent of your bone density—basically, your body thinks you're in menopause. For this reason, anorexics as well as athletes and women who exercise so much that they miss periods are all at high risk for osteoporosis. Breastfeeding women whose periods have not yet resumed can also lose bone quite rapidly, which is why I always recommend they take a calcium/magnesium supplement in addition to continuing their prenatal vitamin for as long as they nurse.

SURGICAL MENOPAUSE. Women who have had their ovaries removed, either alone or as part of a hysterectomy, are at serious risk of bone loss unless they are put on hormone replacement therapy immediately. When fifty women who had gone through surgical menopause without hormone replacement were compared with fifty perimenopausal women over a ten-year period, the former group was found to have significantly lower bone mineral density, especially in the hip and spine.

PREMENSTRUAL SYNDROME. When I prescribe calcium/magnesium supplements to my PMS patients, their symptoms—including irritability, depression, anxiety, headache, bloating, and cramps—are remarkably improved. In fact, the latest thinking is that PMS may be associated with calcium deficiency. If this proves to be the case, wouldn't it make sense for there to be a connection between PMS and osteoporosis? A few recent studies, including one that showed significantly lower bone density in a group of women who had PMS than in a group of controls, seem to bear out this hypothesis.

If you suffer PMS, make sure to take a calcium and magnesium supplement daily—it will help alleviate your symptoms today and protect your bones tomorrow.

SMOKING. Ever wonder why, in candid photos, supermodels are frequently caught with cigarettes dangling from their elongated fingers? It's because smoking speeds up your metabolism and suppresses your appetite, helping you lose weight and stay skinny. Of course, there's a price to pay: severe damage to your skin, your heart, your lungs, and your bones. Women who smoke a pack of cigarettes a day lose an extra 5 to 10 percent of their bone density.

Smoking increases the liver's metabolism of oestrogen, therefore decreasing the amount available to your body. Lowered oestrogen means bone deterioration, plain and simple. Smoking also decreases the oxygenation of your blood, and without adequate oxygen your bones, like your skin, will become less supple and healthy. Furthermore, because cigarette smoking suppresses the appetite, you may not be taking in adequate calcium and vitamins to maintain your bones. And if you're smoking to stay supermodel thin, you put yourself further at risk for osteoporosis because you lack the fat stores needed to keep up your oestrogen levels.

ALCOHOL ABUSE. Alcoholism is a major risk factor for osteoporosis in women as well as men. A study of 96 men between ages 24 and 62 who were chronic alcoholics found that 31 percent of the men under age 40 already had osteoporosis. What's the connection? First, alcohol

CAN I HAVE A CUP OF COFFEE?

Yes, but don't drain the whole urn. Although studies have shown that caffeine causes us to excrete calcium in our urine, in moderate doses the effect is minimal, especially if we get enough calcium in our diet. One cup of coffee reduces our calcium balance by only 2 to 4 mg, a loss that can be made up by an extra 2 tablespoons of milk. I tell my patients it's okay to have a couple of cups—but even better, have a latte.

is toxic to bone. It inhibits osteoblast activity and doesn't allow for new bone formation. Second, people who drink a lot tend to neglect their nutrition and not get enough calcium. And even if they do eat enough calcium, their bodies don't benefit from it, as alcohol reduces the stomach's production of hydrochloric acid, which is needed to help absorb calcium from food.

THYROID DISEASE. Like parathyroid hormone, thyroid hormone stimulates osteoclasts to resorb bone, therefore increasing serum calcium levels. In the presence of excessive amounts of thyroid hormone, parathyroid hormone levels go down, because the thyroid hormone takes over regulating the amount of calcium in the blood. With inadequate parathyroid hormone, your vitamin D level declines as does your intestinal absorption of calcium.

Women with untreated hyperthyroidism (Graves' disease) are therefore at increased risk of osteoporosis. Women being overtreated for hypothyroidism are also at risk—the synthetic supplement they are taking, thyroxine (Synthroid), can build up if it is not carefully monitored and cause bone loss. To make sure you are being treated with the minimum dose necessary, have your TSH (thyroid-stimulating hormone) levels tested regularly; at different times in your life you may need different amounts of thyroxine. If you have any kind of thyroid problem it is crucial that you receive treatment and have annual bone densitometry scans so that if bone loss does become an issue it can be addressed quickly.

CALCIUM DEFICIENCY. Calcium deficiency isn't just a matter of not getting enough calcium in your diet because of poor eating habits, anorexia, or bulimia. It can also occur when you don't absorb calcium properly from the food you do eat or when you excrete calcium in your urine. Even though vitamin D and hydrochloric acid are both essential for good calcium absorption, excessive protein and salt draw calcium out of the bones, into the bloodstream, and ultimately into the urine. Fiber and diuretics can also leach minerals, including calcium, from your body.

VITAMIN D DEFICIENCY. When the ultraviolet rays found in sunshine interact with a molecule called oergosterol, found in the skin, they convert it to vitamin D. Fifteen minutes a day of sunlight are all you need to produce adequate levels of vitamin D. Because vitamin D is critical for calcium absorption, if you suffer a deficiency your blood level of calcium will be low and your body will have to break down bone to restore it to normal.

Unlike our ancestors who were out every day plowing fields or feeding chickens or tending sheep, most of us spend most of our time indoors, out of the sun. And when we do go outside, we cover up or wear UV-protecting sunblock. Vitamin D deficiency is thus a side effect of modern life (or of living at a very high latitude), one that we can remedy through diet and, if necessary, supplements.

HYPERTENSION. When you have high blood pressure, you lose calcium in your urine. If you have hypertension, you are therefore susceptible to osteoporosis and should do everything in your power to keep your blood pressure under control (see page 221) and take a calcium supplement.

DRUGS. If you are taking a prescription drug, discuss its effects on your bones with your doctor, as a number of medications can cause bone loss. Ones to be especially concerned about are steroids such as prednisone, anticonvulsant drugs such as phenobarbitone and phenytoin, anticoagulants such as Coumadin and heparin, lithium, tetracycline, digoxin, methotrexate, GnRH agonists, and excessive amounts of thyroid hormone (Thyroxine). As I discussed in Chapter 7, use of Depo-Provera for birth control can also lead to bone loss of up to 8 percent a year, making it a poor choice for perimenopausal women. Even over-the-counter drugs such as antacids containing aluminum, fiber preparations such as Metamucil, and certain diuretics can interfere with calcium absorption.

KILLING TWO BIRDS WITH ONE STONE

Recent rat studies have shown that a class of anticholesterol drugs called statins may actually help build bone. In the experiments, lovastatin and simvastatin appeared to increase osteoblast activity, promoting new bone formation. Other researchers have observed that osteoporosis patients taking statin drugs have greater bone density than those who are not. Statin drugs are also associated with a 50 percent reduced risk of fracture. Although statin drugs are not currently being used to treat bone loss, who knows what the future will bring!

DIAGNOSING BONE LOSS

According to a survey done by the Centers for Disease Control and Prevention, a shocking 93 percent of oestrogen-deficient women who were found to have osteoporosis were previously unaware of their condition. Why? *Because they didn't have bone densitometry scans!*

Bone densitometry is a technique for measuring bone mineral density. It is based on the fact that ionizing radiation is absorbed in proportion to the density of bone: the greater the bone density, the greater the absorbed energy. There are several machines that perform this measurement, but the top-of-the-line test is called dual-energy x-ray absorptiometry, or DEXA. DEXA involves only one-tenth the amount of radiation you would get in a normal chest x-ray and takes only a few minutes. It can measure the density of bones in the wrist, spine, or hip, and it is noninvasive—you don't even need to get undressed.

Bone densitometry is the only way to assess the condition of a person's bones—you cannot make a judgment based on appearance alone. I have patients who look like a strong wind could blow them away but have bones as hard as steel. I also have patients who look like football players but have lost one-third of their bone. Fortunately, bone densitometry is an extremely accurate test, and its results are an excellent predictor of osteoporosis—far more accurate than, say, cholesterol measurement is at predicting heart disease.

Your "score" on a bone densitometry scan is calculated as a number of standard deviations (S.D.s) away from zero, which corresponds to the peak density of an average woman's bones—usually that of a 35-year-old. If you score within 1 S.D. of normal, you have lost less than 12 percent of your bone mineral density and are considered healthy. If you score between 1 and 2.5 S.D.s below normal, you are considered to have *osteopenia,* a precursor to osteoporosis. Osteoporosis itself is diagnosed if you score -2.5 S.D.s or less.

If possible, it is important to have all three major fracture sites—your spine, hip, and wrist—tested when you go for a bone densitometry scan. Because bone turnover is more rapid in the trabecular bone of the spine than the cortical bone of the hip, you could score within 1 S.D. of normal for the hip but have osteopenia or even osteoporosis in your spine. Also, have both hips checked—there can be as much as a 25 percent disparity between the two.

Hyperparathyroidism along with other disorders of calcium metabolism can cause extreme deterioration in the wrist but not so much in the spine or hip. With hyperparathyroidism, the parathyroid gland is working overtime, releasing lots of parathyroid hormone. As you recall, parathyroid hormone increases blood levels of calcium by stimulating osteoclasts to break down bone. Hyperparathyroidism is confirmed by a blood test; if the condition is present, the test will show an elevated calcium level. Other disorders of calcium metabolism could show a normal calcium level. Hyperparathyroidism is treated surgically at present, and in the near future medical treatments will also become an option.

In a fascinating new study, low bone mineral density of the spine has been associated with increased hardening of the arteries. Although the biochemical connection is not 100 percent clear, it seems that the same enzymatic pathways may be involved in bone breakdown and blood vessel deterioration. In light of this information, I now refer patients with low spine scores on their bone densitometry scans to cardiologists so they can be screened for subclinical vascular disease.

YOU ARE WHAT YOU EAT

Nowhere is this more true than in relation to your bones. Throughout this chapter I've been touting the benefits of calcium and vitamin D for maintaining healthy bones, and while they're the most important single mineral and vitamin, there are several others that are also good for your bones. Make sure you get enough of the following.

CALCIUM. Calcium plays an essential role in a variety of life processes, including muscle contractions, cell division, and intercellular communication. During our adult lives we need at least 1,200 mg per day of

---

WARNING: LEG CRAMPS MEAN MORE THAN LOST SLEEP

A lot of my perimenopausal patients complain about joint pain and nightly leg cramps, both potential warning signs of declining oestrogen, which might also be affecting your bones. Diminished oestrogen levels cause you to lose both bone density and muscle mass, putting increased pressure on your joints. Because oestrogen facilitates calcium absorption, less circulating oestrogen can lead to a calcium deficiency that causes leg cramps, as calcium is necessary for muscle contractions.

If your joints ache or you suffer nocturnal leg cramps, mention it to your doctor and ask whether she thinks a bone densitometry scan would be a good idea. Meanwhile, take a calcium/magnesium supplement and incorporate into your daily routine the preventive strategies outlined in this chapter. Osteoporosis is a silent disease. By the time you begin feeling back pain because of fractured vertebrae, bone loss is already advanced.

---

calcium in order not to deplete our bone stores. (Pregnant women need 1,500 mg.) After age 50 this requirement increases to 1,500 mg per day because calcium is absorbed less efficiently as we age and our oestrogen levels decline. If you are over age 50 and on oestrogen replacement therapy, however, your requirement remains 1,200 mg. My patients often tell me they're confused when they look at a bottle of calcium supplements, because they're not sure whether it's the total or elemental calcium they should pay attention to. The important number is the amount of elemental calcium.

There are lots of different calcium compounds available—calcium citrate, calcium carbonate (the active ingredient in antacids), calcium gluconate, bone calcium (which I don't recommend, as it may contain impurities), and others. A recent study found that most over-the-counter preparations are poorly absorbed, and it singled out Tums, Os-Cal 500, and Citracal as the most effective.

Along with many of my patients, I get stomach cramps and constipation from calcium supplements, so I have not been as conscientious as I should about taking them all these years. Recently, however, I discovered Viactiv chewables—candy-like supplements that come in three yummy flavors, mochachino, chocolate, and caramel. Each contains 500 mg calcium citrate, and the best part is that they don't cause

HOW DO I GET ENOUGH CALCIUM IF I CAN'T DRINK MILK?

If you're lactose intolerant, vegan, or just prefer not to eat dairy, you'll have to work a little harder to meet your daily calcium requirement. It's not impossible, however. The following foods are good alternative sources:

- calcium-fortified orange juice
- calcium-fortified soy milk
- calcium-fortified tofu
- canned sardines, with bones
- canned salmon, with bones
- almonds
- turnip greens
- broccoli
- kale
- okra
- beet greens

gastrointestinal problems. For best absorption take no more than 500 mg elemental calcium at a time with food.

MAGNESIUM. Calcium and magnesium have an interdependent relationship, which is why I always recommend a combination calcium/magnesium supplement with the elements in a 2:1 ratio (1,200 mg calcium and 600 mg magnesium, for example). Together they work to relax nerves and muscles. Bones contain as much as 50 percent of the total amount of magnesium in the body. If you don't get enough magnesium, abnormal calcium crystals will form in your bones, increasing your risk of fracture, especially of trabecular bone.

BORON. This trace mineral plays a major role in calcium and magnesium metabolism. It is also needed to help vitamin D stimulate the absorption and utilization of calcium. Three mg of boron taken daily has been shown to reduce calcium excretion by 44 percent and increase blood levels of the most biologically active form of oestradiol. Check your multivitamin—you may need to take an additional supplement.

EAT GLOBALLY

You've heard about how good a Mediterranean diet is for your heart? Well, it's great for your bones, too. In a study done in Athens, Greece, 36 men and 118 women were interviewed about their diet. When bone densitometry scans were then performed, a positive correlation was found between consumption of monounsaturated fats—i.e., olive oil (remember, we're talking Greece)—and bone mineral density.

The Asian diet also has health benefits for your bones. In earlier chapters we discussed how the phytoestrogens contained in soy can help relieve perimenopausal symptoms such as hot flushes and mood swings. They can also help prevent osteoporosis. When rats that had been made surgically postmenopausal were given soy phytoestrogens, the mass of their weight-bearing bones increased significantly.

VITAMIN D. While it's possible to get adequate vitamin D from eating enriched foods and spending time outdoors, I recommend taking a 400 IU supplement because rainy days and northern winters keep sun exposure sub-par.

VITAMIN K. The Harvard University Nurses' Health Study found that women with low blood levels of vitamin K had an increased risk of hip fracture, suggesting that vitamin K supplements may help protect your bones. A daily dose of 100 mcg vitamin K is necessary for adequate production of osteocalcin, the raw material of bone, and prevention of calcium loss. Women with Candida, a systemic yeast infection, or other bacterial infections in their gastrointestinal tract often have vitamin K deficiencies because they cannot absorb vitamin K from their gut.

VITAMIN A. Vitamin A is needed to regulate bone remodeling. If you're deficient, new bone cells will be formed more quickly than the old cells can be destroyed, and you will experience painful, abnormal bone formations. The recommended dose of 5,000 IU daily should be easily attainable if you eat a good assortment of fruit and vegetables.

VITAMIN B$_6$. As I mentioned earlier, adequate levels of hydrochloric acid must be maintained in the stomach for proper calcium absorption. Vitamin B$_6$ is necessary for the production of hydrochloric acid. Your multivitamin should contain 50 to 100 mg, but never take more than 200 mg.

VITAMIN C. C is for collagen—vitamin C helps produce collagen, the connective tissue that holds so much of our body together, especially our bones. Make sure to get at least 1,000 mg a day.

OTHER VITAMINS AND MINERALS. Make sure your multivitamin also contains:

- 25 mg zinc
- 400 to 800 mcg folic acid
- 5 mg manganese
- 3 mg copper
- 3 mg silicon

TREATING BONE LOSS

If your bone densitometry scan shows osteopenia, I recommend trying a combination of weight-bearing and aerobic exercise, healthful eating, vitamins, and, if you like, herbal supplements. After a full year, have another scan and see whether or not you need to take more aggressive measures. If so, or if your bone densitometry scan shows osteoporosis, waste no time in discussing treatment options with your doctor. Fortunately, there are several excellent choices: hormone replacement therapy, drug therapy, and combinations of the two. The sooner you begin, the better your chance of restoring some, most, or even all of your lost bone.

Be aware that it is not uncommon for your bone scan to show a *loss* of bone during the first year of treatment. If this happens, do not stop or change your medication. In many cases this loss reflects variations in measurements or your body's adjustment to the medication. After two years you will probably see an increase in bone mineral density.

Hormones

OESTROGEN. One of the easiest and best ways to halt bone loss is to go on oestrogen replacement therapy, which has the added benefit of alleviating many other perimenopausal symptoms as well. Interestingly, oestradiol seems to have a much stronger effect on bones than oestriol. Taking 1 mg per day of oestradiol (natural oestrogen) or 0.625 mg per day of synthetic conjugated equine oestrogen (Premarin) has been shown to increase bone density by between 3.5 and 6 percent over three years and decrease the risk of fracture of the spine, hip, and wrist by 50 percent. Of course, in women with an intact uterus, this dose of oestrogen must always be combined with progesterone to mitigate the risk of uterine cancer.

My patient Doreen is a walking advertisement for oestrogen therapy. At age 35 she had a hysterectomy in which both ovaries were removed and was immediately put on oestrogen. Now age 55, she comes in for an exam and I send her for a bone densitometry scan. Her bones are absolutely perfect! Because she has taken hormone supplements from the time of her peak bone density and has been spared the normal perimenopausal fluctuation and ultimate decline in oestrogen levels, her bones have been preserved 100 percent.

I find standard dosages of natural oestrogen taken with natural progesterone are well tolerated by my patients. Recent studies have shown that even the low-dose transdermal patch, which only delivers 0.025 mg oestradiol (E_2) daily (comparable to 0.3 mg conjugated oestrogen), has a restorative effect on bones—although not quite as much as the higher dose. In general, low-dose oestrogen has been shown to increase bone mineral density of the lumbar spine by 2 to 3 percent within two years. I prescribe it with a low dose of progesterone, to protect the uterus.

If you're in perimenopause and have not yet developed osteoporosis, low-dose oestrogen over a long period of time can be enough to sustain your bones. It's only if you've had accelerated bone loss or have developed postmenopausal osteoporosis that you need the big gains that can be provided by standard oestrogen replacement therapy.

One thing to be aware of is that taking oestrogen to fortify your bones is a lifelong proposition. If you stop, within a few years your bone mineral density will decline until it is at the level it would have been had you never taken hormones at all. This is another reason I recommend low-dose oestrogen whenever possible, because there are as of yet no proven health risks to taking it long term.

NATURAL PROGESTERONE. Combining oestrogen and progesterone therapy can have an even stronger effect on bone than taking oestrogen alone. This makes perfect sense, because we know that progesterone increases osteoblast activity. Bone-building osteoblasts are busiest during the second half, or luteal phase, of the menstrual cycle, which is when the ovaries release progesterone. To give my patients the maximum bone benefit and protect their uteri against the effects of unopposed oestrogen, I prescribe a natural progestogen along with oestrogen. (Cyclic progesterone doesn't help bone.)

Patients who are nervous about taking oestrogen can still build bone by taking natural progesterone alone. Oral micronized progesterone taken 100 mg twice a day and topical progesterone (5 percent cream) have both been shown to build bone. Note, however, that the synthetic, medroxyprogesterone (Provera), seems to have little effect—and possibly even a negative effect—on bone.

ORAL CONTRACEPTIVES. The evidence isn't conclusive, but it looks as if yet another benefit of going on the Pill in perimenopause is that it may protect you against bone loss. Indeed, taking oral contraceptives in your forties has been shown to reduce the rate of hip fracture later in life by 25 percent. The longer you take oral contraceptives, the more they can help your bones.

TESTOSTERONE. Here's a fascinating fact: height loss in postmenopausal women seems to be more directly related to their diminishing testosterone levels than to their oestrogen depletion. Adding natural or synthetic testosterone to oestrogen therapy can increase bone mineral density by twice as much as taking oestrogen alone. Not only does testosterone have a stimulating effect on osteoblasts, but it also increases muscle strength. Stronger muscles give bones more of a workout, keeping them supple and healthy.

DHEA. If blood or saliva testing has shown you to have low DHEA levels and you have other risk factors for osteoporosis, you may want to consider taking a 25 to 50 mg daily supplement. Only take DHEA under a doctor's supervision.

Medications

BISPHOSPHONATES. Alendronate (Fosamax) is the first drug in this category to be approved for treatment of osteoporosis. For women who can't take oestrogen, because of side effects or breast cancer, a daily 10 mg dose of Fosamax has proven a godsend in terms of preserving bone mass. Like oestrogen, it inhibits osteoclasts from breaking down bone. Its effect is just as strong as oestrogen, too, increasing bone density up to 2 percent a year for the first three years. If you're not building enough bone on Fosamax or oestrogen alone, you can combine the two for an enhanced effect. Fosamax may also benefit your cardiovascular system: a recent study showed that rats who were given Fosamax had less arterial and heart valve calcification than rats who were not.

But, as they say, there's no free lunch. Fosamax can cause irritation of the stomach and oesophagus. To minimize this effect, you have to take it on an empty stomach first thing in the morning with an 8-ounce glass of water and remain upright for at least 30 minutes afterward. You also cannot eat or drink anything but water for at least 30 minutes, as food or other beverages reduce its bioavailability to zero. If you're going to have side effects, they'll manifest within the first couple of months. If you have osteopenia and can't handle the 10 mg dose, try 5 mg—although you won't build as much bone as you would on the higher dose, you will be protected from losing more. One more caveat: if you have kidney problems you cannot take Fosamax, because it is cleared through the kidneys and if it builds up it can be toxic.

For women who can't tolerate the side effects of Fosamax or who don't want to go through such a production every morning, alternatives are on the horizon. Two other bisphosphonates currently undergoing clinical trials for treatment of osteoporosis are Skelid (tiludronate), which is already approved for treating Paget's disease, and Actonel (risedronate).

IS MY TREATMENT WORKING?

Apart from having bone densitometry scans every other year, how can you tell whether the hormones or drugs you're taking to stop your bones from thinning are doing their job? To monitor their effectiveness and determine your optimal dose, your doctor can test your urine for a variety of biochemical markers of bone turnover. To my mind, the quickest and most reliable test currently available is called Osteomark NTx, which measures a product of bone breakdown called cross-linked N-telopeptides of Type I collagen. After you begin treatment, the amount of these markers you excrete should be reduced by at least 50 percent within one to three months. Other urine tests on the market include OsteoCheck, which measures a bone breakdown product called deoxypyridinoline (D-Pyd).

RALOXIFENE. Marketed as Evista, raloxifene is one of a new family of drugs called selective oestrogen receptor modulators, or SERMs. SERMs are designed to imitate the beneficial effects of oestrogen in certain tissues, such as bones and heart, without affecting others, such as the breast and uterus. Evista is great for preventing and treating osteoporosis in postmenopausal women, but it has not yet been tested on perimenopausal women. Personally, I am concerned about prescribing it to my perimenopausal patients because it seems to increase hot flushes substantially—by approximately 35 percent—as well as leg cramps.

FLUORIDE. We've all grown up hearing how good fluoride is for your teeth, so why not for your bones? Sodium fluoride does stimulate bone formation to a remarkable degree—one study showed an increase in bone density of 8 percent a year in women who took it for four consecutive years. The problem is that in the presence of fluoride, osteoblasts use fluoride to make new bone instead of calcium. Unlike calcium, fluoride is inflexible, so although your bones become more dense, they also become more brittle, making you just as susceptible to fractures should you fall as when your bones were thin.

COMPARING TREATMENTS FOR OSTEOPOROSIS

TREATMENT	DECREASES FRACTURE RATES?	APPROXIMATE INCREASE IN BONE MINERAL DENSITY OVER 2 TO 3 YEARS
CALCIUM	No, unless your prior calcium level was low	1–3%
OESTROGEN	Yes	5–6%
ALENDRONATE (FOSAMAX)	Yes	5–6%
ALENDRONATE (FOSAMAX) AND STANDARD OESTROGEN	Yes	8%
CALCITONIN	Yes	1–2%
RALOXIFENE (EVISTA)	Yes	1–2%
FLUORIDE	Yes/no, depending on dose	8%

Phytoestrogens

SOY. Japanese women have half as many hip fractures as American women, and it looks as if soy is the reason. *Genistein,* the phytoestrogen in soy, protects against loss of bone mineral density and increases osteoblastic activity. It can also inhibit osteoclast activity and therefore prevent bone resorption. A recent study showed that consuming 40 g soy protein a day for six months increased bone density by 2.2 percent. I recommend incorporating up to 50 mg soy isoflavones into your diet daily from food sources such as tofu, soy milk, or soy nuts (see Appendix B).

DO'S AND DON'TS FOR PREVENTING OSTEOPOROSIS

Do...   get a bone densitometry scan if you're age 45, have had hot flushes, or have a number of the risk factors for osteoporosis.

make sure you're not too thin: you should have a body mass index of no less than 22. (See page 349.)

get 30 minutes of strength training twice a week to build bone and 30 minutes of aerobic weight-bearing exercise three times a week to keep your bones oxygenated. (See Chapter 13 for more details on exercise.)

consume adequate calcium—1,200 mg a day—and magnesium—600 mg a day—from either food or supplements.

get enough vitamin D, either by spending time in the sun or taking a 400 IU supplement daily.

moderate your protein intake (no more than 0.8g/kg body weight per day). A certain amount of protein is good for bones, as it provides the building blocks for collagen. Too much, however, leaches calcium from your body.

cut back on salt, as it causes you to excrete calcium in your urine.

DON'T...   overexercise or lose so much weight that you stop menstruating.

smoke—at all!

consume more than one alcoholic beverage a day.

consume more than two cups of a caffeinated beverage a day.

drink soda or seltzer water—the phosphorus contained in carbonated drinks weakens your bones.

take antacids with aluminum, fiber preparations, or diuretics without consulting your doctor.

ORAL IPRIFLAVONE. This is a synthetic isoflavone-derived compound that inhibits osteoclast activity. It is not a true phytoestrogen, however, because it has no oestrogenic activity. Taken by itself in three 200 mg doses at mealtimes or with low-dose oestrogen in two 200 mg doses at mealtimes, it can slightly decrease bone turnover and increase bone density, providing a small amount of protection against vertebral fracture. Its effect is strengthened when it is taken with calcium. Just be careful—the pure form comes from Italy and is hard to find in the United States.

On The Horizon

PARATHYROID HORMONE. One of the most exciting new treatments in development for bone loss is parathyroid hormone. This may seem like a strange way to build bone, as parathyroid hormone normally stimulates osteoclasts to break down bone when blood levels of calcium are low. In the presence of oestrogen, however, it appears that parathyroid hormone stimulates osteoblasts instead. When thirty-four women with osteoporosis who were already taking oestrogen replacement were given parathyroid hormone, they had an average overall increase in bone density of 8 percent. Parathyroid hormone also seems to build bone in the presence of Fosamax, making this combination a potential treatment for women who cannot take oestrogen.

CHAPTER 9

Beating the Odds: Your Heart

One of the major reasons women of our generation are refusing to put up complacently with the discomforts of perimenopause is that unlike many of our mothers, we have big plans for the years ahead. We don't want symptoms like hot flushes or fatigue or more serious medical problems to prevent us from fulfilling our dreams, whether they be to trek the Himalayas, sail the Galápagos, take up tennis or golf or scuba diving, write poetry, learn to paint, or just sit back and relax for a change. But unless we act now, in our perimenopause, to protect ourselves against heart disease, those dreams could disappear overnight.

Most of us are still under the false impression that heart disease is a man's problem and that women don't get heart attacks. *Wake up and smell the coffee!* Although we're generally protected from heart disease by oestrogen during our reproductive years, as our oestrogen levels decline we begin to lose that protection. After menopause our advantage disappears altogether, and later in life our prognosis is even *worse* than men's. Here are a few facts that will knock your socks off:

- Cardiovascular disease is the number-one killer of women in the United Kingdom. Each year in the United States, 2.5 million women are hospitalized for coronary artery disease and 500,000 die of it—*that's more than all other causes of women's death combined,* including lung, breast, ovarian, and uterine cancer.

- Women have a 2.5 times greater risk of heart disease than men, and since 1984 more women than men have died of heart disease annually.

- One in nine women between the ages of 45 and 64 has some form of cardiovascular disease (one in three over age 65), and approximately 20,000 women under the age of 65 die of a heart attack each year.

- Women fear breast cancer more than twice as much as a heart attack, but they're mistaken: 50 percent of women will die of heart disease or stroke; less than 4 percent will die of breast cancer. To put it another way, each year nearly 11 times more women die of cardiovascular disease than do of breast cancer.

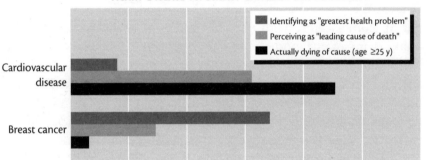

HEART DISEASE VS. BREAST CANCER: FEAR VS. REALITY

- Heart attacks are much more deadly for women than for men. Women under age 50 are more than twice as likely to die of them than men—in or out of the hospital. Of the 625,000 women in the United States who suffer heart attacks annually, 44 percent—275,000—die within a year, compared with 27 percent of men. Women are also 35 percent more likely to suffer a second attack within six years of the first than are men.

- Women are less likely than men to be given screening tests for heart disease, are treated less aggressively than men when they have a heart attack, and are more likely than men to die in the hospital after they have a heart attack.

- Black women of African origin are 38 percent more likely to die of a heart attack and 76 percent more likely to die of a stroke than are Caucasian women.

- Women account for 60 percent of deaths from stroke, which is the third leading killer of women overall.

THE LANGUAGE OF THE HEART

People throw around a lot of terms when they're talking about heart disease, and it's not always clear what they mean. In brief, *cardiovascular disease* or *heart disease* is an umbrella term that includes:

- *Atherosclerosis (arterial sclerosis)*, which means hardening of the arteries due to cholesterol plaque buildup. It can occur in the arteries of the heart *(coronary artery disease)* or in other vessels *(peripheral vascular disease)*.
- *Stroke*, which occurs when the brain is deprived of oxygen, usually because of a blood clot but sometimes because of a haemorrhage.
- *Myocardial infarction* or *heart attack,* which occurs when heart tissue is deprived of oxygen because of hardened arteries or a blood clot, usually leading to permanent scarring or heart damage.
- *Hypertension* or *high blood pressure*, which can cause any or all of the above.
- *Angina (angina pectoris)*, which is chest pain or symptoms resulting when heart tissue is temporarily deprived of oxygen because of hardening of the arteries or a blood clot *(myocardial ischemia).*
- *Congestive heart failure (CHF)*, which occurs when damaged heart tissue does not pump blood effectively and fluid backs up into the lungs, causing shortness of breath, coughing, and fatigue.

Even though your chance of developing heart disease is still low in your perimenopausal years, now is the time to start taking note of your risk factors and doing everything in your power to control them. Cardiovascular disease is like the wolf in "Little Red Riding Hood." He's already eaten up Grandma; now he can't wait to get his fangs into you. But you can outsmart him: dump the cookies out of your basket and substitute fruits and veggies instead; keep on skipping through the woods; and don't smoke—it causes forest fires, among other things.

OESTROGEN: THE HEART OF THE MATTER

My mother has this old saying, "Men work from sun to sun, but women's work is never done." The same could be said of the oestrogen your body produces naturally. In addition to controlling our reproductive functions, keeping our brains and bones healthy, giving us beautiful skin and hair, and helping to regulate our metabolism, it influences just about every aspect of our cardiovascular system—quite a job! This makes perfect sense in evolutionary terms: it wouldn't be too smart for Mother Nature to have us dying of heart attacks during our prime childbearing years. She's a fickle friend, however. Once we can no longer be of service to her by perpetuating the species, it seems she could care less what happens to us.

But we *do* care. Understanding exactly how oestrogen affects your heart, blood vessels, and blood will help you focus your energies on compensating for your declining levels of this essential hormone through diet, exercise, vitamins and minerals, and, if desired, hormone supplements.

How does oestrogen benefit your heart and circulation? Two-thirds of oestrogen's protective effect is a result of direct action on the vascular system. As I explained in earlier chapters, there are oestrogen receptors on the surfaces of blood vessels. In the presence of oestrogen, blood vessels dilate; in the absence of oestrogen, they constrict.

When your blood vessels constrict, your blood pressure rises, damaging the linings of the vessels. When the lining of a blood vessel is scraped or roughed up, blood flow over that spot slows down and it becomes a magnet for fatty deposits, or plaques. Plaque buildup hardens and further narrows the *lumen,* or interior of the blood vessel. When the lumen is constricted, the blood (heart) has to pump harder to force its way through, leading to even higher blood pressure. A narrowed artery also becomes a trap where clots can form. Furthermore, chunks of plaque can break off and cause a heart attack or stroke— one of the leading causes of sudden death in perimenopausal women.

Blood vessel linings are also damaged by the oxidized form of LDL cholesterol. The damaged walls not only make the vessel inflamed and vulnerable to atherosclerosis, but also produce less of the vasodilating and anticlotting agents nitric oxide and prostacyclin. Oestrogen stimulates the release of nitric oxide, thereby keeping the blood vessels supple. Oestrogen is also a powerful antioxidant, soaking up dangerous free radicals produced when LDL cholesterol is oxidized, thereby protecting the vessel walls from damage and reducing the risk of blood clots. Two other ways in which oestrogen prevents blood clotting are by making platelets—the cells responsible for forming blood clots— less sticky and by decreasing levels of fibrinogen, an important clotting factor.

Oestrogen relaxes not only blood vessels but the walls of the heart itself. When women are treated with oestrogen, the pumping, or contractibility, of their left ventricle improves. The heart can therefore take in more blood with each beat, improving circulation overall and decreasing the risk of heart failure.

The remaining third of oestrogen's beneficial effect comes from its influence on lipid metabolism. Put simply, oestrogen keeps your overall cholesterol level down. It also helps you maintain a favorable balance of "good" (HDL) cholesterol over "bad" (LDL) cholesterol. When your oestrogen levels decline, the balance is inverted: your HDL cholesterol levels go down and your LDL cholesterol levels go up, putting you at greater risk for cardiovascular disease.

Last but not least, a very important component of oestrogen's effect on your heart is its insulin-lowering property. Oestrogen lowers your circulating insulin and therefore keeps your central body fat at a minimum. And we know that elevated insulin levels are associated with elevated cholesterol, which is bad news for your blood vessels. Because of this insulin-oestrogen connection, postmenopausal women treated with oral oestrogen have lower fasting insulin levels, decreased insulin response to glucose, and a 20 percent decreased risk of non–insulin-dependent diabetes (the eventual outcome of increasing insulin resistance) than women who don't take oestrogen. As I'll discuss shortly, diabetes is one of the major contributing factors to heart disease in women.

WHAT YOUR CHOLESTEROL NUMBERS MEAN

I sit at the manicurist and overhear women trading stats: "Mine was over 200, but since I stopped eating cheese I got it down to 180."

"Mine's still over 200, but my doctor says I have lots of the good ones so I don't need to worry." Nowadays it seems as important to know your cholesterol levels as your name, address, and Social Security number. But how many people really understand what all the terms on their lipid profile mean? Let me explain.

As anyone who has made gravy knows, fats are not soluble in water-based solutions. Blood is water-based. So to be transported through the circulation, fats such as cholesterol and triglycerides need to be bound to proteins, which are water-soluble. When these proteins bind lipids (fat), they form complexes called *lipoproteins*. The more cholesterol and triglycerides are bound to a particular protein, the higher the density of the lipoprotein complex.

There are three major kinds of lipoproteins:

VLDL (very low density lipoprotein) is made in the liver and mainly transports triglycerides, which increase the risk of blood clots. It is converted to LDL in fat tissue.

LDL (low density lipoprotein) mainly transports cholesterol, which is needed for the formation of hormones, including oestrogen and testosterone. Excess LDL is cleared by the liver; but if there is more LDL than the liver can handle, it begins building up in the bloodstream, leading to higher circulating cholesterol levels and increasing the risk of atherosclerosis. That's why LDL cholesterol is considered "bad."

HDL (high density lipoprotein), which is produced in both the liver and the intestine, mops up excess cholesterol from the circulation as well as from cells lining the blood vessels and transports it back to the liver, where it is broken down. HDL therefore reduces the risk of atherosclerosis and is considered "good."

When you have your cholesterol levels tested, as you should once every five years if they're in the normal range, the results come back in four categories: total cholesterol, LDL, HDL, and triglycerides (VLDL). Even though the total number is important, it doesn't tell the whole story. If you have a high total but also high HDLs, you may be in better shape than someone with a low total but high LDLs. There are gender differences as well. Whereas men's cardiovascular systems seem to be more sensitive to LDL levels, women's are more sensitive to HDL levels. This means that it's worse for your HDL level to drop than it is for your LDL level to rise, whereas it's worse for a man's LDL

YOUR CHOLESTEROL LEVELS AT A GLANCE			
	NORMAL/LOW RISK	BORDERLINE	HIGH RISK
TOTAL CHOLESTEROL	below 200 mg/dL	200–239 mg/dL	above 239 mg/dL
LDL	below 130 mg/dL	130–159 mg/dL	above 159 mg/dL
HDL	above 60 mg/dL	35–59 mg/dL	below 35 mg/dL
TRIGLYCERIDES	below 200 mg/dL	200–400 mg/dL	above 400 mg/dL

level to rise than it is for his HDL level to drop. Elevated triglycerides are also a risk factor for heart disease in women, but only when they are associated with low HDL cholesterol levels.

Incidently, the way you have your cholesterol levels tested may be changing in the not too-distant future. An exciting new product is hitting the market that measures your cholesterol levels by sampling the outer layer of your skin. Apparently, the higher your levels of skin cholesterol, the greater your risk of cardiovascular disease. The test only takes three minutes and doesn't involve any needles. Plus, it may be an even better indicator of the condition of your arteries than the traditional blood test.

Oestrogen regulates our cholesterol levels by acting directly on the liver and intestine, where cholesterol-binding proteins are made. Pre-menopausally, oestrogen protects our hearts, helping keep our LDL levels down and our HDL levels about 10 mg/dL higher than men's. When our oestrogen levels decline in perimenopause, however, our HDL levels begin to drop and our LDL levels begin to rise until they eventually exceed that of men. So much for our advantage. That's why perimenopause is the critical moment to take stock of your heart health and do everything you can to lower your risk of cardiac disease.

RISK FACTORS FOR HEART DISEASE

Many people have a strangely resigned attitude toward heart disease. "Everyone in my family has high blood pressure and both my parents died of heart attacks in their sixties, so I figure I've got about twenty more years," a patient in her forties recently told me.

"Are you out of your mind?" I responded. "We know so much more than our parents knew about heart disease and what you can do to fight it." True, there are hereditary factors that can make you more or less susceptible, but there are also a host of risk factors that are well under your control, through either lifestyle choices or medication.

Since scientists began identifying risk factors such as smoking and hypertension as part of the legendary Framingham Heart Study, the rate of heart disease in the United States has dropped by nearly two-thirds. The key is to be aware of your vulnerabilities, discuss them with your doctor, and take whatever preventive strategies you need to in order to preserve your heart health.

MENOPAUSE. For women, this one tops the list. Women who are menopausal have four times the risk of cardiovascular disease as women the same age who still get their periods. Up to now, oestrogen has kept you from having a heart attack in spite of your crappy diet, your smoking, your couch-potato tendencies. But as soon as you lose that oestrogen, either surgically or naturally, all these risky behaviors are going to come back to haunt you, causing blood clots, hardening of the arteries, heart attack, and stroke. Fortunately, the cardiovascular system is somewhat forgiving: if you mend your ways in perimenopause, you can significantly reduce your chances of developing heart disease in your postmenopausal years.

AGE. Before age 60, one in seventeen women die of heart disease; after age 60, the number rises to one in four. Although much of the difference has to do with women's menopausal status, plain old age is also a factor. After decades of exposure to free radicals, our arterial walls become damaged, making them vulnerable to plaque formation. As the endothelial cells lining our blood vessels grow older, they produce less nitric oxide, which is necessary for dilating blood vessels. This vasoconstriction makes our blood pressure rise, which also contributes to hardening of the arteries and puts us at risk of stroke. Basically, everyone has some degree of atherosclerosis by middle age; the trick is to keep it from getting so bad that it becomes a health hazard.

GENETICS. Even though you're not entirely doomed if your parents had heart disease, you should be especially vigilant about trying to protect yourself. A number of risk factors such as high blood pressure and cholesterol, diabetes, and age at menopause are hereditary. In addition, the vulnerability of your entire cardiovascular system to various risk factors may be genetically determined. As a rule of thumb, *tell your doctor* if your mother or sister had a heart attack before age 65, or if your father or brother had a heart attack before age 55. If so, you are at increased risk of heart disease and should be monitored carefully.

RACE. As mentioned previously, black women have a far higher rate of heart attack and stroke than do white women. This is because they are more likely to suffer hypertension, diabetes, and obesity, all serious risk factors for heart disease.

SMOKING. April, a longtime patient and even longer-time smoker—a pack a day for thirty years—came in to see me complaining of hot flushes, insomnia, memory problems, and nonexistent sex drive. She'd already tried Remifemin (black cohosh), but it wasn't working anymore. I told her she needed oestrogen.

"N-O," she replied. "I have two friends who went on hormone replacement therapy and were diagnosed with breast cancer a year later. I refuse to take oestrogen."

"I understand your worry about breast cancer," I said, "but let's put this in perspective. For one thing, you don't know that hormones caused your friends' cancer. It could have been a coincidence—likely as not they were going to get breast cancer anyway. The hormones probably just spurred it on. To be honest with you, you're much more likely to die of heart disease or lung cancer, the way you smoke."

"If I've told you once, I've told you a hundred times, I cannot give up smoking. I've tried and failed over and over again. Besides," she said defensively, "I enjoy it."

"You're not going to enjoy having a heart attack or a stroke," I responded severely. "Listen to me, April. The five-year survival rate for women with breast cancer is *97 percent; one in two* who have heart attacks don't make it a year. By smoking, you increase your chance of dying from heart disease by *70 percent!* Smoking is the number-one cause of death for women and for men. It's like committing suicide!" I continued to barrage her with statistics and didn't let her out of the examining room until she promised me she'd try quitting one more time.

Smoking accounts for one in five deaths from heart disease, making it the most significant controllable risk factor. Among participants in the extraordinary Harvard University Nurses' Health Study (which in 1976 enrolled 121,700 women between ages 30 and 55 and has followed them for the past quarter-century), smoking caused more than half the heart attacks. Cutting down helps, but even smoking just one to four cigarettes a day doubles your chance of having a heart attack or stroke. The reason is that smoking increases blood clotting; deprives cells of oxygen, which causes the heart to beat faster and weakens the arteries; and impairs the function of the endothelial cells lining the vessel walls, constricting the blood vessels and inviting formation of atherosclerotic plaques.

The culprit in cigarette smoke that facilitates hardening of the arteries is nicotine. Cells lining the blood vessels have receptors for acetylcholine, a molecule that helps them keep their shape and connection to each other. When nicotine is present in the bloodstream, it aggressively binds the acetylcholine receptors, jamming them up and preventing acetylcholine from doing its job. The cells, which are normally flat and rectangular, then bunch up. The irregularly shaped cells and spaces between them become prime target sites for cholesterol deposition. Whether you get your nicotine from cigarettes or from patches or gum, it seems likely that the negative effect on your cardiovascular system will be the same. And remember, secondhand smoke will also affect you, so talk to your partner about kicking the habit.

Smoking is an especially important issue for women, as they tend to be heavier smokers than men, to start smoking younger, and to have a tougher time quitting. Back in 1955, twice as many men smoked as women; today the gap has narrowed to the point at which we're almost neck and neck: 28 percent of men over age 18 smoke, and 22 percent of women do. And in that interval, the death rate from lung cancer among women has increased by more than 400 percent.

Fortunately, the body is somewhat forgiving: within three to five years of quitting, your cardiovascular risk will go down to that of a nonsmoker and your lungs will repair themselves as well. So if you smoke, make this cigarette your last.

OBESITY. Here's a shocker: 33.5 percent of white women and 49.6 percent of black women in the United States are clinically obese— that is, 20 percent or more over their ideal body weight. And this excess fat is killing them. A mere 25 to 30 extra pounds can raise your risk of a heart attack by 80 percent! Obesity puts a strain on the heart, contributing to high blood pressure. Also, fat is associated with insulin resistance, which raises LDL cholesterol levels and causes hardening of the arteries.

But all fat is not created equal. Women who are bottom-heavy have an advantage over their middle-heavy sisters. As discussed in Chapter 6, fat in the hips and thighs does not adversely affect your cholesterol profile, whereas abdominal fat can lower HDL cholesterol levels and raise triglyceride levels, making you more prone to heart disease. "Apple-shaped" women with a waistline of more than 35 inches or a waist-hip ratio (see page 349) of greater than 0.80 are at particular risk.

In the best of all possible worlds, we would all remain within ten pounds of what we weighed at age 18 (providing we were at a healthy weight at that time). While this is only a pipe dream for most of us, nevertheless we must do all we can to keep our weight under control, especially in our perimenopausal years. These days, the preferred measure for ideal weight is called the body mass index (BMI), a number that represents the relationship between your height and your weight (see page 350 to figure out how to calculate your BMI). Ideally, the number should be between 22 and 25. Women with a BMI of between 25 and 29 have nearly double the risk of heart disease as do women with a BMI of less than 21. And women with a BMI of greater than 29 have three times the risk! In Chapter 13 you'll find my suggestions for a sensible eating plan to take off or maintain weight and avoid the gain-and-loss rollercoaster that is so damaging not only to your morale but to your heart as well.

SEDENTARY LIFESTYLE. Addiction to soap operas and an otherwise slothful existence is as great a risk factor for heart disease as are smoking, high blood pressure, or high cholesterol levels. Physical exercise is essential to heart health: it trains your heart muscle to work more efficiently, reducing your resting pulse; it oxygenates all the tissues in your body including your blood vessels, keeping them supple and dilated; and it burns fat and builds muscle, raising your metabolism and making it easier to keep your weight under control. Furthermore, aerobic exercise increases your HDL cholesterol level, the most important measure of a woman's heart health.

Women who don't exercise are three times as likely to die of a heart attack than those who exercise regularly. Simply walking for thirty minutes three times a week halves your risk of dying of heart disease; more aggressive aerobic exercise has an even greater beneficial effect. So get out there! If you can't find a half hour, try three ten-minute sessions. And if you can't miss your soaps, invest in a stationary bicycle, StairMaster, or NordicTrack and work out while you watch (an added plus—it'll keep you from raiding the fridge during commercials).

THE LONG AND THE SHORT OF IT

According to the Harvard University Nurses' Health Study, the largest and longest ongoing study of how lifestyle factors influence women's health, tall women have a lower rate of heart disease than shorter women. (The same happens to be true of tall men when compared with shorter men.) Likely as not, this is because they have larger arteries and are at less risk for atherosclerosis.

ALCOHOL ABUSE. Excessive consumption of alcohol—more than one drink a day—can elevate blood pressure and stimulate the formation of blood clots, increasing the risk of death from a heart attack or stroke. Also, people who fill up on alcohol tend to consume less food and therefore less vitamins and minerals needed to maintain their well-being, including their heart health.

DISTRESS. "Calm down! Do you want to have a heart attack?" We've all said it a million times, but is it true? Although *stress* does compromise the immune system, studies have not been able to prove that stress puts people at risk for cardiovascular disease. Fortunately for me, we "Type A" personalities are no more susceptible than our more laid-back cousins, although we are more prone to chest pain.

*Dis*tress, on the other hand, including depression and social isolation, is a proven risk factor. The reason is probably that people who are down and lonely are less likely to exercise or eat well and more likely to abuse alcohol and smoke than the general population. Also, a recent study showed that people who are depressed after having a heart attack have a decreased chance of survival.

HYPERTENSION. Called "the silent killer," hypertension is rampant among women. More than one in five between the ages of 20 and 74 have high blood pressure; one in two over age 55. Among African-origin women the rate is an astonishing four out of five—epidemic proportions! It's also high for Latin Americans. The scariest part to me is the fact that of the 50 million people with high blood pressure in the United States, only 34 million are aware of it, only 27 million seek

> ## TAKE A TEA BREAK
>
> Black tea, with or without caffeine, contains lots of flavonoids, the antioxidants found in soybeans that protect the arteries from hardening. In a study of nearly 700 women and men in Boston (a Boston Tea Party, if you will), those who drank no tea had nearly twice the risk of heart attack as those who drank one or more cups of black tea a day. Green tea (which has as much caffeine as black tea) and oolong tea share this beneficial effect, but herbal tea does not.

treatment, and only half of them get their pressure under control. In addition to contributing to heart attack and stroke, hypertension can lead to kidney disease and congestive heart failure.

The problem is that hypertension rarely exhibits any symptoms. The only way to know you have it is to *get your blood pressure checked regularly—at least once a year.* A reading of 140/90 mm Hg or higher signifies hypertension; below 120/80 is considered optimal; 120–129/80–84 is normal; 130–139/85–89 is high normal and bears monitoring, especially if it is on the rise. (In case you've ever wondered, the top number, or systolic pressure, is measured when the heart is contracting; the bottom number, or diastolic pressure, is measured when the heart is relaxing between beats.)

Hypertension may be caused by any number of factors. Age, a high-fat and high-salt diet, sedentary lifestyle, obesity, alcohol abuse, smoking, diabetes, and other risk factors for atherosclerosis can all contribute to the problem, as can a genetic predisposition. Take Lydia, for example. When she first came to me, at age 30, she was five-foot-five, weighed 135 pounds, and was in great shape. Her blood pressure was 120/80—normal. Now at age 37 she's pushing 200 pounds and her blood pressure is 150/90. What's the problem? She's in a rotten marriage (her husband is a notorious cheat) and is so depressed about her life that she overeats and doesn't take care of herself. "Lydia, you've got to get a grip," I said. "You've got to look at what you're eating— your fats, your carbs, your protein, and start exercising—you need to lose some weight. Your blood pressure is creeping up and you're basically volunteering for a heart attack."

THE MOST COMMON MEDICAL TREATMENTS FOR HYPERTENSION

DIURETICS. "Water pills" such as hydrochlorothiazide (HCTZ) and Lasix are often the first treatment doctors prescribe. These diuretics stimulate the kidneys to flush excess salt and water from the circulation, lowering blood volume and relieving the heart. They can reduce the risk of stroke by as much as 40 percent and of heart attack by as much as 14 percent. You'll spend a lot of time in the bathroom and may have to take a potassium supplement in order to prevent muscle weakness and a calcium/magnesium supplement to protect your bones, but it's worth it. Just make sure that your doctor monitors your blood sugar and cholesterol levels—if they begin to rise, you may need to try a different treatment.

BETA-BLOCKERS. Drugs like Inderal and Tenormin reduce nerve impulses to the heart, slowing and relaxing it so that it pumps less strongly, thereby lowering blood pressure and helping prevent chest pain and heart arrhythmias. You have to watch out that these drugs don't slow your pulse down too much—they also can cause weakness and insomnia. Beta-blockers should be used with caution in older people and in people with lung disease or diabetes. They are an excellent choice for women in their perimenopausal years or for anyone who has already had a heart attack.

"Can I tell you something?" she asked, looking up at me with tears in her eyes. "I really don't care. Sometimes I think I'd rather be dead than live with this humiliation."

"Then divorce the creep."

"I just don't have the energy. Isn't that pathetic?"

"Honey, you're depressed. I'm giving you the name of a psychiatrist. When you leave this room, go to the reception desk and have Joanie make you an appointment." I was afraid that if I sent her home with the number she'd never call. "I'm not a shrink, but I have a feeling you could use an antidepressant. Then, once you feel up to it, I want you on a strict diet and doing some exercise."

"Dr. Corio, sometimes I think you're the only one who really cares what happens to me."

CALCIUM CHANNEL BLOCKERS. Muscle cells need calcium in order to contract. By preventing calcium from entering the smooth muscle cells of the heart and arteries, drugs such as verapamil (Cordilox and Securon) and diltiazem (Cardizem and Verelan) keep the heart and blood vessel walls relaxed. They also can relieve chest pain and abnormal heart rhythms, and they may lower the heartbeat. Unfortunately, calcium channel blockers can affect muscle cells elsewhere in your body, leading to fatigue, constipation, and swollen legs or ankles.

ACE (ANGIOTENSIN CONVERTING ENZYME) INHIBITORS. Angiotensin is a protein that constricts blood vessels. By inhibiting the formation of angiotensin, drugs such as enalapril (Innovace) and lisinopril (Zestril) relax the blood vessels. One peculiar side effect that affects women twice as much as men is a dry cough. Other side effects include a rash, weakness, and reduced kidney function. ACE inhibitors are the drug of choice for diabetics or those with congestive heart failure. They cannot be taken by women who are considering pregnancy or are already pregnant.

ANGIOTENSIN BLOCKERS. Vasodilators such as losartan (Cozaar) directly block the effect of angiotensin on blood vessels. They do not cause a dry cough like the ACE inhibitors do.

"I do care," I said. "But you should, too." We talked some more and then I told her to jog over and see me again in one month for a blood pressure check. "If it continues to go up, you may need medication."

Certain medications, including steroids, nasal decongestants, and bronchodilators, can also cause high blood pressure. Also, be careful about combining drugs and herbs, or more than one herb. Taking ginseng and Saint John's wort together, for example, can raise your blood pressure. *Be sure to tell your doctor about any medications—prescription or over-the-counter—and/or supplements you are taking.*

Controlling hypertension is crucial for maintaining heart health—lowering the top number of your blood pressure just 10 mm mercury or lowering the bottom number just 5 mm mercury reduces your risk of dying of heart disease by 28 percent! For mild cases in patients with no other risk factors, diet and exercise are the first line of defense. In addition to keeping your sodium intake below 1,200 mg daily, make sure you are getting at least 1,200 mg calcium and 600 mg magnesium a day. Stop smoking, reduce your alcohol intake, keep your weight under control, and try to manage your stress. If after one month there is no improvement or if other risk factors are present, however, medication is warranted.

Even though there are 65 different drugs and 29 combination pills available to treat hypertension, the most common ones either relax blood vessels or decrease blood volume. The key to having your medication work is that you have to take it *every day*. This may seem like a simple prescription, but only one out of three people follow it. Part of the problem has to do with the side effects some of the drugs can cause, such as headaches, palpitations, frequent urination, dizziness, rash, lowered sex drive, or an annoying cough. Unfortunately, many doctors fail to tell their patients to hang in there—side effects usually go away within four to six weeks. And if they don't, your doctor can change your dosage or have you try a different drug. The important thing is, *don't just stop taking your pills if you have side effects; discuss them with your doctor.*

DIABETES. Women with diabetes have as much as seven times the risk of heart disease and double the risk of heart attack as women without diabetes. This is far greater an increase than men with diabetes have over their nondiabetic counterparts. The difference is that hyperinsulinemia, or non–insulin-dependent diabetes, which is the eventual outcome of insulin resistance, affects serum cholesterol and blood pressure in ways that are particularly harmful to women.

Excess insulin causes sugar to be stored as fat, particularly in the abdominal region, which is a risk factor in and of itself for women. It also prevents the burning of fat as energy, making it difficult to keep your weight down. Most important, it stimulates the liver to produce LDL cholesterol and triglycerides, and it depresses HDL cholesterol—a dangerous combination of events for women. Finally, insulin also raises blood pressure by stimulating plaque formation and causing arterial smooth muscle cells to proliferate, therefore narrowing blood vessels.

HYPERLIPIDEMIA (A FANCY TERM FOR HIGH CHOLESTEROL). Cholesterol is a type of fat found naturally in the body that is needed

CALLING ALL CHOCOHOLICS!

Believe it or not, chocolate is relatively benign—and may even be beneficial— when it comes to your arteries. Stearic acid, the main fat found in chocolate, does not raise LDL cholesterol and may even lower it. Plus, a 1.5 ounce morsel of dark chocolate has as much of the heart-protecting antioxidant phenol as a glass of red wine and *four times* the amount of catechins (other antioxidants) as black tea! Like aspirin, chocolate reduces the activity of platelets that contribute to blood clotting and arterial plaque formation. Of course, that doesn't mean you should celebrate by gulping down a pound of dark chocolate. Any type of chocolate is full of sugar, which raises your insulin levels and packs on the pounds. But if you're desperate for a sweet fix, choose a variety of dark chocolate (which contains more cocoa than milk chocolate, and cocoa is particularly high in stearic acid) rather than a jam doughnut.

to build cell walls and make certain hormones, including the sex hormones. In excess, this waxy substance can build up on the interior walls of the blood vessels, raising your blood pressure and putting you at risk for a heart attack.

On page 215 I've included a table showing normal, borderline, and high-risk levels of total cholesterol, LDL, HDL, and triglycerides. If any of your lipid levels is in the borderline range and you have other risk factors such as high blood pressure, smoking, a family history of heart disease, diabetes, or obesity, you are actually considered high risk.

Although "high cholesterol" is generally not good for your health, there's one number that actually should be high, especially for women: the HDL cholesterol level. Women with HDL cholesterol levels lower than 46 mg/dL have six times the risk of heart disease as women whose HDL cholesterol levels are higher than 67 mg/dL. Every increase of 10 mg/dL of HDL cholesterol in women decreases the risk of heart disease by 50 percent. In contrast, LDL cholesterol ideally should be low, as every decrease of 11 percent of LDL cholesterol reduces the risk of heart disease by 19 percent.

When a patient's blood test shows high LDL cholesterol, the first thing I do is ask a few questions to rule out any other possible cause. Diabetes, hypothyroidism, kidney disease, liver disease, and drugs such as corticosteroids, anabolic steroids, and certain antihypertensives can all cause elevated LDL cholesterol. If none of these factors is present, we then have a serious talk about diet and exercise.

VEGGIE STIR-FRY, ANYONE?

Here's a great recipe for a heart-healthy dish. Stir-fry some onions, garlic, and ginger in a little olive oil. Then add heaps of your favorite high-fiber veggies and, if you like, a little tofu or tempeh. Flavor with some low-sodium soy sauce, then spoon the whole works over brown rice.

What's the magic in this meal? Olive oil is full of "good" monounsaturated fat that will not break down upon heating, as will its polyunsaturated cousins such as peanut, safflower, sunflower, corn, soy, and cottonseed oils. Garlic, onions, and ginger have been proven to reduce cholesterol. Brown rice is a great source of fiber, which helps flush cholesterol out of your system, as are vegetables, which also contain antioxidants that prevent-plaque buildup in your arteries. And tofu and tempeh all contain cholesterol-lowering phytoestrogens and antioxidant flavonoids that protect your arteries.

Gail, my office manager for twenty-five years, is a poster child for successful non-drug cholesterol management. Last September I ran a routine blood test on her and was shocked when the results came back: her total cholesterol was 274 mg/dL, her triglycerides were 210 mg/dL, and while her HDL cholesterol was a respectable 45 mg/dL, her LDL cholesterol was a whopping 187 mg/dL. Her weight had also gone up to 160 pounds—far too high for her five feet, three inches. "Gail, this is terrible," I said to her. "It's like you're standing in front of a freight train marked 'Heart Attack.' We've got to do something about this." I immediately put her on a high-protein, moderate-carb, low-fat diet and prescribed thirty minutes of aerobic exercise at least three times a week. Seeing as she works in my office, it was easy to keep an eye on her and encourage her when her willpower flagged.

Two months later we ran another blood test. Her total cholesterol had gone down *thirty-six points* to 238 mg/dL. Her LDL cholesterol was down to 156 mg/dL, and her triglycerides had plummeted to 73 mg/dL. Her HDL cholesterol had jumped up to 67 mg/dL. And best of all, she'd lost 15 pounds! "Way to go, Gail," I congratulated her, giving her a high-five. "You've now significantly lowered your risk."

"Thank goodness," she replied. "You had me scared to death."

MEDICAL TREATMENTS FOR HIGH CHOLESTEROL

If diet and exercise aren't sufficient to bring down your cholesterol levels, drugs may be warranted.

HMG CoA REDUCTASE INHIBITORS (STATINS). A new and very popular type of drug, statins are the first choice for lowering LDL cholesterol. Drugs such as cerivastatin (Lipobay), pravastatin (Lipostat), simvastatin (Zocor), and atorvastatin (Lipitor) inhibit HMG CoA reductase, a key enzyme in cholesterol production. One study found that statins reduced LDL cholesterol levels by 25 percent and triglycerides by 15 percent, and raised HDL cholesterol by 6 percent, decreasing the risk of a heart attack by 36 percent overall. Statins can also decrease your risk of stroke and reduce your risk of venus thrombosis (blood clots) by 50 percent.

BILE ACID SEQUESTRANT DRUGS. These types of drugs, such as cholestyramine, facilitate cholesterol's excretion along with bile acid through the intestine. They also stimulate the liver to produce new LDL receptors to remove LDL cholesterol from the bloodstream. Primarily used to lower LDL cholesterol levels and raise HDL cholesterol levels, they may raise triglyceride levels as well.

NICOTINIC ACID (NIACIN). This water-soluble B vitamin prevents fatty acids from reaching the liver, therefore decreasing the amount of triglycerides the liver produces. It also lowers LDL cholesterol levels and raises HDL cholesterol levels, making it the drug of choice when your HDL levels are low. It can cause flushing and stomach pain, but there is now a newer, long-acting form called Niaspan that causes fewer side effects.

FIBRIC ACID DERIVATIVES. Drugs such as gemfibrozil (Lopid) are prescribed mainly to lower triglyceride levels, although they also lower LDL cholesterol levels and raise HDL cholesterol levels. They work by inhibiting the production of cholesterol and bile acids and encouraging the secretion of cholesterol in bile through the intestine. Do not take these if you have a history of gallbladder disease.

NUTS FOR NUTS

Need a nosh? Grab a handful of nuts. In the United States, the Harvard University Nurses' Health Study found that women who ate a little more than 5 ounces of nuts a week had one-third fewer heart attacks than those who rarely or never ate nuts. Why? Nuts are cholesterol-free and full of "good" monounsaturated fat that lowers the levels of harmful LDL cholesterol and triglycerides. Nuts contain powerful antioxidants including vitamin E. They also contain folic acid, which lowers the blood levels of homocysteine. Furthermore, nuts lower the blood pressure by increasing your nitric oxide and relaxing your blood vessels. Be careful not to overdo it, though, as nuts are a high-calorie snack food. Also, avoid salted nuts, as salt raises blood pressure.

"*You* had *me* scared to death!" (P.S. Gail continued to stay on her diet and over the next six months lost another 20 pounds. She now looks and feels terrific.)

ELEVATED HOMOCYSTEINE. Recently a new awareness has developed of the link between elevated circulating levels of homocysteine and cardiovascular disease. Homocysteine is a result of the incomplete metabolism of methionine, an amino acid found in animal protein. It scrapes arterial walls and then combines with LDL cholesterol to form plaques on the damaged surfaces and promotes blood clotting. High homocysteine can be as dangerous as high cholesterol: a rise of only 5 micromoles per liter of blood plasma can raise your risk of heart disease as much as a 20 mg rise in cholesterol. To keep homocysteine in check, lower your intake of animal protein and saturated fat. Also, eat foods rich in folate, such as legumes, dark green leafy vegetables, oranges, and orange juice; and consider taking B_6, B_{12}, and folic acid supplements, as these vitamins are necessary for the completion of methionine metabolism.

ELEVATED C-REACTIVE PROTEIN. It has just hit the news that a recently identified molecule called C-reactive protein may be a more accurate indicator of heart disease than cholesterol levels in healthy men and women. C-reactive protein triggers the inflammation response that stimulates plaque formation in coronary arteries. A simple and inexpensive blood test can predict your risk of a heart attack up to ten years in advance.

ELEVATED FIBRINOGEN AND LIPOPROTEIN (A). Fibrinogen is a protein found in the blood that promotes clotting and increases plasma viscosity, contributing to plaque buildup. One of the many ways in which oestrogen maintains your heart health is by keeping your fibrinogen levels down. It does so by means of an intermediary known as lipoprotein (a), or Lp(a), which inhibits fibrinogen breakdown and is itself an independent risk factor for atherosclerosis in women. As long as your oestrogen levels are high, your Lp(a) and fibrinogen levels will be low. But when your oestrogen levels decline in perimenopause, your Lp(a) levels will rise and so, consequently, will your plasma fibrinogen. Other factors that increase plasma fibrinogen are age, smoking, and body mass index.

Know Your ABC's

The American College of Obstetricians and Gynecologists has come up with a nifty list they call the "ABC's" of common symptoms of heart attack in women. If you are experiencing *any one* of these, see a doctor immediately:

Angina (or chest pain)—back pain or deep aching and throbbing in the left or right bicep or forearm

Breathlessness—or waking up having difficulty catching your breath

Clammy perspiration

Dizziness—unexplained lightheadedness, even blackouts

Oedema—swelling, particularly of the ankles and/or lower legs

Fluttering (or rapid) heartbeat

Gastric upset (or nausea)

Heavy fullness—or pressure-like chest pain between breasts and radiating to left arm or shoulder

SYMPTOMS OF A STROKE

Even though the *risk factors* for a heart attack and a stroke are similar, the *symptoms* are not. If you experience any of the following, call your doctor or 999 immediately:

- sudden loss of feeling or weakness in your face, an arm or a leg, or on one whole side of your body
- sudden loss or dimming of vision, especially in one eye
- difficulty talking or understanding speech
- out-of-the-blue severe headache with no obvious cause
- lightheadedness, unsteadiness, dizziness, or a sudden fall
- TIAs (transient ischemic attacks) or fleeting strokelike symptoms, including muscle weakness on one side, impaired vision in one eye, or slurred speech

HOW DO I KNOW IF I'M HAVING A HEART ATTACK?

Many women have memorized the signs of a heart attack so they will know if their husband is having one. Unfortunately, they could very well miss their own. Why? Because the symptoms of heart attack may be different for men than for women. For example, although heart pain, or angina, is the most frequent initial complaint for both sexes, men tend to experience it brought on by physical exertion (typical angina), whereas women are more likely to experience it at rest (atypical or unstable angina).

In general, women's symptoms tend to be more subtle than men's, and as a result they tend to be taken less seriously by doctors and by women themselves. Indeed, approximately 35 percent of heart attacks in women go unnoticed or unreported. Even if a woman does recognize her symptoms and seek medical attention, the diagnostic tests her doctor will most likely use—such as the treadmill stress test—are not as accurate in women as they are in men.

It is interesting that studies of women under age 65 who've had heart attacks have shown that they have less narrowing of the coronary arteries than do older women or men. Although most premenopausal heart attacks are caused by blood clots, a certain amount are caused by spasming of the coronary arteries, a condition that may be genetic.

Just as fluctuating oestrogen levels can cause blood vessels in your brain to spasm, leading to migraine headaches (see Chapter 4), the waxing and waning of your hormones can also cause your coronary blood vessels to spasm. The spasm can reduce blood flow to the heart muscle, causing a heart attack directly without any of the classic symptoms seen with atherosclerosis. In these cases coronary angiography, the gold-standard for detecting clogged arteries, would not be of any help in predicting a heart attack, as it would in older women and in men.

If you do feel any symptom of a heart attack, call 999 and *swallow a crushed or chewed aspirin with a glass of water as soon as possible*. Aspirin can prevent the formation of additional blood clots, giving you extra time to get to the emergency room.

Unfortunately, 45 percent of women who die of sudden heart attacks have no symptoms at all. That's why it's critical to do everything in your power to try to keep your heart in shape.

INGREDIENTS FOR A HEALTHY HEART

Your heart works hard. If your resting pulse is 70 beats per minute, your heart beats at least 100,800 times a day, 36,792,000 times a year. By the time you reach age 55, we're talking more than two trillion contractions! To keep up this relentless pace, your heart needs the energy that comes from a well-balanced diet. In addition, certain vitamins and minerals are critical for maintaining the health of your blood and blood vessels. Phytoestrogens, herbs, and hormones can also greatly benefit your cardiovascular system.

Vitamins and Minerals

VITAMIN B_6, VITAMIN B_{12}, AND FOLIC ACID. As discussed previously, adequate levels of vitamins B_6 and B_{12} and folic acid help keep homocysteine under control, thus protecting your arteries. Make sure you get 400 mcg folic acid, 50 to 100 mg vitamin B_6, and 50 to 100 mcg vitamin B_{12} daily, either through your diet or from a supplement.

VITAMIN C. Vitamin C is great for the heart. First, it relaxes blood vessels, thereby reducing angina pain and lowering the risk of heart attack and stroke. Second, it is a powerful antioxidant, meaning that it mops up the free radicals that can oxidize molecules such as LDL cholesterol. In its oxidized form, LDL cholesterol sticks to the walls of blood vessels, forming atherosclerotic plaques. And third, vitamin C reduces blood pressure—one study found that taking 500 mg vitamin C a day reduced the blood pressure of 45 people with hypertension by an average of 9 percent. So the more vitamin C the merrier, right?

Wrong. As with so much in life, you can have too much of a good thing. Megadoses such as those promoted by the dearly departed Nobel laureate Linus Pauling have not been proven to have any health advantage and can even cause problems. Excess vitamin C is excreted in the urine. Doses over 1,000 mg can contribute to kidney stones and may interact adversely with high levels of iron. They can also cause gas and diarrhoea.

So what's the optimal dose? I tell my patients to get between 500 and 1,000 mg a day, preferably through diet, although supplements are okay if necessary. While the recommended daily allowance of 60 mg saturates your blood by 72 percent, that's only enough to prevent scurvy. To saturate your blood by 86 percent, you need 200 mg—about two 8-ounce glasses of orange juice. Doubling that brings your saturation level up five percentage points, to 91 percent. Full saturation occurs at 1,000 mg. Basically, if you eat five or more servings of fruit or vegetables a day, that's plenty to protect your heart and lower your risk of stroke. A study of 2,400 Finnish women showed that only half as many of those who consumed at least 90 mg a day died of heart disease as those who consumed 60 mg a day or less.

For optimal absorption take a 500 mg tablet of ester vitamin C, the mineral salt of ascorbic acid, twice a day. If you take more than 500 mg at a time, the excess will go out in your urine.

NATURAL VITAMIN E. Also an antioxidant, natural vitamin E can counter LDL cholesterol oxidation if taken in a daily dose of 400 to 800 IU—an amount virtually impossible to attain through diet alone. It can also protect against stroke and heart attack by inhibiting clotting, especially if taken in conjunction with a daily aspirin. Indeed, the World Health Organization found that low levels of vitamin E were a stronger predictor of heart disease than high cholesterol was. Studies in America by researchers at both Boston's Brigham & Women's

Hospital and the Harvard School of Public Health confirmed that a daily supplement can reduce the risk of heart disease by 25 to 50 percent.

I always recommend natural vitamin E, derived from soy and other plant products, as it is far more bioactive than the synthetic. Look for the *d*-alpha-tocopherol, not the *dl*. People who have bleeding problems or hypertension should not take vitamin E supplements, however, as it can raise blood pressure and interfere with clotting.

MIXED CAROTENES. The combination of alpha, beta, and other carotene supplements may reduce your risk of heart disease. Taking mixed carotenes is a more natural approach than taking each one and/or vitamin A (which mixed carotenes are broken down into) individually. An optimal dose is 3 to 6 mg daily, which can be attained through a well-balanced diet if you eat five servings of fruit and vegetables daily. Unfortunately, most of us don't get the recommended daily amount from their diet and therefore need to take supplements.

CALCIUM. Without adequate calcium, muscles tend to cramp up. This applies equally to the muscles of your calves and the muscles in your arterial walls. The recent federally financed DASH (Dietary Approaches to Stop Hypertension) study in the United States found that raising calcium levels was even more beneficial to lowering blood pressure than was reducing salt intake. It also decreases the risk of stroke. We women need at least 1,200 mg calcium per day (1,500 mg if we're pregnant or over age 50 and not on oestrogen replacement therapy), not only to maintain vascular flexibility and avert hypertension but also to maintain our bones (see Chapter 8).

MAGNESIUM. Magnesium deficiency has been linked to hardening of the arteries, hypertension, and angina pain. Because magnesium prevents calcium from crystallizing abnormally and causing kidney stones, it ought to be taken along with calcium in a combination calcium/magnesium supplement, with a calcium-to-magnesium ratio of 2:1. Therefore, if you're taking 1,200 mg calcium, you should also be taking 600 mg magnesium. If you're taking a diuretic, it's especially important to take a magnesium supplement (unless your diuretic is designed not to deplete magnesium), as magnesium is also needed to promote absorption and use of other minerals, to metabolize proteins, and to activate essential enzymes.

An Aspirin a Day . . .

In addition to eating an apple a day (a great source of cholesterol-lowering fiber), women over age 50 with one or more cardiovascular risk factors should take an aspirin a day to ward off heart attack and stroke. The recommendation applies to anyone with diabetes, hypertension, or elevated LDL cholesterol, as well as to smokers or those who don't exercise—*unless* they have contraindications, such as bleeding disorders or gastric ulcers. Your doctor will suggest an optimal dose, anywhere from 80 to 325 mg daily, but generally a simple baby aspirin (75 mg) a day is sufficient. *Do not begin this treatment without consulting your physician!*

Late-breaking news from the Baylor Medical School in Texas suggests that Paracetamol may also have a beneficial effect on the heart, reducing fatty streaks that can clog the arteries. But don't start taking Paracetamol just yet—studies thus far have only been performed on rabbits.

POTASSIUM. Bananas, oranges, tomatoes, and cantaloupes are all rich sources of potassium, a mineral essential to keeping blood pressure in check. One reason why those of African origin may have a higher rate of hypertension than Caucasians may be because their diet is generally deficient in potassium. Unless you are on certain diuretics, you don't need to take a supplement; just make sure to get enough in your diet.

COENZYME Q10. CoQ10 is a fatty, vitamin-like substance needed by mitochondria, the small intracellular bodies that generate the energy required for cells' activity. The highest concentrations of CoQ10 are in the heart muscle. Doses of 90 mg to 150 mg have been shown to increase the heart's efficiency and decrease resistance to blood flow in peripheral arteries. Patients with angina who took daily doses of 150 mg for four weeks had half as many attacks as those who didn't. I recommend a 50 mg daily CoQ10 supplement or 100 mg daily if you are at risk for heart disease. If you're taking nicotinic acid or a statin drug, discuss CoQ10 supplements with your doctor, as those medications tend to lower your CoQ10 levels.

NIACIN. A member of the vitamin B family, niacin can be taken as a supplement to help lower cholesterol (see page 227). The problem is that in high enough doses to lower cholesterol, niacin can cause annoying flushing. For that reason, the recommended form is a special type of niacin called inositol hexaniacinate (IHN) or "no-flush" niacin. If you have high cholesterol, take 500 mg three times a day.

Phytoestrogens

Foods—not supplements—that contain phytoestrogens have been shown to improve cardiovascular health.

SOY. Rich in isoflavones, soy reduces LDL cholesterol by affecting its synthesis and metabolism in the liver. Consuming 25 g of soy protein a day can lower your total cholesterol by 10 percent, your LDL cholesterol by 13 percent, and your trigylcerides by 11 percent; it also slightly raises HDL cholesterol levels. Genistein, another phytoestrogen found in soy, may prevent clot formation by inhibiting platelet aggregation. It also seems to dilate blood vessels, thereby reducing the risk of heart attack and stroke and relieving angina pain. As if that weren't enough, soy may also prove to be a means by which to lower levels of lipoprotein (a), an independent risk factor for heart disease in women.

FLAXSEED. Rich in lignans, flaxseed also should be part of a healthy heart diet. Eating 50 g of flaxseed daily has been shown to lower LDL cholesterol levels by 8 percent. Eating 1 to 2 teaspoons of flaxseed oil a day also has beneficial cardiovascular effects. It's easy to add ground flaxseed and flaxseed oil to your diet—sprinkle some powder on your cereal, into batter, or into a shake, or use the oil to make salad dressing.

Herbs

HAWTHORN. An excellent heart herb, hawthorn contains numerous flavonoids, or natural antioxidants, that prevent LDL cholesterol from building up on artery walls. It also acts as a natural ACE inhibitor (see page 223), keeping blood vessels dilated and flexible and improving blood flow to the heart. The recommended dose is 100 to 250 mg three times a day. Hawthorn may increase the effects of other heart medications, so make sure to check with your doctor before taking it.

CHINESE RED-YEAST-RICE. Also called Cholesterin, this herb has been getting a lot of press recently. It's a natural product that contains the same cholesterol-lowering compounds as synthetic statin drugs. Because it is classified as a dietary supplement and not a drug, however, it is not subject to regulation or quality control, which has a lot of us in the medical community worried. Like statin drugs, it can have harmful side effects such as liver and muscle damage if not taken in controlled doses under medical supervision. *I urge you not to explore this option without first consulting your healthcare provider.*

Foods

Like flaxseed, oily fish, which also contain omega-3 fatty acids, are extremely good for your heart. They decrease platelet aggregation (thereby reducing blood clots), prevent arrhythmias, and lower triglyceride levels. Dark-fleshed fish, such as salmon, tuna, sardines, mackerel, bluefish, and pompano, are much higher in omega-3 fatty acids than are white-fleshed fish.

Sautéing that fish in a little garlic will make it even more heart-healthy. Garlic lowers blood pressure, reduces blood clots, and lowers cholesterol levels. But if you are on bloodthinners, don't overdose on garlic or omega-3 fatty acids or take supplements of either, as they can cause bleeding problems.

Hormones

I've been in favor of using hormone supplements to treat perimenopausal and menopausal discomforts for years. But it wasn't until I began reading up on the vast benefits oestrogen provides to the cardiovascular system that I decided that perimenopausal women should not be denied this great opportunity. Questions still remain, however. What type of oestrogen works best? Do progestogens diminish oestrogen's effect? How about designer oestrogens—synthetic oestrogens that affect some parts of the body but not others? Here's some information that I hope will help you make up your own mind.

EFFECTS OF DIFFERENT TYPES OF OESTROGEN ON BLOOD LIPIDS

TYPE OF OESTROGEN	TOTAL CHOLESTEROL	LDL	HDL	TRIGLYCERIDES
ORAL	↓↓	↓↓	↑↑	↑
TRANSDERMAL	↓↓	↓	—	↓
PHYTOESTROGEN (25 G SOY PROTEIN)	↓	↓	↑	↓

OESTROGEN. No matter how you slice it, oestrogen does wonders for your cardiovascular health, lowering your risk of heart disease by approximately 50 percent. (Low-dose patches or pills are about half as effective as the standard dose, reducing your risk of cardiovascular disease by 20 to 30 percent.) Oestrogen improves your lipid profile, keeps your blood vessels from hardening, reduces blood clotting, and increases your heart's pumping capacity. But all oestrogens are not created equal.

Oral natural oestrogen—oestrogen that is identical to that which the body produces—is the preferred choice for cardiovascular protection over transdermal natural oestrogen, but in certain circumstances a natural patch or gel might work better. This is because oestrogen absorbed through the skin does not pass through the liver and therefore does not influence cholesterol metabolism as much as oestrogen absorbed through the intestine. Before deciding which type of oestrogen to go on, it is important to know your blood lipid profile so you can make the best choice.

In a randomized controlled study done in Milan, Italy, 120 women were given either a 0.05 mg/day patch or 0.625 mg daily oestrogen supplement. Though both lowered total cholesterol and LDL cholesterol, the patch did not lower LDL cholesterol as much as the oral oestrogen did. Also, oral oestrogen raised HDL cholesterol levels, whereas the patch lowered them slightly. Because high HDL cholesterol is the best indicator of protection from heart disease in women, this difference is significant.

My recommendation for lowering cardiovascular risk is oral natural oestrogen—oral because it raises HDL cholesterol, and natural

BUT I READ SOMEWHERE THAT
HORMONES WERE BAD FOR YOUR HEART . . .

There's been a lot of talk recently about the Heart and Oestrogen/Progesto-gen Replacement Study, which found that synthetic hormone replacement therapy (HRT) increased the risk of blood clotting in some women. The fine print to note here is the word "synthetic." This large study looked at 2,763 postmenopausal women with established heart disease and found that nearly three times as many on synthetic hormone therapy suffered blood clots as those on a placebo (34 versus 12). In the first year, those on synthetic hormones suffered more coronary events, but by years 4 and 5 they suffered fewer. These studies were not done on natural hormones and they did not make clear whether the synthetic oestrogen or progestogen was the culprit.

The recommendation that has come out of this study is that synthetic hormone replacement should not be given to patients with coronary artery disease. But if someone with heart disease is already on HRT, they should stay on it rather than quit, in order to reap the benefits of long-term use.

This is still a controversial issue. The final decision as to whether or not a patient with heart disease should take oestrogen replacement therapy should be made on a case-by-case basis in consultation with both her gynaecologist and her cardiologist, and take into consideration the option of taking natural rather than synthetic hormones.

because the natural preparation will exactly replace what your body is losing and provide identical protection to what you've been enjoying up till now. However, if you have elevated triglyerides, using an oestro-gen patch may be preferable, especially if your HDL levels are good. Adding testosterone to your oestrogen will lower your triglycerides. It will also lower your HDL cholesterol, but not to dangerous levels. Birth control pills may reduce the risk of stroke and heart attack. Specifically, the new third-generation pills such as Cilest, Marvelon, and Femodene have been shown to lower cholesterol levels.

PROGESTOGENS. Here there's a big difference between synthetic progestogens and natural progesterone. The progestogen medroxy-progesterone (Provera) negates the positive effects of oestrogen on the cardiovascular system. Women who take pure oestrogen or oestrogen and natural progesterone experience numerous benefits, including dilated blood vessels and reduced plaque formation. Women taking oestrogen and Provera do not show any of these improvements—it's as if they aren't taking anything at all.

Across the board I recommend natural progesterone over Provera, not only because of the cardiovascular advantage but also because of Provera's side effects, which include bloating, weight gain, and mood swings.

RALOXIFENE. One of the new selective oestrogen receptor modulators (SERMs), raloxifene (Evista) has been proven to have some cardiovascular benefits, but not nearly as much as oestrogen. Both lower total and LDL cholesterol, but raloxifene has no effect on HDL cholesterol, whereas oestrogen raises it. And as you now know, raising HDL cholesterol is the most important way to protect your arteries.

Evista has been approved only for postmenopausal prevention and treatment of osteoporosis; research is currently under way to determine its cardiovascular benefits. Because of its tendency to cause hot flushes, I don't recommend it to my perimenopausal patients.

Do's and Don'ts for Maintaining a Healthy Heart

Now that you know the risk factors for heart disease, it should be clear that there are certain things you should and shouldn't do to protect yourself from a heart attack or stroke:

Do... aerobic exercise for at least 30 minutes at least three times a week to raise your HDL cholesterol. Women who walked briskly (a 20-minute-mile or faster) for a minimum of three hours a week or exercised vigorously for at least 90 minutes a week have been shown to have a 30 to 40 percent reduction in their risk of heart disease. (See Chapter 13 for more details on exercise.)

have your blood pressure checked annually, your lipid profile checked every five years or more often if it's abnormal, and if you're on medication, take it as directed.

eat a low-fat, low-cholesterol diet. If you must eat fats, make sure they're unsaturated, such as olive, canola, sesame, peanut, and walnut oils; avocados; and nuts.

increase your intake of soluble fiber to between 20 and 35 g a day. Fiber aids the excretion of cholesterol, reduces blood pressure, helps you keep weight off, lowers your insulin levels, and wards off blood clots. A daily half-cup serving of bran cereal containing 5 g of fiber is associated with a 37 percent decrease in risk of heart disease and can lower your cholesterol level by 8 points.

enjoy fish at least three times a week, as the omega-3 fatty acids in fish, especially oily fish like salmon, lower triglyceride levels and reduce the risk of atherosclerosis.

drink one—and only one—glass of red wine or purple grape juice a day. The skins of red grapes contain (1) resveratrol, a compound that reduces cholesterol in the body and helps prevent blood clots and hardening of the arteries, and (2) quercitin, which dilates blood vessels and breaks up clots.

incorporate soy protein into your diet—consuming 15 to 30 g soy protein daily for four weeks can lower high total cholesterol, LDL cholesterol, and triglycerides by 10 to 20 percent.

Do...   experiment with flaxseed, either by cooking with flaxseed oil or by sprinkling ground flaxseed onto cereal or yogurt, or adding it to pancake batter or bread dough. Flaxseed contains omega-3 fatty acids as well as cancer-fighting substances called lignans.

consume at least five to seven servings a day of fruits and veggies— they're full of fiber, antioxidants, and phytochemicals that make your heart sing.

Don't...   smoke—ever again.

mess around with cocaine or marijuana. Within the first hour after taking the drug, cocaine users have *24 times* the rate of heart attacks of the general population. Cocaine increases the number of red blood cells, causing blood to thicken, and increases amounts of a protein that promotes platelet aggregation, causing blood to clot. Marijuana increases a middle-aged person's risk of heart attack five times within the first hour of use. Smoking marijuana raises the heart rate by about 40 beats per minute, elevating blood pressure and therefore damaging the lining of the blood vessels and setting the stage for clot formation.

overindulge in sugar and refined carbohydrates, as they can lead to insulin resistance.

eat too much salt, as it can raise your blood pressure.

consume excessive amounts of animal fat, so that you keep your homocysteine levels down.

let your weight get out of control: you should aim for a body mass index of no greater than 25 (see page 350). Losing just 10 pounds can lower your serum cholesterol by as many as 30 points.

ride the elevator if you can take the stairs; drive if you can walk or bike; drag your heels if you can pick up the pace.

ignore symptoms that could indicate a heart attack (see page 229).

sit home alone and vegetate. An active life and an active social life are both good for your health.

CHAPTER 10

Bosom Buddies:
Your Breasts

Day after day I'm struck and saddened by how many of my patients are living in mortal terror of breast cancer. They lie on the examination table with stricken looks on their faces as I palpate their breasts, holding their breath until they hear me say, "Everything feels perfectly normal."

Why is there all this anxiety in the air? Part of the reason is that everywhere we turn, it seems, someone in the news or someone in our lives is being diagnosed with breast cancer. After having been "outed" as a disease in the late 1970s, breast cancer has gotten a lot of press and breast cancer research has benefited from many fundraising efforts. Practically each week there's an announcement of some new finding related to risk or treatment of the disease. It's the perfect example of how women have successfully made the personal political.

All the publicity about breast cancer has done wonders to heighten awareness, promote mammography, identify genes that predispose women to the disease, and put on the fast track approvals for drugs that can treat and may even prevent breast cancer. But it has also made a lot of women paranoid. Every day at least one patient brings up the statistic that one in nine women gets breast cancer. "That number represents *lifetime risk*—if you live past age 85," I explain. "At age 45, only 1 in 93 are afflicted. I want you to take all this energy you're wasting worrying about breast cancer and use it to eat well, exercise, and enjoy life."

That's not to say that breast cancer isn't a devastating disease for the

ODDS OF DEVELOPING BREAST CANCER BY AGE

By age 25 .... 1 in 15,000

By age 30 .... 1 in 1,900

By age 40 .... 1 in 200

By age 60 .... 1 in 23

By age 70 .... 1 in 15

By age 80 .... 1 in 11

By age 85 .... 1 in 10

Lifetime .... 1 in 9

many women who contract it each year (38,000 in the UK in 1997). But it is more so psychologically than physically. For one thing, I think that women's fear and anxiety about breast cancer treatment is worse than the actual procedure. Although chemotherapy is a challenge, most of my patients report back to me that breast surgery and radiotherapy are not as bad as they feared.

For another, while it's true that breast cancer risk for women rises with age, it is not nearly as deadly a disease as most women think. A full 97 percent of women diagnosed with localized breast cancer survive at least five years—up from 72 percent in the 1940s—and most of them will not have any recurrence in their lifetime. Even if the cancer spreads to the surrounding tissue, the five-year survival rate is still 76 percent. Including cases detected in the advanced stage, 65 percent of women with breast cancer will survive ten years and 56 percent will survive fifteen years.

Yet the damage breast disease wreaks on our sense of security and femininity can be severe and longlasting. Not only do we live in a society obsessed with the female breast as a sex object, but we are also biologically programmed to reverence our breasts as symbols of our power to nurture our children. We tend to identify so closely with our breasts that when something happens to them, it cuts to the core of who we envision ourselves to be.

The fact of the matter is, however, that breast cancer is by far *not* the biggest threat to women's lives. In the race to put us six feet under, heart disease leaves breast cancer in the dust. By age 50, only 1 in 50 women in the United States will have been diagnosed with breast cancer, whereas 1 in 2 will have heart disease. And as far as cancers are concerned, in 1987 lung cancer pulled into the lead as the primary cause of cancer death among women and now kills twice as many women each year as breast cancer does. But fewer women worry about lung cancer and heart disease. The difference is, when you look in the mirror each day your breasts are right there in front of you. By contrast, you don't see your lungs or your heart, so you don't worry about them as much, even though they're more likely to do you in.

None of this is to say that we should ignore breast cancer. Rather, we should focus rational attention on it and not become victims of irrational fears. And the time to begin paying attention is now, in our perimenopausal years. So make yourself a cup of tea, get your glasses, and put your feet up on the couch, because I'm going to tell you how you can help protect yourself against breast cancer and, should you have a suspicious finding, make informed choices about dealing with it.

MEET YOUR BREASTS

Remember what a big deal it was to develop breasts? How we teased but secretly envied the girls who got them early? How we begged our mothers to let us graduate from undershirts? How we complained but often really enjoyed when boys snapped our bras?

Breasts play a large role in our sense of ourselves as women. But most women are surprisingly uninformed about the anatomy of their breasts. Here's a brief overview of what they're all about.

The primary function of female breasts is to produce milk. This takes place in the fifteen to twenty lobes, or milk glands, found within each breast and the numerous lobules found within each lobe. The lobes and lobules are connected to each other and to the nipple by a network of thin tubes called ducts through which milk passes. Fat and connective tissue surround the lobes, and a network of blood vessels

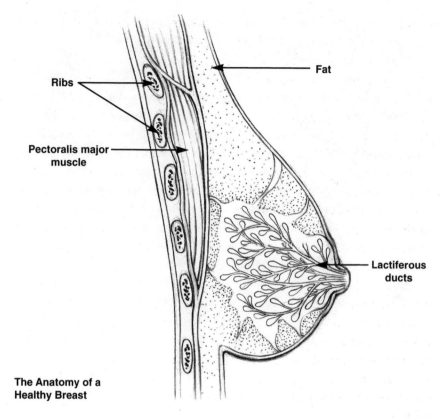

Ribs

Pectoralis major muscle

Fat

Lactiferous ducts

The Anatomy of a Healthy Breast

keeps the cells well oxygenated. The breasts themselves are attached to the pectoral muscles, which overlie the rib cage.

A little bit of breast tissue known as the tail of Spence extends out into the armpit. The armpit is also where a series of lymph nodes is located into which fluid from the breast tissue drains. That's why when you do a breast self-exam, which I'll describe shortly, you should make sure to feel under your arms.

Breasts are hormonally sensitive organs. Oestrogen stimulates the ductal cells of the breast tissue, causing them to proliferate and retain fluid. When babies are born—boys as well as girls—their breasts are a little bit puffy because of all the oestrogen they were exposed to in the womb. Later on, it's the increasing production of oestrogen that makes girls' breasts develop in puberty. Ever wonder why overweight men tend to have breasts? It's because their fat tissue produces oestrogen, which enlarges their breasts.

Other hormones have a similar effect. Progesterone, for example, which is present in high levels in the second half of the menstrual

THE PERIMENOPAUSAL SAG

Patients are often surprised that their bra size goes up as they approach menopause. "In my twenties, all I wanted was to wear a C-cup," sighed Lois, a happily married mother of three. "A lot of good it does me now!" What's happening is that just as your waist is enlarging, your breasts are growing as fat deposits shift up from your hips and buttocks to your chest and abdomen.

Unfortunately, these new C-cup boobs won't look quite the way you envisioned them in your twenties. Rather, they'll be a bit droopy because the collagen fibers that have kept them firm and perky up till now are breaking down as your oestrogen levels decline. And don't believe any of those advertisements for collagen-enriched skin creams that claim they'll restore your breasts to their youthful silhouette. Collagen can't be absorbed through the skin. My prescription? A trip to a department store selling both sexy and supportive bras.

cycle, stimulates glandular breast tissue. That's why your breasts become swollen and sore right before you get your period. Many women on birth control pills find their breasts become tender and enlarged because of the extra oestrogen and progesterone. Progesterone also makes your breasts grow during pregnancy; as does prolactin, the hormone that stimulates milk production.

BUMPS AND LUMPS

In addition to becoming larger under hormonal influences, your breasts may undergo fibrocystic changes in which they become lumpy and sore. These lumps are normal—they're just inflamed tissue or benign fluid-filled cysts. Some women are more prone to developing them than others. Through regular breast self-exam, you should familiarize yourself with how your breasts feel so you know which cysts, bumps, and areas of sensitivity are normal for you.

Fibrocystic changes can affect women at any time of life. Approximately 10 percent of women in the United States have them in adolescence; this rises to 25 percent during the reproductive years and to *at least 50 percent* during perimenopause. Whereas premenopausal women may only experience fibrocystic changes during the week or so before their periods, in perimenopause your breasts may feel lumpy and tender more often than not because your hormones are constantly in flux. I've had patients beg me not to do manual breast exams on them or weep with pain as I've palpated their breasts because they're so sensitive. "I feel as if I'm premenstrual all the time—I have to hold my boobs to my chest whenever I walk down stairs, they hurt so much!" one woman recently complained. "When my husband tries to touch them, I'm like, 'Don't even *think* about it!' "

The symptoms of fibrocystic breasts vary from woman to woman. Some may only experience swelling and increased tenderness in the outer quadrant of their breasts. Others, who are predisposed to cysts, may feel lumps ranging from 3 mm to 3 cm in size. Still others whose fibrocystic changes include thickening of the ducts into which the nipples drain may experience swelling, nodules, or puckering of the skin around the areola and a bloody or greenish-brown discharge from the nipples. Breast pain is also a possibility, as nerve endings in the breast can become irritated when fluid builds up in the tissues.

My patients with fibrocystic breasts are constantly asking me whether their condition predisposes them to breast cancer. I reassure them that study after study has failed to prove any connection. If we have any doubts about a particular lump, however, I send them straight off for a mammogram and ultrasound scan. Draining the fluid from the cyst with a fine needle guided by one of these technologies can provide us with even more information and collapse the cyst, relieving the discomfort.

If your breasts are becoming a pain, here are several things you can do to relieve the discomfort:

- Make sure your bra is giving you adequate support.

- Lower your salt intake.

- Ask your doctor about prescribing a mild diuretic. I recommend taking 25 mg daily of spironolactone (Aldactone) beginning as soon as your breasts feel sore for no more than seven days. It is a potassium-sparing diuretic, so you won't need to take potassium supplements with it.

- Restrict your consumption of caffeine (methylxanthines): coffee and tea (decaffeinated still contains a slight amount of caffeine), cola (diet and regular), and chocolate. A case-controlled study of 1,700 women found that those who consumed 250 mg of caffeine (2½ cups of coffee) a day were 1.5 times more likely to have fibrocystic changes as those who consumed none, and those who consumed 500 mg of caffeine (5 cups of coffee) a day were 2.3 times more likely.

- Take 1,000 to 3,000 mg a day of evening primrose oil—it contains gamma linoleic acid (GLA), an essential fatty acid that decreases inflammation and provides relief within 24 hours.

- Take vitamin E, vitamin B$_6$, and Vitex (chasteberry) supplements.

- If you're in agony, take an over-the-counter pain reliever such as aspirin, ibuprofen, or acetaminophen.

- Consider oral contraceptives. By evening out your hormone levels, birth control pills can provide relief for fibrocystic breasts.

- If you are already on hormone replacement therapy or oral contraceptives, talk with your doctor about switching to a lower dose or different formulation, as the hormones may be the source of your problem.

AND NOW, LET'S TALK ABOUT BREAST CANCER

Fibrocystic and aesthetic changes are the most common things that happen to perimenopausal breasts. Far less common, but far more serious, is breast cancer.

Patients desperate for information about this frightening disease often ask me how breast cancer happens. While we can't answer this question completely at present, a brand-new model suggests that there are three critical windows of vulnerability during the life of your breasts: prenatal, prepubescent, and perimenopausal. If your breasts are assaulted by hormonal or environmental carcinogens during one or more of these windows, your chances of developing breast cancer rise significantly.

According to this theory, breast cancer may start in utero. Long before we have breasts, the cells that are going to become our breast tissue are nourished with a cocktail of proteins, nutrients, and hormones extracted from our mothers' blood. In some pregnant women—overweight women, women who eat a lot of hormone-supplemented food, women who are exposed to environmental hormones—the concentration of oestrogen in that mixture may be especially high.

The primordial breast cells in these women's foetuses become hypersensitized to oestrogen, meaning that when they encounter oestrogen later in life they will overreact, proliferating excessively. Increased proliferation means increased risk of breast cancer, because every time a cell divides there's a chance that a mistake will be made in copying the DNA that may lead to a cancer-causing mutation. The net result is that women whose breast tissue has been sensitized in utero will be especially vulnerable to other risk factors for breast cancer.

Mutations during cell replication occur more frequently when we're exposed to carcinogens, which include pollution, cigarette smoke, and radiation. When your breast cells are most actively proliferating—during the undershirt-to-bra transition—they are particularly vulnerable. If you were exposed to radiation or began smoking during your prepubescent years, you are at a greater risk of developing breast cancer than if you were exposed to the same amount of radiation or began smoking later in life.

The third window of vulnerability is perimenopause. Starting as early as age 30 to 35, when your oestrogen levels begin to wane, your breasts undergo a process called *involution*. The glandular tissue begins to shrink, or atrophy, and is gradually displaced by fat and connective tissue. This protects the breast by reducing the number of lobular and ductal cells at risk of assault by hormonal or environmental agents. Delaying this process or subjecting your breasts to stimulation by getting pregnant or gaining weight when they are trying to quiet down increases your risk of breast cancer. There is still some question as to whether hormone replacement therapy in the perimenopausal years constitutes a risk because it increases the oestrogen level during this window. As I'll discuss shortly, I believe the benefits far outweigh whatever slight increased risk there might be.

AM I AT RISK FOR BREAST CANCER?

The scary thing about breast cancer is that it seems so random—80 percent of women who get it have no common risk factor other than the fact that they're all female. Of course that doesn't mean that certain things don't elevate your chance of getting breast cancer. Because oestrogen exposure can transform precancerous cells into actively growing tumors, anything that increases your circulating oestrogen level—early onset of your period, late menopause, not having children, being overweight, ingesting oestrogenic substances such as excessive alcohol—increases your risk.

Ideally, we'd all get our period at age 16, go through menopause at 45, and have no relatives with breast cancer. Unfortunately, these matters are not in our hands. Even those that are may not be reasonable options—for example, having your first child before age 20 reduces your risk of breast cancer, but I'd be the last one to advocate teenage pregnancy as a public health measure. The best you can do to reduce your chance of developing breast cancer is to raise your awareness of the risk factors that aren't in your control, and identify the ones that are so you can manage them wisely. Let's start with the givens:

AGE. As you've seen from the table on page 243, the incidence of breast cancer increases with age. Even after menopause, when your exposure to oestrogen declines, your risk of breast cancer still increases. Why? Because with age our cells replicate less perfectly, so there is more chance of a mutation that could lead to a cancerous growth. Also, the negative effect of carcinogens such as pollution, radiation, and chemical exposure is cumulative, so that the older we get, the more likely they are to cause problems.

RACE. It's not clear whether race is a risk factor for breast cancer, even though there are differences of the incidence of the disease among the racial groups. In the United States white women over age 45 are more likely to be diagnosed with breast cancer than are black women of the same age, but this may be because white women are more likely to go for regular mammograms. (Similarly, wealthier women are more likely to be diagnosed than less well-off women.) Black women who get breast cancer tend to develop it at a younger age and to have the oestrogen-negative type, which is known to have a poor survival rate. Asian women have a substantially lower incidence than white women, but this seems to be more an issue of diet than of genetics. Numerous studies have shown that when Japanese women immigrate to the United States and begin consuming less sushi and tofu and more hamburgers and fries, their breast cancer risk increases until it eventually matches that of American women.

BIRTHWEIGHT. A high birthweight, especially over 9 pounds, is associated with increased risk of breast cancer. At first glance this may seem an odd correlation, but if you think about it in terms of the windows of vulnerability, it makes sense. One of the three major windows is in utero, when exposure to high levels of oestrogen can sensitize the developing breast tissue to oestrogen stimulation. The uterine environment becomes more oestrogenic if a pregnant woman has elevated oestrogen levels from being overweight or eating foods pumped up with growth hormones. In addition to having sensitized breast tissue, foetuses growing under these conditions tend to put on more weight; hence the connection between birthweight and breast cancer risk.

EARLY MENARCHE AND LATE MENOPAUSE. Women who get their periods at an early age and go through menopause at a late age are exposed to more oestrogen during their lifetime and are therefore at increased risk of breast cancer. Furthermore, they are exposed to more oestrogen at critical windows in their lives, such as adolescence and perimenopause, when their breast tissue is vulnerable to overstimulation. Women who experience menarche before age 14 have a 30 percent higher risk than women who get their first periods after age 16. This may help explain the increase in breast cancer over the past century: with better nutrition, the average age of menarche among American girls has dropped below age 12 from age 16 in the past 130 years.

Similarly, women whose periods stop at age 55 or later have a 50 percent higher risk than women whose menopause begins before age 55. Surgical menopause before age 40 confers an especially protective effect, which is why prophylactic oophorectomy (having both ovaries removed) is considered a reasonable option for women carrying one of the two "breast cancer genes" (see page 258).

NO CHILDREN OR LATE FIRST CHILD. Having no children increases your risk of breast cancer for two reasons. First, you are exposed to more unopposed oestrogen than a woman whose cycle has been interrupted by nine months at least once in her reproductive life. Second, it seems that carrying a baby to term causes changes in the breast tissue that somehow "fix" the cells, making them less vulnerable to cancer.

Because you miss more periods the more times you're pregnant, it makes sense that protection against breast cancer would increase with the number of pregnancies you have. This is true up to a point. Pregnancy after age 35 can have a negative effect on your breasts, because they become stimulated during that critical window when they're trying to involute. In fact, having your first baby after age 35 increases your risk even more than having no children at all.

Overall, it has been estimated that late pregnancies and not having children—two trends that are on the rise—could account for 30 percent of postmenopausal breast cancer cases in the United States. Whereas in 1975, 11 percent of women age 35 or older were childless, in 1991, 21 percent of women age 35 or older had not had a child.

FAMILY HISTORY OF BREAST CANCER. Those of us with a first-degree relative with breast cancer (mother, daughter, or sister) have a two to three times higher risk than other women. While some of this may be attributed to environmental factors, it's becoming apparent that genetics have a great deal to do with familial clusters (see page 258).

PERSONAL HISTORY OF BREAST CANCER. If you've had breast cancer, you must be extra vigilant about doing breast self-exams and getting regular mammograms. Women who have already had breast cancer have a fivefold greater chance of developing a tumor in the opposite breast than do women in the general population. Even if you've had radiotherapy, you're still not fully protected against new breast cancer because the radiation only kills the cancer cells present at the time of treatment. And women who've had a mastectomy can still develop cancer in the residual breast tissue left behind on the same side as the original cancer.

A history of breast biopsies also increases your risk of breast cancer, especially if any of them showed atypical lobular or atypical ductal hyperplasia or a lesion known as radial scarring.

RADIATION. That adolescent window is also an especially dangerous time to be exposed to radiation. Take my patient Serena, for example. Always a fit freak, she eats well, stays trim, and doesn't smoke or drink. She has no family history of breast cancer or any type of cancer, for that matter. And yet, at age 36, with two children and a thriving interior decorating business, she was diagnosed with breast cancer. It turns out that when she was 13 years old she had pneumonia and developed an abscess in her lung, for which the standard treatment at that time was radiation. That insult to her actively proliferating breast tissue set the stage for her cancer to develop twenty-three years later.

As I'll discuss shortly, the risk of cancer from the radiation used in mammography is so small as compared to the risk of breast cancer that it's just plain foolhardy not to have a mammogram for fear of radiation.

CHEMICAL EXPOSURE. In today's world, it's nearly impossible to avoid being exposed to a variety of chemicals that can adversely affect your hormonal balance or are outright carcinogens. Farm animals are routinely fed growth hormones, including diethylstilbestrol (DES) and other oestrogenic compounds. In the United States, for years tons of polychlorinated biphenyls (PCBs)—which have been associated with increased breast cancer risk—were dumped into the Hudson River, contaminating it to the point at which it became dangerous to eat the fish. And then, of course, there's the classic case in which startlingly high breast cancer rates on Long Island were likely linked with the routine spraying of the insecticide DDT throughout suburban neighborhoods in the 1950s and 1960s.

While there's little you can do to avoid environmental carcinogens altogether, you can reduce your risk of exposure by eating organic meat and produce and living in a relatively unpolluted area. For those of us who can't just pick up and move to a mountaintop, however, there's still hope: consuming foods with lots of antioxidants (such as a Mediterranean diet of fish, nuts, fruits, and vegetables) or taking antioxidant supplements can fortify our cells against assault.

WHAT YOU CAN DO TO PREVENT BREAST CANCER

WATCH YOUR WEIGHT. To my mind, the most important thing you can do in your perimenopausal years to reduce the risk of post-menopausal breast cancer is to keep your weight down. Study after study shows that women with a high body mass index, especially if it's associated with a high waist-hip ratio, have an increased chance of developing the disease. I see it in my practice—most of my patients with postmenopausal breast cancer are overweight. It's not just the extra 10 pounds you may have put on during your perimenopause that's the culprit; it's the baby fat you may not have shed since, well, you were a baby!

Let's start at the beginning. You're born and, through no fault of your own, you're on the heavy side. That's risk one (see "Birthweight," above). Even if you have an average or low birthweight, let's say you start to plump up in childhood. This brings on your period at an earlier age—risk two (see "Early Menarche," above). Girls who experienced puberty during the great Norwegian famine of World War II were protected for life against breast cancer. Overweight adolescents tend to become overweight adults—one-third of all obese adult women were obese as teenagers—and the longer you're overweight, the greater your chance of developing risk three, insulin resistance.

Insulin resistance (see Chapter 6) is extremely hazardous to your breasts during the perimenopausal years. It increases your levels of insulin-like growth factor-I (IGF-I), which, in the presence of oestrogen, stimulates precancerous cells in your breast. It also decreases your levels of sex hormone binding globulin (SHBG), leading to higher levels of unbound, or biologically active, oestrogen in your system. Meanwhile, the extra fat you're carrying around is busy producing extra oestrogen, thereby bombarding your breasts with stimulation at a time when they're trying to quiet down and involute.

Finally, risk four, obesity, delays menopause by an average of five years, and late menopause, as I've explained, is yet another contributing factor to breast cancer. And to top it all off, once they've been diagnosed, obese women have a worse prognosis for recovery than slim women do.

EXERCISE. Lifelong exercise can have a lifelong positive effect on your breasts. A Harvard study showed that adult women who were sporty as students had a significantly lower incidence of breast cancer later in life than women who hadn't participated in athletics as adolescents. Pre- and perimenopausal women who do three hours of moderate exercise a week have a 30 percent lower risk of breast cancer than their sedentary contemporaries, and those who do four or more hours a week have a 50 percent lower risk. So get moving!

KEEP YOUR ALCOHOL INTAKE LOW. There's some controversy as to how much alcohol is safe to drink without increasing your risk of

THE FAT FALLACY

One of the great myths of women's health is that a high-fat diet leads to breast cancer. Population studies such as those comparing Asian and American women's diets and rates of disease seemed to support this theory. But a 1999 article in the *Journal of the American Medical Association* based on a fourteen-year observation of 89,000 women in the Harvard University Nurses' Health Study reported that dietary fat has no direct impact on breast cancer risk. Rather, *the fat on your body*—which may very well result from intake of high dietary fat, but just as likely comes from a diet high in sugar and carbohydrates—is the problem.

Indeed, some dietary fats may even lower your risk of breast cancer. Women in the Arctic North and in the Mediterranean, whose diet is made up of approximately 40 percent fat, have lower rates of breast cancer than American women. It seems that the unsaturated fats such as those found in fish and olive oil can have a protective effect.

breast cancer. A recent analysis of several studies that tracked more than 300,000 women showed that just one drink a day could increase a woman's risk by 9 percent over nondrinkers. Yet the decades-long Framingham Study suggests that breast cancer risk may be even slightly lower for women who consume one and a half drinks a day than for women who don't drink at all. Two or more drinks a day *does* seem to increase breast cancer risk: women who begin drinking before age 25 and consume more than one drink a day are two and a half times more likely to develop breast cancer, and women consuming two to four drinks a day have a 30 to 40 percent higher risk of developing breast cancer than nondrinkers.

Alcohol adversely affects liver functioning; and because the liver is responsible for breaking down oestrogen, drinking results in higher levels of circulating oestrogen, which is a breast cancer risk. Also, ethanol itself is directly oestrogenic. Furthermore, alcohol may have a carcinogenic effect on breast tissue by increasing the permeability of the cell membranes to other carcinogens, activating precancerous cells and inhibiting the detoxification of the cells.

So what's a woman to do? My advice is to relax and enjoy a glass of wine with dinner. The cardiovascular benefits of a drink a day far outweigh the potential risk of breast cancer. Indeed, several studies have suggested that light consumption of alcohol can lower the overall death rate among women by 5 to 20 percent.

DON'T SMOKE. You'd be shocked to know how much money cigarette manufacturers have pumped into breast cancer research. Don't kid yourself—it's not to prove their strong commitment to women's health. Rather, it's because they've hoped to be able to show that cigarette smoking can protect against breast cancer. After all, cigarette smoking lowers circulating oestrogen levels, and oestrogen is associated with breast cancer. Moreover, smokers go through menopause earlier than nonsmokers, and early menopause protects against breast cancer.

Well, let's just say it hasn't turned out to be such a wise investment. Research has shown that cigarette smoking not only increases breast cancer risk overall, but it especially increases the risk of the far more serious oestrogen-negative type (see page 276). There are several theories about how this happens. One is that smoking has a directly carcinogenic effect on breast tissue, causing mutations that can transform normal cells into cancer cells. Another is that smoking causes a hormone imbalance that has been associated with breast cancer. Finally, chemicals in tobacco smoke may interact negatively with oestrogen receptors on the breast cell surfaces.

The more and longer you smoke, the greater your risk of breast cancer. According to a large Danish study, women who have smoked for more than thirty years face an increased risk of 60 percent. The Harvard University Nurses' Health Study reports that women who smoke more than twenty-five cigarettes a day and who started smoking before age 16 face an increased risk of 80 percent. Starting to smoke in adolescence is especially dangerous, because it exposes the breasts to carcinogens during one of the major windows of vulnerability. Passive smoking also puts you at risk—a fact that may help you to persuade that special someone in your life to kick the habit.

BREASTFEED. Like pregnancy, breastfeeding suspends your menstrual cycle, protecting your breasts from oestrogen stimulation. The Carolina Breast Cancer Study of nearly 1,500 women concluded that having breastfed cuts the risk of breast cancer by 20 percent in premenopausal women and by 30 percent in postmenopausal women. The longer you breastfeed, the better, and the effect is cumulative: breastfeeding one child for two years is as good as breastfeeding three children for eight months each.

SLEEP IN THE DARK. Using a nightlight or sleeping during the day and working at night inhibits production of the hormone melatonin by the pineal gland in the brain, which is connected by nerve pathways to the eye. Melatonin, among other things, dampens the effects of oestrogen. Studies of blind women show that those with complete light insensitivity have 60 percent fewer breast cancers than do women with normal sight. The answer is *not* to take melatonin supplements, the effectiveness and safety of which are dubious, but to buy thick blinds and get lots of sleep.

WILL TAKING HORMONES PUT ME AT RISK?

Every time I discuss hormone replacement therapy with one of my perimenopausal patients, the question arises: "Won't it increase my risk of breast cancer?"

My reply is always the same: "There may be a small risk. But the benefits to your heart and bones and brain far outweigh it."

Study after study has been conducted over the past fifty years to try to find some connection between the most common types of breast cancer and hormone replacement therapy. Some say there's a slight increased risk, others show a decreased risk, still others show that hormones can exert a protective effect. It's an extremely controversial issue and the jury is still out. However, based on more than twenty years of experience and a thorough review of the research, I still feel confident in recommending HRT to most of my patients.

A 1999 article in the *Journal of the American Medical Association* seemed to clarify the situation when it reported that the only increase of any significance is of a few unusual kinds of more easily treatable breast cancer. These rare types of invasive cancer are slow growing, rarely metastasize, and have a good prognosis. In fact, women undergoing hormone replacement therapy actually have a lower mortality rate from breast cancer than women who don't take hormones. This is probably because they see their doctors regularly, making it likely that any abnormality will be detected at an early stage.

Then in early 2000 the *Journal of the American Medical Association* published another article that stirred up a lot of anxiety and confusion—the day it was released I got phone calls from at least twenty panicked patients. The study concluded that taking hormone replacement therapy increased the risk of breast cancer—and this was all that was reported on the news. But if you actually read the article, it showed only a *slight, not statistically significant* increase in breast cancer. In a questionnaire, patients were asked to recall what hormones they had been on and how long they had taken them. Some women had tried many different products over the course of several years. Personally, I can't remember what I ate for dinner a week ago, much less what medication I took seven years ago.

It also turns out that only synthetic hormones were tested and that synthetic progestogen is the culprit. Patients taking a combination of synthetic oestrogen and progestogen had higher rates of breast cancer than those taking just synthetic oestrogen, who in turn had only a slightly higher rate of breast cancer than those not taking any hormones at all. This study only confirms my preference for natural progesterone.

Oral contraceptives seem unlikely to cause breast cancer. Unlike the megadoses of oestrogen that used to be prescribed for contraception, today's oral contraceptives are low-dose and balanced with progestogens. Even long-term use has not been linked with any increased risk of breast cancer.

SHOULD I BE TESTED FOR THE BREAST CANCER GENE?

I'll never forget the day back in 1990 when the *New York Times* announced the discovery of the first BRCA (BReast CAncer) gene. "Isn't it exciting? They found the gene for breast cancer!" my 8:30 A.M. appointment greeted me. For the rest of the week the phones were ringing off the hook with patients asking how they could have their DNA tested. Hopes were high that with a simple blood test women could find out whether or not they were at risk for breast cancer. Unfortunately, as with all matters biological, it could never be so simple.

First, there is no single "breast cancer gene." BRCA1 and BRCA2, which normally direct cells to make proteins that suppress tumors, account for 80 percent of all inherited cases; p53, H-ras, and several other genes are responsible for the remaining 20 percent. Second, only be-tween 5 and 10 percent of all breast cancers have a genetic basis—that means nine out of ten cases are in women with no hereditary predis-position whatsoever. And finally, *even if you have a mutation in one of the "breast cancer genes," it's not a death sentence.* Although women with a sig-nificant mutation in one of the two BRCA genes have an 82 percent risk of developing breast cancer by age 80, advances in cancer detection and treatment are such that they still have a far better chance of surviving than not.

When a patient asks me about getting tested, I first sit down and take a complete medical history, including finding out if any first-degree female relative has had breast cancer and if so, when she got it. The more who have had it and the younger the ages at which they got it, the greater the risk. I also ask about any family members on ei-ther the mother's or the father's side with cancer (the mutant BRCA genes are dominant, which means that you only need one copy to be at risk). The BRCA genes are not only associated with breast, ovarian, and colon cancer in women, but also with colon and prostate cancer in men. BRCA2 is also linked with male breast cancer. Finally, I ask if the patient has any Ashkenazi (Eastern European) Jewish ancestry on either side of the family. BRCA1 and BRCA2 mutations occur in 2.5 percent of Ashkenazi Jews—over 800 times more frequently than in the population at large.

If it turns out that my patient is a candidate for genetic testing—that is, she has a strong family history of cancer, including breast and/or ovarian cancer in her close female relatives, or she has a per-sonal history of breast or ovarian cancer and is of Ashkenazi Jewish ancestry—we ask: "Why do you want to be tested?"

"Because I want to know if I'm going to get breast cancer" is the usual response. When I explain how little predictive value genetic test-ing actually has, my patient usually begins to rethink her decision. Certainly, if worrying about whether you're a carrier is causing you great anxiety, it may be worth finding out simply to put your mind at rest. But if finding out you are a carrier is going to make your life a living hell, why put yourself through the agony?

The women I feel most comfortable referring to a genetic coun-selor for further conversations are those who have a definite idea of what they will do should the tests come back positive. Their options include making certain lifestyle changes to minimize further insult to their breast tissue, or joining a trial of one of the latest hormone therapies, or considering a prophylactic oophorectomy—which reduces the risk of breast cancer by 63 percent—or even a bilateral mastectomy.

This last choice, while radical, may seem wisest—after all, if you don't have breasts, you can't get breast cancer, right? Unfortunately, it's not so simple. Even a radical mastectomy doesn't remove every last bit of breast tissue, which can be found all the way up to the collarbone, into the armpit, and down the abdominal wall. So there's still a slight chance—about 10 percent—of developing breast cancer even if you've had both breasts removed.

BRCA screening isn't for everyone. Genetic analysis is extremely time consuming and expensive. Considering that only 0.003 percent of the general population carries a defective BRCA1 or BRCA2 gene, it is not worth doing across the board.

ALL BREAST CANCER IS NOT CREATED EQUAL

In spite of how people talk about it, breast cancer isn't just one big scary "C." It's more like a lot of little "c's," some of which are mild and easily treatable, and some of which are more serious and require aggressive intervention. Here are some common terms it's useful to know.

ATYPICAL HYPERPLASIA. This refers to cells that may be precancerous—cells that look abnormal under the microscope. In breast tissue, we find abnormal cells either in the ducts (ductal) or in the glands (lobular). Because these cells do not pose a threat on their own and may indeed never turn into cancer, we leave them alone. But they do increase the risk of developing breast cancer, so we monitor them carefully through mammograms and ultrasound scans.

DUCTAL CARCINOMA IN SITU (DCIS). Also known as *intraductal carcinoma of the breast*, DCIS is diagnosed when cancerous duct cells are entirely localized. Entirely asymptomatic and detectable only by mammogram, this early stage of breast cancer accounts for 30 percent of all breast cancer diagnoses. With increased screening, doctors are seeing more and more DCIS. This doesn't necessarily mean that breast cancer is on the rise; rather, it probably indicates that breast cancer is being detected more often at an earlier stage.

DCIS turns into invasive cancer in 30 to 50 percent of cases. Fortunately, it is curable more than 95 percent of the time. Treatment options include lumpectomy alone, in which only the affected area is removed; lumpectomy plus radiotherapy (clinical trials are under way to see whether, in the future, hormone therapy should be added to the protocol); and total mastectomy. If mastectomy is not chosen, the risk of recurrence of either DCIS or invasive carcinoma is on average 10 percent after five years and 30 percent after ten years. The recurrence may be in the same breast or, infrequently, in the opposite breast. The risk of recurrence is higher in women who are still menstruating, are taking hormone replacement therapy, or are obese, and lower if they have radiation along with lumpectomy surgery. After mastectomy, the risk of recurrence is 1 to 2 percent.

LOBULAR CARCINOMA IN SITU (LCIS). This is not considered breast cancer, but women who have it have a 25 percent chance of developing invasive cancer in either breast over the next twenty-five years. Of course, that means that 75 percent of women with LCIS do not go on to develop breast cancer, so most doctors do not recommend surgery. Rather, after the abnormality appears on mammogram and diagnosis is confirmed through biopsy—LCIS, like DCIS, is asymptomatic—patients are followed closely with yearly mammograms and check-ups. (Clinical trials are under way to determine whether treating LCIS patients with tamoxifen, an antioestrogen used to treat breast cancer, can prevent later development of breast cancer, but the jury is still out.) In rare cases, a woman may find a one-in-four chance of getting breast cancer too high to live with and opt for voluntary removal of both breasts. This radical procedure does substantially reduce the risk of developing breast cancer, but not all the way to zero, as I explained on page 260.

INVASIVE CARCINOMA. True breast cancer, accounting for 70 percent of all breast cancer diagnoses, occurs when abnormal cells in either the ducts or the milk-producing glands begin to multiply and invade the surrounding tissue. In order to discuss a particular woman's condition and formulate a treatment plan, a system of descriptive stages has been developed. The stages range from I to IV, I being small and entirely localized and IV being fully metastasized (spread to other parts of the body). Depending on the number and severity of the tumors, either a lumpectomy or some form of mastectomy will be recommended, in addition to radiation, chemotherapy, and/or hormone therapy. Some lymph nodes from under the arm on the same side as the cancer are removed to see if cancerous cells are found in them as well.

BREAST SELF-EXAMINATION—TAKING MATTERS INTO YOUR OWN HANDS

Giving your breasts a good feel once a month is the best thing you can do to reduce your chance of developing serious breast cancer. (Follow the instructions on pages 264–265.) Ninety percent of lumps are first detected by women performing breast self-examinations.

The first few times you perform a breast self-exam you'll probably be pretty freaked out. Our breasts are naturally quite lumpy. But as you become more familiar with your breasts' unique topography, you'll find the normal lumps less frightening and be better prepared to notice an abnormal one. Remember, tumors are usually quite hard, like gravel. If you feel something different from what you usually feel, bring it to the attention of your doctor. She may want to check you right away and/or ask you to wait a month to see if it goes away by itself.

In the United States (although not in the UK) a manual breast exam is part of your regular gynaecologic check-up. Usually I spend at least five minutes palpating my patients' breasts. It's a great chance to catch up with them about their lives. Of course, by the end they're in agony—one woman told me she was still sore ten days later! In spite of the pain, they always end up thanking me.

MAMMOGRAMS—YOUR BEST DEFENSE

Recently a 40-year-old patient came in for an exam. At the end of the visit I said I was going to write her a prescription for a mammogram. "I don't need a mammogram," she replied. "I have no family history. I'm not at risk for breast cancer."

"Sweetie," I replied, writing out the prescription, "we're all at risk."

If you ask me, the institution of routine mammographic screening is one of the most significant advances in women's health in recent times. These very low radiation x-rays detect 85 percent of breast cancers in women under age 50 (93 percent in women over age 50), many of them when the tumors are too tiny to be seen or felt. Because of mammograms, one out of every four cancers diagnosed today is smaller than 1/3 inch and hasn't spread beyond the breast. Before mammographic screening became widespread, these cancers were rarely identified. Mammography has been shown to reduce breast cancer mortality by 30 percent—that means one in three women who have breast cancer survives it simply because her tumor was detected early by mammography. And if all women over age 40 were screened annually, that number could be as high as 40 to 50 percent.

Why anyone would drag her heels about having a mammogram is beyond me. Yet in a 1993 survey by the American College of Radiology, 60 percent of women age 40 and over had never had one! In my own practice I have plenty of patients who procrastinate and procrastinate. "I hate having my breasts smushed in that clamp," they complain. All right, I'll admit it's not the most pleasant experience in the world. But isn't the possibility of finding an abnormality before it becomes life-threatening worth a little discomfort?

Some patients tell me they refuse to have a mammogram because they believe the radiation it exposes their breasts to will actually give them cancer. "The amount of radiation you're exposed to in a mammogram is less than what you're exposed to flying to Europe," I reply. The chance of getting cancer from mammography is tiny.

I'm such a big believer in the value of mammography that I recommend a baseline mammogram at age 35 (age 30 in women with a strong family history) and then yearly screens for all women age 40 and above. Now this is a somewhat controversial stance (and it is not one that has been adopted in the UK). While everyone in the medical community agrees that annual screening should be recommended from age 50 on, there is some debate as to whether it's more cost-effective for women in their forties to go every year or every other year. My response? It's saving lives, not cost, that counts.

I've been sending women every year and I've never regretted it for a number of reasons. First, women in their forties represent 18.1 percent of new breast cancer cases annually in the United States—that's about 30,000 cases a year. Second, the effect of mammography is cumulative: after twelve to fourteen years, you reduce your risk of dying from breast cancer by 25 percent. Third, the earlier tumors are picked

HOW TO EXAMINE YOUR BREASTS

The best time to do a self-exam is right after your period ends, when your breasts are least sore and cystic. Begin by lying down with a pillow under your right shoulder and your right arm behind your head. Then take the three middle fingers of your left hand and use the flat parts—not the tips—to firmly massage your breasts.

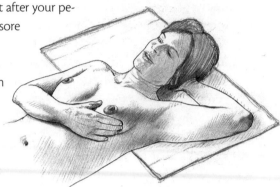

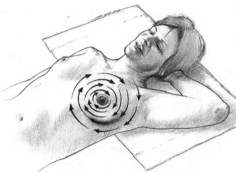

Some women like to go in a circular pattern starting on the outside and moving in.

Others like to divide their breasts into quadrants and move from the outside to the nipple in each quadrant.

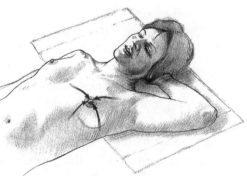

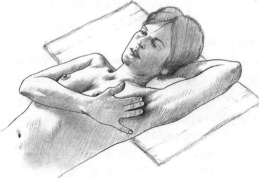

Make sure to incorporate a wide circumference and include the tail of Spence in your armpit, as about half of all breast cancers are found there.

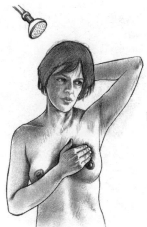

When you're done with your right breast, repeat the procedure with your left. Then, repeat the entire process on both breasts while standing (I usually recommend doing this part in the shower, as the soap helps your fingers glide smoothly over your breasts).

When you're done, stand in front of a mirror and look at your breasts. Is there any change in the way they look? Are they asymmetrical?

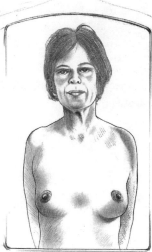

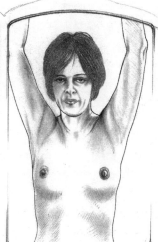

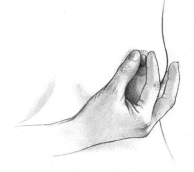

Is there any abnormal swelling, redness, or puckering of the skin on your breasts? Any swelling under your arm or in your upper arm? Is one of your nipples dimpled or puckered in an unusual way? Gently squeeze your nipples—is there any discharge?

TIPS FOR A SUCCESSFUL MAMMOGRAM

- Don't schedule your mammogram right before your period. Rather, schedule your mammogram right after your period, the time of the month when your breasts are least cystic.
- Take a mild over-the-counter pain reliever an hour or so before the test if you're worried about discomfort.
- Be prepared to discuss any family history of breast cancer and any current or past problems with your breasts, such as pain or nipple discharge.
- Do not use deodorant, talcum powder, or lotion under your arms or near your breasts on the day of your screen, as they can show up on the x-ray and make it difficult to read.
- Tell the technician if you're taking birth control pills or hormone replacement therapy because they may make your breasts dense and your mammograms more difficult to read.
- If the doctor is not going to check your mammogram while you wait, find out exactly when she will be sending a report to your gynaecologist so you can follow up.
- If you go to a new radiologist to have a mammogram, make sure to bring copies of your previous mammograms so the doctor can compare them.

up, the smaller and less developed they are, and the less chance there is of lymph node involvement. Mammography reliably detects tumors less than 1.5 cm in diameter, when the cure rate is 90 percent. Finally, breast tumors in premenopausal women grow much more rapidly than those in postmenopausal women because they are still under the influence of oestrogen. You could conceivably have a clean mammogram one year and a tumor greater than 1.5 cm two years later. It is therefore critical that too much time not elapse between screenings in your perimenopausal years.

BREAST ULTRASOUND SCANS

"But my old doctor said my breasts are too dense for mammography to do any good," a new patient in her mid-forties told me. "In fact," she continued with a smile, "he said I have the breasts of a 20-year-old!"

Although it's certainly nice to have firm, youthful breasts, that perkiness comes with a price. Dense or glandular breast tissue can make it more difficult to detect abnormalities by mammogram. Younger women, whose breasts have not yet involuted, and women with fibrocystic breasts may benefit from having ultrasound scans of their breasts as well as mammograms. On a mammogram, glandular tissue shows up all white, as do tumors, making them hard to distinguish. On a sonogram, which uses ultra-high-speed sound waves instead of radiation, tumors show up black against the white tissue. A recent study of more than 16,000 women found that ultrasound plus mammography detected 93 percent of cancers in women with the densest breasts, whereas mammography alone detected only 55 percent of cancers in the same group of women. Ultrasound alone is not as good as mammography alone, however, so if you have an ultrasound scan, make sure it is *in addition to* and not *instead of* your regular mammogram.

OTHER SCREENING TECHNOLOGIES

Even though mammography is considered the gold standard when it comes to early detection, it isn't foolproof. Especially in younger women with denser breasts, there are occasional false-negative results (1 out of 4 in women age 40 to 49, and 1 out of 10 in women age 50 to 69) in which the test fails to pick up a tumor. False positives, which occur in about 1 in 10 cases, are also more common in the under-50 set. As I mentioned earlier, mammography picks up a lot of things that are not cancer, leading to a number of unnecessary biopsies being carried out each year. Also, mammography is not designed to distinguish between benign and malignant tumors. For these reasons, radiologists are always on the lookout for new tools that could improve the accuracy of the screening process. Here is a brief look at some of the latest technologies.

MAGNETIC RESONANCE IMAGING (MRI). MRI, which takes pictures using high radio frequencies, is currently being investigated as an option for women who have dense breasts, breast implants, or scarring from previous biopsies that may make mammograms difficult to read. The drawbacks are that it involves being injected with a special dye that highlights tumors, it does not distinguish between cancerous and noncancerous tumors, it requires patients to lie in a claustrophobic tube, and it's costly and time consuming. There are, however, no side effects.

MRI will not replace mammography, but it may become an adjunct in difficult cases. It is also recommended for women at high risk of breast cancer who must begin annual screening at a young age when their breasts are dense and hard to image on mammogram.

IMMUNOSCINTIGRAPHY IMAGING. Carcinoembryonic antigen (CEA) immunoscintigraphy is a technique already used to detect colon cancer. It is an extremely exciting prospect for breast cancer because it can distinguish between benign and malignant breast disease with virtually no false-positives. In women with suspicious mammograms, it accurately predicts cancer 90 percent of the time. And it can reliably pick up cancers as small as 0.5 cm in diameter. Immunoscintigraphy involves the injection of a radioisotope, followed three to five hours later by imaging in a nuclear medicine lab. There are no reported side effects.

DIGITAL MAMMOGRAPHY. Using digital imaging instead of x-ray film, this is basically a new-and-improved mammogram. Its advantages are that it shows more detail than a traditional mammogram, can be read on a computer, and eliminates the need for retakes caused by over- or underexposure.

DIGITAL THERMAL IMAGING. Because cancer cells reproduce at a rapid rate, they throw off more heat than benign tissue does. Based on that premise, digital thermal imaging is a promising tool for determining whether a suspicious spot on a mammogram is indeed cancerous. In one study, digital thermal imaging prevented unnecessary biopsies in 38 percent of cases. The test takes 15 minutes, and the only discomfort it entails is a 30-second blast of cold air aimed at both breasts.

MICROWAVE RADIOGRAPHY. When cancerous cells emit heat, they do so in the form of microwaves. While not enough to cook by, the microwaves can be detected by the new Oncoscan radiometry system. Whereas digital thermal imaging only senses temperature changes on the surface of the breast, microwave radiography obtains data from roughly 2 cm below the surface of the breast, closer to where tumors are located. When used to follow up abnormal mammograms, it can prevent unnecessary biopsies in 60 percent of cases. The test compares the two breasts without any painful compression and takes only ten minutes.

ELECTROPOTENTIAL ANALYSIS. Another distinctive feature of cancer cells is that their cell membranes become depolarized. Normally the inside of the cell membrane is negatively charged to the exterior. In the new Biofield test, malignant tumors can be identified by placing electropotential sensors on the surface of the skin. As an adjunct to mammography, the test boosts diagnostic accuracy from 56 to 75 percent.

ELECTRICAL IMPEDANCE SCANNING (EIS). Also relying on the characteristic electrical effects of cancerous cells, this technique involves applying a small alternating current across the breast. Malignant tumors distort the electrical field, producing measurable changes in the way the current flows through the breast that appear as bright spots. In a study of 141 women, EIS was shown to be more accurate than mammography; larger clinical trials are in the works.

OPTICAL BREAST IMAGING. Just as cancerous cells distort electrical current, they also change the way light waves flow. Still in the preliminary stages, this technique involves capturing laser light that has passed through breast tissue. Malignant tumors show up as a different color than benign breast tissue.

WHAT IF MY MAMMOGRAM IS ABNORMAL?

Don't panic. Mammography casts a very wide net and picks up all kinds of abnormalities, many of which are benign and some of which are entirely false-positives. Mammograms, for example, cannot distinguish between an innocent cyst and a cancerous tumor.

If your mammogram has a suspicious spot on it, the first step usually is to do a sonogram. The spot might turn out to be a fluid-filled cyst, which can be aspirated (drained) with a fine needle. As long as the cyst collapses and does not recur once the fluid is removed, and the cells are benign, you have nothing to worry about.

A BAD HAIR DAY

Scientists from the University of New South Wales in Sydney, Australia, have reported success in a small trial of a new technique for diagnosing breast cancer: x-ray analysis of a single strand of hair. The procedure, known as synchrotron x-ray scattering, involves bombarding the hair with x-rays and analyzing the resulting scatter pattern on a piece of film. Using pubic hair from 51 women (because of chemical processes like hair coloring or permanents, scalp hair was found to be unreliable), researchers were able to correctly identify the 23 patients with breast cancer. While hair testing probably isn't going to replace mammography anytime soon, it's an intriguing possibility.

If the ultrasound scan indicates something other than a cyst, such as a solid tumor, or if the cyst is bloody or refills after aspiration, a biopsy is in order. You may also need a biopsy if you experience abnormal nipple discharge, puckering of the skin, or swelling of the breast tissue. In general, *every suspicious lump must be biopsied regardless of whether it shows up on a mammogram and/or ultrasound scan.*

Rochelle, a 44-year-old patient, came to me a couple of months ago with a lump she had detected during a breast self-exam. I palpated her breasts and told her I thought it felt suspicious, too. I sent her to a breast specialist who prescribed a mammogram, but nothing showed up. Rochelle went for a second mammogram and a sonogram. Both of these were negative, too, and the breast specialist reassured her that everything was fine. "What should I do?" Rochelle asked me. "I know the tests were negative, but I still can't sleep at night worrying about this lump."

"If I were you, I would go for a second opinion to another breast specialist and demand a surgical biopsy," I advised her and referred her to another doctor.

In a breast biopsy a small amount of tissue is removed so that it can be examined by a pathologist, who determines whether it is benign or malignant. To determine what kind of biopsy to perform, the doctor usually begins with a fine-needle aspiration in which he or she sucks out a few cells and examines them under a microscope. Depending on the results, one of three different types of biopsy can be performed:

- In a ***core needle biopsy*** a large needle with a cutting surface re-moves a tiny slice of tissue. This can be performed with or with-out ultrasound or mammogram (*stereotaxic*) guidance depending on whether or not the mass is palpable. Core needle biopsy is great for diagnosing whether a growth is cancerous and, if it is, determining the type, grade, and stage of the disease. The down-side is that should the lesion be malignant, it does not reveal the margins of the tumor.

- A ***surgical excisional biopsy*** requires cutting through the breast tissue to remove the entire lesion. If the lesion cannot be felt, the area to be biopsied is identified by inserting a needle under mammographic guidance (*needle localization*).

- An ***incisional biopsy*** is identical to an excisional biopsy except that only a sample of the growth is removed, not the whole thing. Incisional biopsies are usually performed for diagnostic purposes in growths that don't look too suspicious or to test large tumors for hormone receptors.

All these procedures can be performed under local anesthesia, al-though some excisional and incisional biopsies may require general anesthesia. The good news is that 70 to 80 percent of biopsies are neg-ative, showing no cancer.

In Rochelle's case, the breast specialist began with a fine-needle as-piration of her lump but was unable to retrieve enough cells to make a diagnosis. The doctor went on to perform an excisional biopsy and re-moved the entire growth. It turned out to be breast cancer. Rochelle called and thanked me for encouraging her not to take "no" for an an-swer.

IF THE DIAGNOSIS IS CANCER...

The other day I got a phone call from the radiologist about a patient, Lucy, who had gone for a routine mammogram. Age 44 and childless, Lucy had a history of endometriosis. "Laura, on mammogram I see a small cluster of calcifications that appear indeterminant," the radiologist told me. This meant that she couldn't decide whether it was benign or malignant. She had also performed a sonogram, which was negative, and she now recommended a biopsy. We discussed it and decided that a stereotactic core needle biopsy should be done the next day.

Lucy returned to the radiologist the following day and for about 30 minutes under mammography the core biopsy was taken. Unfortunately, it turned out to be cancer and I immediately sent her to a breast specialist.

Whenever a patient has a breast problem, the radiologist, the breast specialist, and I remain in close contact throughout her treatment. Not only is it important that I stay informed from a medical point of view, but I also want to be able to provide as much emotional support as I can during this trying time. When faced with an array of treatment choices, my patients often like to call or come in for an appointment to have me help them decide which is best for them.

Thirty or forty-five years ago, when a woman found out she had breast cancer (usually invasive, as mammography was not available to detect in situ), her only option was a radical mastectomy in which she lost her breast, chest muscle, and all of her underarm lymph nodes. This left a dent and a huge scar where the breast used to be, as well as the possibility of swelling, restricted motion, numbness, and loss of strength in the neighboring arm. Reconstruction was also difficult.

Nowadays, radical mastectomies are not performed unless absolutely necessary. Even in cases where breast cancer is advanced, studies have shown that less extensive surgery combined with adjuvant therapies such as chemotherapy, radiation, and/or hormone therapy have the same success rate. You must have adjuvant therapy with a lumpectomy because the whole breast requires treatment: the duct system allows cells to migrate from the tumor throughout the breast. Your choice will depend on many factors, including the type, stage, and size of your cancer; the size of your breast; certain characteristics of the cancer cells themselves; as well as your age, menopausal status, general health, and state of mind.

Throughout the treatment process you will be dealing primarily with a breast surgeon and an oncologist, who will coordinate your follow-up treatment. Nevertheless, as a gynaecologist I feel it's important to stay in the loop. I frequently discuss how my patients are progressing with their breast specialists and, of course, am always available to provide whatever direct support and advice I can.

LUMPECTOMY. This is the treatment of choice by most women who have a choice—that is, women with a small area of DCIS or a relatively small area of invasive cancer that has not spread. In a lumpectomy only the tumor and a small amount of surrounding tissue are removed, leaving a minimal scar and no need for reconstructive surgery. For invasive cancer, lumpectomy is accompanied by removal of one or more lymph nodes for identifying the stage of the cancer and is generally followed by radiation. The need for systemic therapy such as chemotherapy or hormone therapy is based on the stage of the cancer. The long-term survival rate for women who undergo lumpectomy and radiation is the same as the survival rate for those who undergo mastectomy, because a local recurrence in the conserved breast can be treated by surgery later.

Laser lumpectomies, which are still in the early stages of research, may eventually make it possible to destroy tumors with laser heat, leaving no scar or deformity at all. Guided by MRI, a needle will be inserted into the tumor and a thin fiberoptic wire will be threaded through the needle. The wire will be heated for about ten minutes, during which time the tumor will go from being white to black on the MRI. Out of fifteen women in a recent trial who underwent the procedure, two didn't need any painkiller at all, and the other thirteen only took ibuprofen. The problem with laser lumpectomy is that the surgeon doesn't remove any tissue for pathology diagnosis and there's no way to know if the margins around the tumor are clear.

TOTAL MASTECTOMY. In cases of multicentric DCIS or multiple tumors, when a tumor is too big to be excised by partial mastectomy or is centrally located, when there has been a recurrence of cancer after breast-conserving therapy, or when there is a strong family history, total mastectomy is the wisest choice. In addition, some women who are good candidates for lumpectomy or quadrantectomy (removal of a quarter of the breast) opt for total mastectomy because of psychological reasons—they just can't stand living with the worry of a recurrence in the same breast. Total mastectomy involves removal of the entire breast as well as one or more of the lymph nodes.

MODIFIED RADICAL MASTECTOMY. The most common operation for invasive breast cancer, this involves removal of the breast, some of the lymph nodes under the arm, and the lining over the chest muscles.

RADIATION. High-energy x-rays are used to kill cancer cells left in the remaining breast following lumpectomy, and in certain cases

WHAT'S A SENTINEL-NODE BIOPSY?

The fifty to sixty lymph nodes into which your breast tissue drains are like a cluster of grapes resting among nerves and blood vessels in a fat pad that extends out from the edge of your breast, then under your arm and up toward your neck. Now, instead of removing a large number of nodes, which can cause arm lymphedema—swelling and even nerve damage that limits the range of motion in the arm—your surgeon can biopsy the first grape in the bunch, called the sentinel node. A blue dye and/or a radioactive isotope are injected into your breast near the cancer. A few minutes later, the surgeon will make a small incision under your arm to search for the first few lymph nodes. The blue dye and/or radioactivity is found at the sentinel node. If the sentinel node is clean, no further surgery is required. If the sentinel node has cancer cells, more nodes should be removed.

The disadvantage of this procedure is that the pathologist will not be able to determine whether or not the sentinel node is cancerous right away—it may take a few days. To prevent having to reoperate, your surgeon may choose to do a low-node dissection, removing the first few nodes, so you won't have to go back for a second node sampling.

before or after a complete mastectomy. Radiation is applied externally from a machine. You typically receive treatment five days a week for six to seven weeks. Although side effects may include fatigue, skin changes like redness, mild swelling, itching, peeling, and occasionally even blistering, patients of mine who've undergone radiation have sailed through it beautifully.

CHEMOTHERAPY. After surgery, and occasionally before, anticancer drugs can be given either orally or intravenously to kill any cancer cells that may have spread outside your breast. As opposed to radiation, which is localized to the site of the tumor, chemotherapy is systemic, meaning it travels all over your body. This is a good thing in that it allows the drugs to kill cancer cells wherever they may be found; it also means, however, that you may experience side effects—nausea, vomiting, weakness, hair loss, and a lowering of your white blood cell count. In spite of these reactions, chemotherapy has been shown to be safe when carefully given.

Reconstructive Surgery

After a mastectomy—particularly a unilateral one, in which only one breast is removed—most women do not look forward to living life lopsided. Fortunately, there are wonderful plastic surgeons who can perform miraculous reconstructions. If you wish to have your breast or breasts rebuilt, your choices include saline implants (and silicone ones under controlled circumstances) as well as flap reconstruction. In the case of the flap, the surgeon uses fat and skin tissue from another part of your body—preferably the stomach—to create a new breast. The doctor can even tattoo an extremely realistic-looking nipple.

Depending on your body image, your stage of life, and your relationship with your partner, you may or may not opt for reconstructive surgery. If you are leaning toward reconstruction, I recommend doing it at the same time as the mastectomy, as you probably won't want to undergo a second round of major surgery once you've recovered from the first. If you're unsure, however, you can certainly wait, live for a while without one or both breasts, and make your decision at a later date. Often women—especially those who undergo double mastectomy—choose not to have breast reconstruction. One of my patients said it was actually quite liberating not to have to wear a bra anymore!

BONE MARROW TRANSPLANTATION. High-dose chemotherapy with bone marrow and/or stem cell transplantation, is a complex and difficult procedure in which your own bone marrow and/or stem cells are removed and you are subjected to extremely high doses of chemotherapy, which, along with killing cancer cells, wipes out the body's blood cells. Then your bone marrow and/or stem cells are reintroduced into your system. Such transplantation is only considered in serious situations when standard therapy would not be enough. But the results have not been promising. In five out of five recent studies, it has not been shown to increase breast cancer survival rates.

HORMONE THERAPY. Last but not least, there is the brave new world of hormone therapy, which is revolutionizing the treatment of breast cancer. If you are diagnosed with breast cancer, the pathologist will test the cells retrieved during your biopsy to see if they have surface receptors for various hormones. The presence of these receptors means that the cell can be stimulated by the hormone in question—testosterone, progesterone, and, most important, oestrogen.

If your cancer is oestrogen positive, you're in luck, because there is an explosion of research into the so-called designer oestrogens, such as tamoxifen, that are proving to be successful at treating breast cancer and even reducing the risk of getting it in the first place. If your cancer is oestrogen negative, you may not respond to any of these new drugs. Between 45 and 60 percent of cancers in premenopausal women are oestrogen positive; 65 to 80 percent are positive in postmenopausal women. The rest are oestrogen negative. The higher the level of oestrogen receptors in your tumor, the more you will benefit from hormone therapy.

Hormone therapy doesn't kill cancer cells, like radiotherapy or chemotherapy does. Rather, it regulates their growth, ideally stopping them from proliferating altogether. The benefit of hormone therapy is that it is generally tolerated better than chemotherapy. That doesn't mean it's risk-free, however—remember, there ain't no free lunch!

SHOULD I BE TAKING TAMOXIFEN?

Hailed as a knight in shining armor, rescuing thousands upon thousands of women from the evil dragon of breast cancer, tamoxifen has taken the news media by storm. But believe it or not, tamoxifen has been around for nearly three decades! Since 1973 it has been available as a treatment to prevent the recurrence of breast cancer; recently, however, it has been shown to possibly prevent the disease as well.

Women with oestrogen-positive tumors are often given tamoxifen after surgery as it cuts in half the risk both of recurrence of the original cancer and of developing cancer in the opposite breast. The standard course of treatment is five years, with the benefits extending at least an additional five years after you stop taking the drug. Postoperative tamoxifen use is currently responsible for saving 20,000 lives a year. According to researchers at Oxford University, if all the women who qualified to take tamoxifen did, an additional 20,000 women a year would be saved.

Preventing recurrence of breast cancer is a great thing, to be sure. But wouldn't we all like to see a way to stop it from occurring in the first place? Under certain circumstances, it looks as though tamoxifen might do just that. In April 1998, the $68 million National Cancer Institute's NSABP (National Surgical Adjuvant Breast and Bowel Project) Breast Cancer Prevention Trial study of more than 20,000 North American women considered at high risk for breast cancer was abruptly halted fourteen months before schedule. Why? Because thirteen out of 10,000 women in the placebo group got cancer, versus only 7 out of 10,000 in the tamoxifen group. The scientists decided it was unethical not to offer the drug to the placebo group. *This is the first time a drug has been shown to decrease the risk of cancer.*

Tamoxifen, sold as Nolvadex, is one of a class of designer oestrogens known as selective oestrogen receptor modulators, or SERMs, that bind to some cells but not others. Tamoxifen binds to breast cells but not to heart or brain or ovarian cells. In breast tissue it has what's known as an antioestrogenic effect, essentially taking the parking space normally reserved for oestrogen on the breast cell membrane so that oestrogen cannot make contact with the cell and stimulate it to proliferate. Elsewhere it acts very much like oestrogen, helping maintain bone density and keeping cholesterol levels down.

But—there's always a but—tamoxifen does have side effects. Most worrisome is that it increases the risk of uterine cancer by two to three times. It may also increase the risk of gastrointestinal cancers. Other adverse effects include potentially fatal blood clots, cataracts in women age 50 and over, hot flushes in 25 to 35 percent of users, and vaginal discharge in 5 to 10 percent. Women taking anticoagulants or with a history of deep-vein thrombophlebitis or pulmonary embolus should not take the drug for the same reason they should not take oestrogen—because of its clotting effect. Additionally, I was startled to read in a recent article in *Science* that certain women may develop resistance to tamoxifen over time. In these patients, after two to five years of tamoxifen use, their breast cells began to respond to the drug as if it were an oestrogen, not an antioestrogen. In other words, the tamoxifen began to promote growth of their cancer! So if you're taking tamoxifen, you still need to consult your doctor regularly and report any unusual symptoms immediately.

Who are the women who qualify for prophylactic (preventive) tamoxifen use? The National Cancer Institute has conveniently developed software to calculate your five-year and lifetime risk based on your current age, the age at which you began menstruating, the age when you first gave birth, the number of first-degree relatives you have with breast cancer, and the number of previous breast biopsies you've had. Providing this information to women can reduce anxiety, motivate them to take advantage of screening programs, and identify those at very high risk who may wish to take steps to reduce their chances of developing breast cancer. If you are interested, ask your gynaecologist to use this program, called the Gail model, to figure out your risk. (Roche Pharmaceuticals, which makes Nolvadex, has conveniently provided many of us with a special calculator for just this purpose. The software is also available to professionals online.) If your risk seems unduly high, you and your doctor can discuss whether or not you might be a good candidate for preventive tamoxifen therapy.

FORTIFYING YOUR DEFENSES

To help prevent breast cancer you should eat a balanced diet, get plenty of exercise and rest, and even though it's hard, try to keep your stress level in check. Yoga and meditation are great relaxation practices. Personally, I subscribe to the long-hot-bath school of stress reduction. Whatever works!

In addition, make sure you're taking a good multivitamin and getting adequate amounts of the following vitamins, minerals, and phytoestrogens.

Vitamins and Minerals

COENZYME Q10. A 1994 Danish study showed women with breast cancer fared better when given CoQ10 supplements. A more recent study of 200 women diagnosed with breast cancer found a correlation between the extent of CoQ10 deficiency and the extent of the disease. Some studies have shown megadoses, over 300 mg daily, to be effective in shrinking tumors. I'm more conservative, as high doses can cause overstimulation of the breast tissue. For prevention purposes, take a 50 mg supplement in the morning.

VITAMIN C. I always recommend 500 mg ester vitamin C taken twice a day to enhance immunity.

WHAT ABOUT EVISTA?

Raloxifene, another SERM, marketed as Evista, has also been getting a lot of press recently. A huge international study in which women took raloxifene for three years showed it significantly reduced the risk of breast cancer. Unfortunately, the study was designed to investigate raloxifene's effect on bone, as it is right now only approved for postmenopausal treatment and prevention of osteoporosis. The breast cancer findings were a pleasant surprise. Until a study has been done specifically to assess raloxifene's effect on breast cancer, the results are considered anecdotal, not definitive, and raloxifene cannot be approved for prevention of the disease.

Fortunately, such studies are under way. The latest data to emerge indicate that taking raloxifene for four years can reduce the risk of all breast cancers by 72 percent and the risk of oestrogen-positive breast cancer by 84 percent. Plus, the National Cancer Institute is currently sponsoring the STAR (Study of Tamoxifen and Raloxifene) study, a head-to-head comparison of the effectiveness of tamoxifen and raloxifene in preventing breast cancer in high-risk women. It involves 22,000 women and is expected to last five to ten years. If raloxifene turns out to be as effective as tamoxifen, it may become the drug of choice, as it does not pose any added risk to the uterus.

VITAMIN E. To boost your immune system take 400 to 800 IU a day of natural vitamin E, as it's a powerful antioxidant.

MIXED CAROTENES. Be sure to get 3 to 6 mg a day of these excellent antioxidants either through diet or supplement to protect against DNA damage.

SELENIUM. 200 mcg a day can help repair DNA damage from carcinogens.

OMEGA–3 FATTY ACIDS. Found in oily fish and flaxseed, omega–3 fatty acids help boost immune function. They can benefit breast cancer patients in two ways: they are naturally antioestrogenic, and they inhibit tumor growth. If you don't get three servings a week in your diet, take up to six 1,000 mg capsules daily. Don't take supplements if you're on anticoagulants or have a bleeding disorder.

Phytoestrogens

SOY. One of the most significant differences between the Western and Eastern diet is that Asian women consume vast quantities of soy products, whereas we Western women eat very little, if any. Breast cancer is diagnosed nearly five times less frequently in Asian women than in women in the West. Coincidence? Not likely.

Soy foods are chock-a-block full of phytoestrogens, especially the isoflavone genistein, which is structurally similar to oestradiol. But wait, you may ask. Doesn't oestrogen increase the risk of breast cancer? The answer is yes when it comes to endogenous oestrogen—the kind we produce in our own bodies. Phytoestrogens appear to work a little differently, however. At low concentrations genistein mimics oestrogen, which is why soy foods are so effective for treating perimenopausal symptoms. At high concentrations, however, genistein becomes an antioestrogen, inhibiting cell proliferation. Three possible mechanisms for genistein's protective effects have been suggested: (1) it may block oestrogen receptors, much the way tamoxifen does; (2) it may inhibit aromatase, the enzyme that converts androstenedione to oestrone; and (3) it may stimulate production of sex hormone binding globulin (SHBG) in the liver, leading to lower levels of circulating oestrogen.

So does that mean you have to eat a mountain of tofu to get the antioestrogenic effect? Amazingly, no! It seems that breast tissue either naturally concentrates genistein or is more sensitive to it than other tissue, so a reasonable amount of soy can have a beneficial effect. By eating up to 50 mg soy isoflavones daily (see Appendix B) you can get relief from your hot flushes and help protect your breasts.

Genistein is also thought to be present in two other leguminous plants: liquorice and red clover. In vitro studies have shown liquorice and red clover to be potent binders of the oestrogen receptor; studies are now under way to assess their anticancer potential.

FIBER AND FLAXSEED. Fiber-rich foods such as fruits and vegetables, whole grains, and particularly flaxseed contain lignans, another type of phytoestrogen. Flaxseed is also a strong antioxidant that prevents damage by free radicals to cell membranes and genes. Its anticancer properties may also derive from its richness in alpha-linolenic acid, which may block the production of tumor necrosis factor

(TNF), a protein that stimulates the production of the blood vessels necessary to feed tumors. Women who eat at least five servings of produce a day have a 23 percent lower risk of breast cancer than those who eat fewer than two servings a day. Plus, fiber prevents the reabsorption of oestrogen from the intestine, helping to keep circulating oestrogen levels in check. Eating a healthy dose of fiber daily—say, a half cup of whole-bran cereal—is one simple thing you can do to decrease your risk of cancer.

Do's and Don'ts for Reducing Your Risk of Breast Cancer

Even though there are many risk factors for breast cancer that you can do nothing about, there are plenty that are within your control. Indeed, it has been estimated that we could eliminate 85 percent of breast cancer cases if, starting in our youth, we all ate a low-fat, high-fiber diet, exercised, and stayed slim. Don't feel bad if you've let yourself slide in the past, however; it's never too late to make some basic lifestyle changes to help reduce your risk in the future:

Do... slim down and exercise.

eat lots of whole grains, fruits, and vegetables.

develop a taste for soy.

perform a monthly breast self-exam. This is by far the most important tool we have for early detection.

Don't... put off getting a mammogram. It could save your life.

smoke—under penalty of death!

drink to excess, but also don't feel guilty about enjoying a glass of wine with dinner.

obsess about breast cancer. Rather, spend your energy pursuing a healthy lifestyle—it'll benefit your mind and your breasts.

CHAPTER 11

Below the Belt: Your Uterus, Ovaries, Cervix, and Colon

I'll never forget the first day of anatomy class in medical school. We were each assigned a cadaver to dissect. Out of the fifty or so that were female, only one still had pelvic organs; all the others had had them removed.

We've come a long way since then. Twenty-five years ago it was believed that after age 40, all the female reproductive organs should come out, regardless of whether they were healthy or diseased. The common wisdom was that they served no useful function after childbearing and could only be a source of trouble later on. Now we know otherwise, and when a problem arises most of us try as hard as we can to save our patients' reproductive organs.

Using hormones and medications we can now control symptoms that in bygone days would have been "treated" by a total hysterectomy (removing the ovaries and cervix for good measure). When surgery is required, minimally invasive techniques can often get you in and out of the hospital on the same day. And if a patient does need a hysterectomy, I try to leave the ovaries and cervix if at all possible. If I can't, then I immediately offer the patient hormone replacement therapy so she doesn't have to suffer the often debilitating side effects of surgical menopause.

Unfortunately, perimenopause is a time when problems do tend to arise in the reproductive organs. Why? Because all the tissues in your pelvic region are extremely sensitive to oestrogen and have been since they were a single undifferentiated blob in the womb. In perimenopause, these tissues start being exposed to high levels of unopposed endogenous oestrogen (oestrogen your body produces), often for the first time. Anovulatory or irregular cycles are one source; increasing abdominal fat is another. When oestrogen is not opposed by progesterone, it can activate hormonally sensitive tissue, causing it to proliferate. With increased proliferation comes increased chance of mutation, making perimenopausal women vulnerable to cancer of the uterus, ovaries, and colon. Perimenopause is a time of increased noncancerous problems as well, such as fibroids, polyps, endometriosis, adenomyosis, and ovarian cysts. Although some of these conditions can be managed through diet and hormone therapy, they often require surgery.

The most important thing you can do to reduce your chances of having gynaecologic surgery is to know and minimize your risk factors for these conditions. And if you do develop one or more of these problems, inform yourself of the available options so you can be an active participant in your treatment. Don't be shy about voicing your opinions to your doctor! He or she shouldn't be offended (and if your doctor is, it's time to change doctors). In fact, nothing pleases me more than when a patient has an educated opinion about her illness and we can work together to develop an effective treatment plan.

UTERINE FIBROIDS

The physical problem I see most among my perimenopausal patients is fibroids: benign tumors of the uterine smooth muscle. More than half of all women get fibroids, or *uterine myomas,* and their incidence increases with age. Because they respond to both oestrogen and progesterone stimulation, they tend to act up when your hormone levels become imbalanced. The good news is that they usually begin to regress once you reach menopause. Fibroids can be totally asymptomatic—some women never know they have a fibroid until their doctor picks it up upon exam—or they can cause symptoms such as pain in the pelvis or lower back, cramping, bladder pressure, constipation, bloating, pain on intercourse, or heavy bleeding.

Bobbi, a 49-year-old patient, came in complaining of severe pain in her pelvis and lower back. "Is it cyclical?" I asked.

"No, it's pretty much all the time," she responded.

"And how are your periods? Regular?"

AM I GETTING A THOROUGH PELVIC EXAM?

It is not uncommon for a new patient to come to me and express surprise when, as part of her routine pelvic exam, I insert a well-lubricated finger into her rectum. "My other doctor never did that!" she usually exclaims, wide-eyed. Well, he or she should have. A thorough pelvic exam, technically called a *bimanual rectovaginal pelvic exam*, involves putting fingers inside not only the vagina but the rectum as well. When I'm in the vagina, I put gentle pressure on the belly with my other hand, which allows me to feel the surfaces of both ovaries and the uterus. But the only way to feel the space behind the uterus, known as the cul-de-sac, is via the rectum. Pelvic organs can fall into this space and may be missed if a doctor doesn't use the bimanual approach. A bimanual rectovaginal pelvic exam also gives me the chance to perform a digital rectal examination and faecal blood test for colon cancer (see page 312).

"Yes, but incredibly heavy with lots of disgusting clots."

I examined her and told her I felt a fibroid. "Oh my God!" she cried. "I'm turning into my mother!" It turned out that her mother had had a hysterectomy at age 50 because of severe uterine fibroids. Mere coincidence? Not likely.

Fibroids tend to run in families, suggesting a genetic factor in their development, although we're not exactly sure what that genetic factor may be. Basically, fibroids develop when a uterine muscle cell mutates and begins proliferating excessively, eventually forming a noncancerous tumor.

There are three major types of uterine fibroids, depending on where in the uterine wall they occur. *Intramural* fibroids, the most common type, are found within the wall. *Submucosal* fibroids, which account for 5 percent of all fibroids, are in the inner lining of the uterus and protrude into the uterine cavity. Either intramural or submucosal fibroids are usually the culprit when heavy bleeding is a symptom. *Subserosal* fibroids originate in the outer lining of the uterus and grow outward into the pelvic cavity. They can become quite large without causing any kind of symptom. Submucosal and subserosal fibroids can migrate away from the wall of the uterus *(pedunculate)*, remaining attached by a thick stalk of tissue.

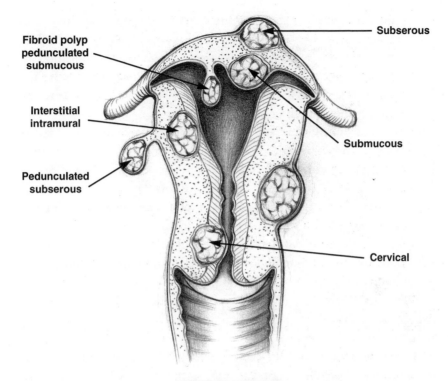

Fibroid polyp pedunculated submucous

Interstitial intramural

Pedunculated subserous

Subserous

Submucous

Cervical

TYPES OF FIBROIDS

I've found that patients who suffer painful fibroids often have a history of other gynaecologic problems. Take Julianne, for instance. At age 44 she's in full-fledged perimenopause, experiencing memory loss, mood swings, and weight gain. Five years earlier I had removed a cyst from her right ovary and during the operation discovered that she had endometriosis, which I cauterized. (Ovarian cysts and endometriosis are discussed later in this chapter). Now she reported constant lower back pain and a feeling of having to urinate all the time. "I've been living on Motrin because my cramps have become unbearable," she told me. Her periods were also extremely heavy.

Upon examination, her uterus was the size of a 12- to 14-week pregnancy and very tender. Her sonogram showed fibroids and adenomyosis (also discussed below). After a long discussion we decided that a hysterectomy, leaving her ovaries intact, was her best option because her fibroids were quite large and she wasn't going to have any more children. "There's one thing that worries me about having a hysterectomy, though," Julianne said hesitantly. "I mean, will I be able to enjoy sex afterward?"

"If anything, you'll enjoy it more," I replied. "For one thing, I'm going to leave your cervix, which will not only support your bladder and rectum but also maintain the shape of your vagina. For another, you won't have any more cramps, back pain, heavy bleeding, or feeling like you have to go to the bathroom all the time. Last but not least, no more worries about birth control!"

If you have fibroids but still want to have a baby, you should know that fibroids can complicate pregnancy. Because they distort the uterine and pelvic cavities, they can cause problems with conception or, down the line, lead to miscarriage. Fibroids grow rapidly during pregnancy, stimulated by the high levels of oestrogen, and can outgrow their blood supply (degenerate), causing irritability to the uterus and contractions. Because women with fibroids are also at high risk for premature delivery, I usually recommend removing submucous fibroids before conception to prevent any complications. But if a fibroid does flare up during pregnancy, bedrest, hydration, anti-inflammatory drugs, and if necessary, anti-contraction medications (tocolytics) are the treatments of choice.

There's not a lot you can do to prevent fibroids, as the risk factors are mostly out of your control. One of the biggest is race: for unknown reasons, black women are two to three times more likely than white women to suffer fibroids. Another is age: the older you are, the more opportunities your cells have to mutate, and up until menopause those mutated cells can be stimulated by oestrogen. Your risk also increases the more you are exposed to unopposed oestrogen—if you are obese, began menstruating at an early age (before age 10), never had children, have suffered infertility because of anovulation, or are experiencing anovulatory cycles as part of your perimenopause.

There are several techniques for diagnosing the type, size, and number of fibroids. The simplest is a transvaginal sonogram (TVS). Another option is a hysterosalpingogram (HSG), in which a radiologist injects dye into the uterus and takes a picture to show if an abnormal growth such as a fibroid or polyp is protruding into the cavity. In a similar procedure, the sonohysterogram, saline is injected into the uterus and a sonogram is taken to evaluate the uterine cavity. At the time of a D&C, hysteroscopy, in which a scope is inserted into the uterus through the cervix, is another way to visualize fibroids.

If your fibroids aren't causing any undue symptoms, I usually suggest just keeping an eye on them with visits every three to six months.

THE ANTI-FIBROID DIET

One thing you can do to help control your fibroids is watch what you eat. Because fibroids are hormonally sensitive, you need to try to minimize the hormones you ingest as well as the hormones you produce. As you know by now, fat produces oestrogen, so my first recommendation is to try to get down to a healthy weight (see Chapter 13). In the process, *avoid:*

- animal fat
- hormone-treated meat and poultry
- chicken skin
- butter
- eggs
- high-fat milk (whole or 2 percent)
- high-fat cheese
- soy products and other foods and herbs containing phytoestrogens (see Appendix B)

In the best of all possible worlds, you'll be able to ride it out until menopause, when your fibroids will begin to disappear on their own. If they are starting to grow or cause discomfort or irregular bleeding, however, it's time to explore the various treatment options.

TREATMENTS FOR FIBROIDS

"Does this mean I have to have a hysterectomy?" is the most common response I get when I tell a patient she has fibroids.

"Not at all," I reassure her. There are a number of options—both medical and surgical—available; the important thing is to find one that you feel most comfortable with.

Hormones and Medications

LOW-DOSE ORAL CONTRACEPTIVES. Because fibroids are hormonally sensitive, keeping the amount of oestrogen and progesterone they are exposed to in constant balance may limit their growth. You still need to be monitored, however, because sometimes fibroids grow in spite of birth control pills. Oral contraceptives also reduce the symptoms of fibroids by making your periods lighter and less crampy, thereby correcting your anaemia.

NATURAL PROGESTERONE. Using 5 percent progesterone cream or taking oral micronized progesterone in the second half of your cycle, beginning on day 10 and stopping when you get your period, can help with heavy bleeding from fibroids. Fibroids are a manifestation of oestrogen dominance. By counteracting the effects of oestrogen with progesterone, you can often relieve heavy bleeding.

DEPO-PROVERA. Synthetic progestogens like Provera have traditionally been used to control fibroids because they also oppose excess oestrogen. Because of its side effects, such as acne, weight gain, and migraines, Depo-Provera may be difficult to tolerate.

GONADOTROPIN-RELEASING HORMONE (GNRH) AGONISTS. Drugs such as Zoladex, and Synarel suppress FSH and LH production in the pituitary, so the ovaries never get the message to release oestrogen. Because these drugs diminish circulating oestrogen levels so dramatically, basically putting you into menopause, they are extremely effective at shrinking fibroids and controlling their symptoms. The problem is that they cause menopausal side effects, including hot flushes in 91 percent of women, sleep and mood disorders in 51 percent, joint pain, leg cramps, and vaginal dryness. If the symptoms become severe, we can add back oestrogen and progesterone in small doses. But by far the most serious side effect is loss of bone density: taking GnRH agonists for six months reduces your bone density by 5 to 8 percent, so I prefer not to prescribe them long-term.

If a patient's uterus has grown larger than the size of a twelve-week pregnancy because of fibroids, I may prescribe GnRH agonists for three months prior to surgery. The drugs can shrink fibroids 30 to 50 percent, making it possible to perform a less invasive vaginal or laparoscopic procedure rather than abdominal surgery. A three-month course of GnRH agonists prior to surgery is also great for building up the blood count of patients who are anaemic because of the heavy bleeding their fibroids have caused.

Surgery

MYOMECTOMY. Given the option, I would much rather perform a myomectomy, in which I remove only the fibroids and leave the uterus, than a hysterectomy. Understandably, most of my patients agree with me. When a woman still wants to have children, it is a wonderful choice, although a cesarean section may later be necessary if the integrity of the uterine wall has been compromised by the surgery. The only downside is that in 27 percent of cases, fibroids recur within ten years of the procedure.

Nevertheless, many women opt for a myomectomy because even if they face the prospect of a recurrence, the surgery itself is generally less radical than a hysterectomy. If the fibroid isn't too large and is on the outside surface of the uterus, I can remove it laparoscopically (see "Operating Options" box). If it is on the inside surface and isn't too big, I can vaginally shave the fibroid using a hysteroscope to visualize the interior of the uterus. But if the fibroid is extremely large and on the outside of the uterus or has penetrated the uterine wall, I may need to perform abdominal surgery (laparotomy) to get it out. In the rare case when a woman has multiple fibroids that encompass her entire uterus, a hysterectomy may be preferable to a myomectomy.

HYSTERECTOMY. Historically, hysterectomy has been the recommended treatment for fibroids. Even today fibroids account for one-third of the approximately 567,000 hysterectomies performed in the United States each year. Because there are so many alternatives to hysterectomies now available, however, I find myself performing them less and less often for fibroids. When I do, I leave the cervix, to preserve sexual function and prevent prolapse of the bladder and rectum. I also leave the ovaries, so the patient will not go through menapause. *Regardless of whether or nor the cervix has been removed, patients still need annual smear tests after hysterectomy.*

To my mind, hysterectomy is the last option for treating fibroids, but in some cases there may be no alternative. If your gynaecologist recommends a hysterectomy but you're uncomfortable with the idea, insist that he or she review all possible alternatives with you. If your doctor is unwilling to offer another option or isn't listening to your concerns, get a second opinion.

OPERATING OPTIONS

There are three main approaches for performing gynaecologic surgery:

Laparotomy, the traditional way, requires an abdominal incision. It involves general anaesthesia, several days in the hospital, a longer recovery period, and an incisional scar.

Laparoscopic surgery, or microsurgery, has been a major breakthrough. A small incision is made right below the navel and a camera is inserted so that the surgeon can view the interior of the abdomen. Two or three tiny incisions are made elsewhere, through which the doctor inserts tools and performs the procedure. Although the patient is anaesthetized, she can generally go home on the same day, will only have a few plasters on her belly, will experience little pain, and can get up and move around sooner than if she'd had a laparotomy.

Vaginal surgery is, for certain conditions, another excellent alternative to abdominal surgery. Performed under general anaesthetic, it leaves a scar high up in the vagina and allows the patient to leave the hospital sooner and experience a quicker, less painful recovery than if she'd had an abdominal incision.

EMBOLIZATION. A relatively new technique, *thromboembolization* or *uterine artery embolization* involves injecting sand-sized plastic particles into the uterine artery. Because this cuts off the blood supply to the fibroids, they shrink, usually by about 50 percent. Symptoms such as pelvic pain and heavy menstrual bleeding should diminish. The uterus remains healthy because it receives blood from many other sources.

The advantage of embolization is that it is minimally invasive and involves a shorter recovery time than hysterectomy, although you may experience severe cramping for the first 24 hours. You can usually leave the hospital on the same day or the next day and be back to full activity in a week or two. There is no guarantee that your fertility won't be impaired, however, so if you're thinking of getting pregnant, I wouldn't recommend embolization. It is also not yet widely available and studies of its effectiveness are under way.

IS AN ENDOMETRIAL POLYP THE SAME AS A FIBROID?

Endometrial polyps are not the same as fibroids. Polyps are soft, benign tumors of the uterine lining present in one out of four women. They can appear as growths attached to the inner lining of the uterus or can be attached to a stalk hanging down into the uterine cavity, even protruding through the cervix. In 18 percent of premenopausal women and 29 percent of postmenopausal women who report abnormal bleeding, uterine polyps are the root of the problem. If they are causing symptoms such as abnormal bleeding, polyps need to be removed by a D&C and inspected by a pathologist. In 0.5 percent of cases they are cancerous.

MYOLYSIS/CRYOMYOLYSIS. These two laparoscopic procedures are in development and could end up transforming the landscape of fibroid treatment if they prove reliable. Myolysis involves using needles or a laser to transmit electricity, which shrinks the blood vessels feeding the fibroid. Cryomyolysis involves using a freezing probe to the same effect. Both are relatively simple operations, requiring little recovery time. The only potential problem may be regrowth of the fibroid.

ADENOMYOSIS

Another uterine problem that I see in my perimenopausal patients is adenomyosis, which occurs when bits of endometrial tissue that normally lines the uterus are found embedded in the uterine wall. This condition is common in women who have had many children. The symptoms are similar to those of fibroids: heavy, painful periods and a gradually enlarging, tender uterus. Adenomyosis frequently occurs in women who also have fibroids, suggesting that some women may have a predisposition for abnormal growths of the uterine lining.

The symptoms of adenomyosis can be severe. Take Ellen, for example, a 46-year-old patient of mine. When she was 38, I did a myomectomy, removing a submucosal fibroid that we thought could have been hindering her attempts to get pregnant. Unfortunately, her infertility persisted. When she was 43, I removed an endometrial polyp. Now she was complaining of extremely heavy periods and such incredible pain that she had actually passed out once in a cinema. "Sometimes it's so bad I just curl up in a ball on the floor and cry."

Upon examination, her uterus felt enlarged—about the size of an eight-week pregnancy—boggy, and soft. It was also tipped backward (*retroverted*). Her sonogram didn't show any fibroids but did show adenomyosis. Because she was no longer trying to get pregnant, I performed a hysterectomy, the treatment of choice for patients with symptomatic adenomyosis, but I left her ovaries so she wouldn't go through menopause.

ENDOMETRIOSIS

Yvette first came to me when she was 38 years old. Totally focused on her career as a producer at one of the network news shows, she had never married, although she practiced what she called "serial monogamy," moving from one long-term relationship to the next. When I asked her what brought her to see me, she told me she'd been having horrendous cramps, nausea, and vomiting before and during her period. "It's so bad I have to stay home from work sometimes, and I really can't afford to miss any time."

"Of course not," I replied. "Are you sexually active?"

"Yes," she answered, "although not as much as we'd like. It's gotten really painful."

I took a medical history and discovered that Yvette had been put on birth control pills at age 16 to regulate her extremely painful periods. She had used them on and off for the next two decades but had been off them for the past two years. "Has anyone ever discussed the possibility of endometriosis with you?" I asked.

"No," she replied.

I proceeded to explain the condition and told her that I thought it might be the root of her problem.

Endometriosis is one of the great mysteries in women's health. No one knows for sure why it occurs or even how frequently it occurs. What we do know is that it's a chronic disease that can affect you at any time during your childbearing years. In perimenopause, your symptoms may flare up in response to your fluctuating hormone levels. Or if you are asymptomatic, you may discover that you have endometriosis during a surgical procedure for another gynaecologic problem.

Endometriosis occurs when bits of endometrial tissue—tissue from the inside of your uterus—make their way out of the uterus and attach themselves to other internal parts of your body. There they sit, still acting like uterine tissue, swelling and bleeding on a monthly cycle, in many cases causing great pain.

Endometriosis is usually found in the pelvic cavity—on the outside of the uterus, the ovaries, the Fallopian tubes, the bladder, and the rectum. This has led researchers to speculate that it is caused by reverse menstruation, that is, when the uterus contracts to expel its lining through the vagina each month, a little bit of tissue flows backward through the Fallopian tubes into the pelvic cavity, where it attaches to nearby structures. But endometriosis has also been diagnosed under the skin, in the lungs, even in the brain! This suggests an alternate pathway of transmission, either through the blood or the lymphatic system, although no one has been able to prove such theories. There's also the notion that tissue anywhere in the body has the potential to change into any other type of tissue, so theoretically endometriosis could result from the spontaneous transformation of normal epithelial tissue into endometrial tissue.

Endometriosis is a democratic disease, affecting women of all races and socioeconomic levels. Some data suggest that almost 100 percent of women will have endometriosis at some time in their reproductive lives. But because endometriosis can only be definitively diagnosed through laparoscopic surgery—it usually looks like black tobacco stains on tissue that is normally pink, although it can also be red or even invisible if it's implanted beneath the surface—we have no way of knowing the exact incidence. We do know that it is especially prevalent among adolescents: among women under age 20, 47 to 65 percent who complain of chronic pelvic pain or painful periods have endometriosis.

So why doesn't every woman have symptoms of endometriosis? Because most cases resolve on their own without causing undue discomfort, either because the body heals itself or because the women go on birth control pills or get pregnant, thereby stopping the cycle of inflammation. Women whose endometriosis doesn't go away by itself may have some kind of immunological deficiency. Their bodies

Say "No" to Soy

Throughout this book I've been touting the benefits of soy for relieving peri-menopausal symptoms. But, of course, there's an exception to every rule. Endometriosis is that exception. Rates of endometriosis among different races and ethnic groups are basically the same except for Japanese women, who experience symptoms twice as frequently. Why? For the same reason they have fewer hot flushes: because they eat a lot of soy products. Because endometriosis gets worse when oestrogen levels are high, you should avoid soy and other foods and herbs that contain phytoestrogens if you suffer from this condition.

mistake the endometriosis lesion for a foreign invader, so they mount a massive attack response. The chemicals released during this attack—prostaglandins, histamines, free radicals, and other toxic substances—further damage the tissue, leading to the formation of painful, fibrous scars and adhesions.

Nevertheless, endometriosis is on the rise. While part of the reason is that doctors are gaining more awareness of the problem and more are likely to diagnose it as laparoscopic procedures become more common, part may also do with our modern lifestyle. In the good old days, women spent most of their reproductive years pregnant or nursing, and therefore not menstruating. They had fewer periods over the course of their lives, giving their endometrial tissue less chance to escape the uterus and, if it did, less opportunity to flare up and cause symptoms.

If you were to come to me complaining of chronic pelvic pain, I'd ask you a series of questions to determine whether endometriosis might be the cause. If the pain is cyclical, that's a tip-off. But that could also indicate PMS. The difference is that PMS symptoms are concentrated in the week or so before your period starts but end when you begin to bleed. Endometriosis intensifies throughout your period.

I'd also ask whether you've experienced any abnormal bleeding, pain on intercourse, constipation, or fertility problems. As I discussed in Chapter 7, endometriosis can cause infertility; indeed, at least 25 percent of infertile women have endometriosis. Other cyclic symptoms, such as headaches, coughing, diarrhoea, or irritation of the urinary tract, can indicate distant locations where endometrial tissue may have settled.

Just because you have a lot of pain doesn't mean you have a severe case of endometriosis. One of the many strange things about this condition is that the severity of the symptoms has nothing whatsoever to do with the extent of the disease. You could be in excruciating agony each month and have one tiny spot. Or you could have spots all over your abdominal cavity and feel perfectly fine.

All of this makes it very difficult to diagnose endometriosis without taking a look inside the pelvic cavity. Although I would rather avoid putting my patients through surgery unless absolutely necessary, in cases when I suspect severe endometriosis, it may be the wisest option. At the same time as I'm confirming my suspicion, I can eliminate as much of the aberrant tissue as possible.

I explained this to Yvette. "You could go back on birth control pills, but because your symptoms are so severe and you've been having them since you were a teenager, I suspect your endometriosis is quite advanced. It would probably be best for me to look inside your pelvis and make a diagnosis. If I do see endometriosis, I can laser off as much as possible during surgery."

"Do I have to decide now, or can I think about it for a few days?"

"Take all the time you need," I said. "Just call me when you've made up your mind."

At the end of the week, Yvette called back and scheduled the operation. I performed laparoscopic surgery and found endometriosis all over her pelvic cavity and adhesions between her large intestine and left ovary. I lasered all the lesions I could see and released all of her adhesions. After surgery I put her on a GnRH agonist called Zoladex for six months. Two months later she was suffering such bad hot flushes that we decided to add back hormones. After the six-month course, I put her on birth control pills and for a while everything seemed fine.

Three years later, still on oral contraceptives, Yvette's symptoms returned. "Dr. Corio, I can't take it! It's not just the cramps and back pain, but I get the worst diarrhoea every time I even taste food before and during my period. What can I do?"

It looked as if Yvette's endometriosis was back. Just to be sure,

however, I sent her for an MRI to rule out any gastrointestinal problems that might be causing her spastic colon. The results were negative. "Excess insulin can aggravate your GI tract," I explained, "so
certain dietary changes may help relieve your diarrhoea. I'd like you to
lower your intake of high-gylcemic carbohydrates such as potatoes,
bread, carrots, and rice, and increase your intake of fatty acids such as
those found in fish. Cut out all caffeine and tyramine, a chemical
found in cheese, wine, and red meat."

"And will that help my menstrual symptoms as well?" she asked.

"It may. If not, we can do another laparoscopy or try more Depo-
Lupron," I told her.

"How many times will I need to go through this?" she moaned.

"That I can't tell you, but let's hope not a lot. Once you hit
menopause and your tissues are no longer exposed to high levels of
oestrogen, your symptoms should improve. So we'll just take it one
day at a time and do whatever we need to do to make you feel better
between now and then."

Treatments for Endometriosis

Fortunately, if you do have endometriosis, there are a number of options for treating your pain. The first four items in the following sections relieve symptoms in 92 percent of cases. The important thing is
to work closely with your doctor to find a treatment that you can live
with long-term, because endometriosis is a chronic condition that
doesn't resolve completely until menopause.

PREGNANCY. If the time is right, go for it! Because your hormone
levels are constant and you're not menstruating, getting pregnant is an
extremely effective way to relieve your endometriosis symptoms.

NONSTEROIDAL ANTI–INFLAMMATORY DRUGS (NSAIDs). If pregnancy isn't in the cards, taking over-the-counter painkillers such as aspirin, ibuprofen (Advil, Neurofen), or naproxen sodium (Naprosyn),
beginning a week before you expect your period *(preloading)* and continuing until you stop bleeding, is the first approach to control symptoms of endometriosis.

LOW-DOSE ORAL CONTRACEPTIVES. If you don't find NSAIDs to
be strong enough, we might try low-dose birth control pills next, as

they relieve pain in 75 to 89 percent of cases. I say low dose—35 mcg oestradiol or less—because too much oestrogen may make your condition worse. If in spite of birth control pills your symptoms are still present and only somewhat abated, I might suggest continuous low-dose pills, breaking only once every three months.

NORETHISTERONE. For those who can't take birth control pills, or if birth control pills aren't helping matters, a daily 5 mg dose of a progestogen called norethisterone may do the trick. In one recent study, 49 out of 52 women reported that norethisterone relieved the pain caused by their endometriosis. Side effects include weight gain, depression, breast tenderness, and breakthrough bleeding.

NATURAL PROGESTERONE. Some patients who suffer endometriosis don't want to take synthetic hormones such as the Pill or norethisterone. In these cases, I prescribe oral micronized progesterone or 5 percent progesterone cream during the second half of the menstrual cycle.

LAPAROSCOPIC SURGERY. If none of the previously mentioned treatments alleviates your pain, the next step is laparoscopic surgery. Through a tiny opening under the navel, I insert a scope to look at your pelvic organs. Through other tiny openings I can then insert instruments to burn off any endometriosis lesions I can find. If I see an endometrioma—an ovarian "chocolate cyst" caused by endometriosis—I can remove it at the same time. Surgery for endometriosis is not a cure. It can relieve your symptoms for a time or reduce their severity to the point where we can control them with medication, but once you have endometriosis, you may not find relief until menopause.

DANAZOL. A modified androgen (male sex hormone), danazol controls endometriosis symptoms by suppressing oestrogen. Unfortunately, it can also cause hair growth, weight gain, and oily skin. In extremely high doses it can even make your voice deeper. I don't use this drug anymore, as there are more effective ones available that don't have such side effects.

GONADOTROPIN-RELEASING HORMONE (GNRH) AGONISTS. As described on page 288, GnRH agonists make your ovaries stop producing oestrogen, sending you into what we call chemical menopause. To minimize their negative effect on bone density, I generally prescribe GnRH agonists to treat endometriosis for six months. When your symptoms are under control, I would then switch you to a low-dose birth control pill for maintenance and to restore your bone density.

HYSTERECTOMY/OOPHORECTOMY. If all else fails and fertility is not an issue, removal of the ovaries is a way to dramatically curtail oestrogen production and treat endometriosis. If you've reached this stage, you've usually suffered severe endometriosis for many years. During the procedure I might find that your uterus and Fallopian tubes are so badly scarred that it makes sense to remove them as well. At the same time, I can destroy any lesions I see elsewhere in your pelvic cavity. After surgery, we can try oestrogen replacement therapy for a few months to make sure it doesn't stimulate a recurrence; if it does, you may only be able to take progesterone.

UTERINE CANCER

Uterine or endometrial cancer is usually considered to be a disease affecting postmenopausal women, but one-fourth of all cases occur in women who are still menstruating. It's the fourth most common cancer in women, with a lifetime risk of 2 to 3 percent. Like breast, ovarian, and colon cancer, it is provoked when your body makes a lot of oestrogen but not enough progesterone to balance it. Prolonged exposure to high levels of unopposed oestrogen causes your endometrial cells to proliferate *(endometrial hyperplasia)*. The more they reproduce, the greater the chance a mutation will occur that can turn into cancer.

Fortunately, uterine cancer is highly curable, with a five-year survival rate of 80 to 85 percent, as most cases can be diagnosed at an early stage. In a postmenopausal woman, any bleeding after one year of stopping her period is cause for concern. In a perimenopausal woman, *any change in bleeding pattern* is a warning sign. Heavy, frequent, or long periods are a red flag indicating high levels of unopposed oestrogen. That's why I always perform an endometrial biopsy, or Pipelle, whenever a patient over age 35 reports periods closer than twenty-one days apart and/or bleeding heavier or longer than usual, or is changing her tampon or pad more than once an hour.

By sampling the endometrium—the lining of the uterus that is shed every month—with a Pipelle, I can diagnose most cases of hyperplasia and determine how serious it is. A sonohysterogram may pick up hyperplasia, and for both perimenopausal and postmenopausal women, a transvaginal sonogram to check for thickening of the endometrial lining is also a useful screening tool. The thicker the lining, the worse the prognosis.

I often see endometrial hyperplasia in perimenopausal patients with anovulatory cycles, who are pumping out excess unopposed oestrogen. In those cases, taking natural progesterone or Provera for the last fourteen days of every cycle for three months can counterbalance the oestrogen and cause the tissue to revert to normal. After two months off the progestogen, I do another Pipelle to make sure the hyperplasia has resolved.

In some cases, however, the cells have begun to mutate. This condition is known as *atypical* hyperplasia and in approximately 25 percent of cases will turn into cancer. After the initial biopsy I schedule a D&C (dilation and curettage), in which I scrape out most of the uterine lining. A pathologist then examines the tissue and determines whether the hyperplasia is localized or whether there is an underlying malignancy. If cancer is diagnosed, the only option is a total hysterectomy, removing both ovaries, both Fallopian tubes, and the cervix as well.

At age 50, Rita was in perimenopause. She had been experiencing irregular periods for more than a year. When she came to see me, she told me she hadn't bled in three months and then had an extremely heavy period that was still going on. I tried to do a Pipelle, but her cervix was stenotic—scarred, perhaps because of a prior abortion—and difficult to penetrate. Instead, I scheduled her for a D&C, which showed severe atypical hyperplasia. I put her on Provera every day with the idea that after three months I'd perform another D&C to see whether the hyperplasia had resolved. Unfortunately, she continued to bleed through the Provera, indicating to me that something was seriously amiss. Together we decided she should have a hysterectomy. It turned out to be the right choice, as she had full-fledged uterine cancer.

Fortunately, there are many ways to prevent uterine cancer. First, have regular gynaecologic exams and report any change in your bleeding pattern to your doctor. Second, have regular physicals and make

RISK FACTORS FOR UTERINE CANCER

Many of the risk factors for uterine cancer are similar to those for breast cancer, as both types of tumor grow in response to stimulation by endogenous oestrogen (the oestrogen your body produces).

AGE. Ninety-five percent of cases of uterine cancer occur in women over age 40. Part of the reason is that older women tend to be heavier and have higher rates of hypertension and diabetes. There is also the fact that older cells are more prone to mutation than younger ones, making age an independent risk factor in all kinds of cancer.

PERIMENOPAUSE. It's no coincidence that the rate of endometrial cancer begins to rise as women enter perimenopause. In perimenopause, you start experiencing anovulatory and irregular cycles, which leave you exposed to unopposed oestrogen.

EARLY MENARCHE/LATE MENOPAUSE. The longer you are exposed to oestrogen, the greater chance there is of adversely stimulating your endometrial tissue. If your periods stop after age 54, you qualify as having a late menopause.

POLYCYSTIC OVARIES. Six percent of women have a condition called polycystic ovaries, in which their ovaries produce multiple follicular cysts but do not ovulate. Because these women never experience the luteal phase of their cycle, they are exposed to a high degree of unopposed oestrogen, which increases their risk of uterine cancer. After childbearing—usually accomplished through fertility drugs—I advise continuing on birth control pills until menopause or having a hysterectomy with removal of ovaries to prevent any future malignancy.

INFERTILITY. Women who have experienced infertility because of anovulation are at an increased risk of developing all types of oestrogen-dependent cancers.

sure to keep hypertension and/or diabetes under control. Third, although I sound like a broken record, I'll say it again: keep your weight under control through diet and exercise, as less body fat means less production of endogenous oestrogen. A high-fiber, low-fat diet rich in fruit, vegetables, and whole grains will help you fight the fat and reduce your risk of endometrial cancer. In addition to helping control

NO CHILDREN. Pregnancy protects you from oestrogen-dependent malignancies because for nine months your hormone levels are balanced. Not having any children means you have been exposed to the unopposed oestrogen of the follicular phase of the menstrual cycle more often than women who have had children and breastfed them.

OBESITY. Because fat cells produce oestrogen, overweight women—particularly those with a high waist-hip ratio—are at a high risk of endometrial cancer. And the heavier you are, the greater your chance of developing it. Being more than 50 pounds overweight is associated with a tenfold increase in risk.

DIABETES AND HYPERTENSION. Both of these conditions are independent risk factors for uterine cancer.

FAMILY HISTORY OF ENDOMETRIAL OR COLON CANCER. As with many cancers, there is a genetic component to uterine cancer. If you have a first-degree relative who had uterine cancer, your risk is tripled; if you have a first-degree relative with colon cancer, your risk is doubled.

RACE. Black women are at greater risk than white women for uterine cancer, and when they get it, they tend to fare much more poorly. The increased incidence seems to be because black women are more likely to be obese and to have hypertension and diabetes. The poorer prognosis has to do with other factors. One is that uterine cancer is not always caught as early in black women, who may not see their gynaecologists as often as white women. Another is that black women tend to carry a mutation in gene p53 twice as often as white women, and that gene has been associated with a decreased risk of survival.

your weight, fiber keeps your oestrogen level down by increasing oestrogen elimination through your bowels.

Boosting your soy and flaxseed consumption also decreases the risk of uterine cancer. Endogenous oestrogen signals endometrial cells to reproduce. When phytoestrogens are competing for the oestrogen receptor sites on uterine cell membranes, less endogenous oestrogen

---

WILL TAKING HORMONES OR TAMOXIFEN GIVE ME UTERINE CANCER?

This is an extremely difficult question. Certainly the unopposed oestrogen prescribed in the early days of hormone replacement therapy did give women endometrial cancer. That's why I never give a patient unopposed oestrogen unless she no longer has a uterus. There is still quite a lot of debate about whether or not the combined oestrogen and progesterone used today puts you at risk for uterine cancer, however. The latest studies show that hormone replacement therapy decreases your risk of uterine cancer to less than that of a postmenopausal woman who never took hormones.

There's no question that tamoxifen increases your risk of uterine cancer by two to three times. There is controversy, however, about what type of endometrial cancer it causes. Some studies have found it to be a low-grade, easily treatable one if it's picked up at an early stage. Other studies have found it to be a more aggressive type of tumor with a worse prognosis. So if you're taking this drug, be sure not to miss your regular gynaecologic exams, and report any abnormal bleeding, spotting, or other symptoms to your doctor.

---

reaches the cell surface, thereby reducing the proliferation of uterine tissue. Phytoestrogens also increase your sex hormone binding globulin (SHBG) levels, consequently lowering your circulating oestrogen.

To regulate abnormal perimenopausal bleeding and keep your endometrial tissue healthy, you can take natural progesterone or progestogen supplements. Another excellent option is the Pill: taking oral contraceptives for only one year reduces your risk of endometrial cancer by 50 percent, and the benefit lasts up to fifteen years after you stop taking the Pill.

SALLY—A PERIMENOPAUSAL OVARIAN CYST

At her annual exam a year ago Sally, a 47-year-old patient, mentioned that she was experiencing irregular periods. We had a long talk about perimenopause and I listed the other symptoms she might experience while her hormones were in flux. Sure enough, at this year's exam she told me she had vaginal dryness, itchy skin, hot flushes, and no sex drive to speak of.

"Aren't you glad we had that discussion last year?" I asked. "Are your periods still all over the place?"

"Yes," she replied. "But what I really want to talk with you about is this pain I've developed recently." She pointed to the right lower portion of her pelvis.

"How long have you been feeling it?" I asked.

"About a month."

"Is it a sharp pain?"

"More like a dull pressure."

"Well, let's begin the exam and see what we find." As I prepared and she got comfortable on the table, we chatted about her children—two boys, ages 13 and 15, whom I'd delivered. Before they were born, Sally had been an organizer for the teachers union; she was now thinking about going back to some kind of community work.

"Dr. Corio, is something wrong?" Sally asked after a pause in our conversation. "You've stopped talking, and you never stop talking."

Indeed, as I was performing her pelvic exam, I felt a mass in the cul-de-sac behind her uterus and in front of her rectum. "Your right ovary is enlarged," I told her. "Let's have you go for a sonogram to see if we can diagnose what's going on."

Sally had a transvaginal sonogram and sure enough, her right ovary was about three times the size of normal. The cause appeared to be what we call a "chocolate cyst," or *endometrioma,* filled with old blood and menstrual detritus, which is characteristic of endometriosis.

I explained to Sally that a cyst of this type and size wasn't going to go away by itself. I would have to remove it surgically.

"Fine," said Sally. "The sooner the better."

Preoperatively Sally met me in my office, where we talked further about her upcoming procedure. "Although I expect your cyst will turn out to be benign, there's always the chance I could discover something cancerous. I'm going to need your permission to do whatever I need to do to take care of this."

"Meaning?" she asked.

"In the best of all possible worlds, I'll be able to remove the cyst and leave your ovary intact. But if the whole ovary is involved, I'll need to remove it entirely and perhaps your right Fallopian tube, too.

The tissue will be examined by a pathologist while you're under anesthetic. If, God forbid, it turns out to be malignant—"

"You mean cancer, right?" she interrupted.

"Yes, cancer," I replied. "In that case I'm going to have to take samples from other parts of your pelvis to determine how much it has spread, in a process called staging. Frankly, since you don't want any more children, I'd recommend a hysterectomy if we're talking cancer."

"Whew," Sally replied, her eyes widening. "That's a biggie. But I trust your judgment. You've seen me through thick and thin over the years, and I know you'll do whatever you think is best for me."

Two weeks later Sally had her operation. Because of the size of the cyst, I made an abdominal incision. The entire ovary was involved, so I removed both it and the right Fallopian tube. Her left ovary and Fallopian tube and her uterus looked fine, and there were no other signs of endometriosis. The pathologist confirmed that the tumor was a benign endometrioma.

After surgery, I put Sally on birth control pills to prevent future endometriosis and ovarian cysts, as well as to treat her perimenopausal symptoms. "Dr. Corio," she said at her follow-up visit three months later, "I have to tell you, I haven't felt this good in over two years!"

OVARIAN CYSTS

Whenever I tell a patient she has an ovarian cyst, I can feel the anxiety level in the room skyrocket. There seems to be a lot of confusion about cysts, and I constantly have to remind my patients that *most cysts are not cancerous.* These abnormal ovarian growths may occasionally require surgical intervention, as Sally's did, but they are often perfectly innocuous.

Ovarian cysts are extremely common and extremely varied, but overall they can be grouped into two categories. *Functional* cysts are fluid-filled sacs that respond to fluctuations in hormone levels. Newborn baby girls, for example, often have small cysts on their ovaries because of the high amounts of oestrogen they were exposed to in utero. These generally regress during the first few months of life. Later on, once menstruation begins, cysts may appear when a follicle fails to produce a mature egg and fills up with fluid instead *(follicle cyst)* or after a mature egg is released and the corpus luteum continues to grow instead of collapsing *(corpus luteum cyst)*. In both these cases the cysts are usually reabsorbed after a menstrual cycle, when oestrogen and progesterone levels go down.

Most women never know they have functional cysts unless their doctor notices them during a pelvic exam. I like to perform a transvaginal sonogram when I suspect a cyst to confirm my diagnosis and determine the size and quality of the growth. If the cyst is less than 6 cm in diameter, moves around easily, is only on one side of the ovary, and isn't causing any pain or fluid buildup in the pelvis, there's a 70 percent chance it will resolve on its own. In this case, I have my patient come back in four to six weeks, after a period, and we do another sonogram.

If the cyst is still there I frequently recommend oral contraceptives, which usually shrink the cyst by preventing ovulation and controlling the amount of hormones in the system. Occasionally a functional cyst will grow big enough to cause discomfort and, if it ruptures or twists, a sharp pain. Very rarely, a large cyst that does not respond to birth control pills will have to be removed surgically. In this case, it may turn out to be a *nonfunctional* cyst, or one that doesn't go away on its own in response to the ebb and flow of hormone levels. Sally's endometrioma is a single example of a nonfunctional cyst, but there are any number of other types.

Recently a patient came to me in agony—she had tremendous pain not only in her right lower pelvis but also in her legs. She was running a high fever, had lost her appetite, and was totally exhausted. On transvaginal sonogram, I saw she had an 8 cm cyst on her right ovary that was leaking into her pelvic cavity. I performed surgery and was able to remove the leaking cyst, clean out the spilled fluid, and preserve her ovary.

If a nonfunctional cyst is more than 6 cm in diameter or if it appears solid or complex, isn't freely mobile, or is accompanied by fluid in the abdomen *(ascites)*, it needs to be investigated surgically. This is a very common procedure; in fact, approximately 289,000 women a year are hospitalized in the United States because of ovarian growths. Depending on the size of the growth and what it looks like on the sonogram, I perform either a laparoscopy or a laparotomy (see page 290).

If the growth appears benign, then I remove it; if multiple growths are present, I may need to take out part or all of the ovary. In most cases this will not affect your fertility, as you only need a small piece—about the size of the last joint on your little finger—of a single ovary to produce eggs. During surgery I carefully inspect the other ovary as well.

For perimenopausal women who don't want any more children and whose risk of ovarian cancer is on the rise, it is sometimes wisest to remove the ovary or ovaries altogether. If both ovaries are removed, you may need to start hormone replacement therapy depending on your symptoms.

OVARIAN CANCER

Next to breast cancer, my patients fear ovarian cancer more than any other. It's not that ovarian cancer is particularly common—it's the fifth most common cancer among American women, affecting only 1 in 70. Rather, it's because ovarian cancer is so deadly that it kills more women than uterine and cervical cancer combined and has an overall five-year survival rate of less than 40 percent. Hearing of famous women such as Gilda Radner and Liz Tilberis, both of whom succumbed to ovarian cancer in their prime, only fuels women's anxiety.

What's scariest about ovarian cancer for me is that there are no specific symptoms, so we often don't catch it until it is advanced. For that reason, 75 to 85 percent of patients with ovarian cancer are not diagnosed until the disease has spread throughout their abdominal cavity, at which point the five-year survival rate is only 25 percent. By contrast, when ovarian cancer is caught in its early stages, the five-year survival rate is 80 to 95 percent. Unfortunately, there is no reliable screening test for early-stage ovarian cancer as there is with breast, uterine, and cervical cancers. The common signs—abdominal discomfort or pain; bloating due to excess fluid or large tumors: gastrointestinal complaints such as nausea, gas, a feeling of fullness, or constipation; and occasionally vaginal bleeding, urinary frequency, or pain upon urination—could be symptoms of a host of different diseases. In spite of all of the available technology, which I've outlined in the following sections, the best tool we have for early detection is still a thorough pelvic exam every six to twelve months.

TRANSVAGINAL SONOGRAM (TVS). A transvaginal sonogram can help your doctor detect early-stage ovarian cancer, although it is not

100 percent reliable. In TVS, the vaginal probe can get closer to the pelvic structures than a traditional pelvic sonogram can, allowing high-resolution imaging of the ovaries. I recommend a transvaginal sonogram every one to two years for women over age 40. If you have a family history of ovarian cancer or carry a mutated form of one of the BRCA genes (see pages 258–260), then you should have one every year starting at age 25.

DOPPLER SCANNING. Based on the principle that malignant tumors generate a lot of new blood-vessel growth, the Doppler scanner works by picking up areas with increased blood flow. Doppler scanning can help distinguish between large malignant and benign tumors but is not great for diagnosing small early-stage tumors.

CA-125. The CA (cancer antigen) 125 blood test is not a useful indicator for most perimenopausal women. A host of noncancerous conditions, including fibroids, benign ovarian tumors, liver disease, adenomyosis, endometriosis, pregnancy, and pelvic inflammatory disease (PID), can all give elevated (more than 35 U per ml) results. And 50 percent of patients with the earliest stage of ovarian cancer have CA-125 levels in the normal range. The only premenopausal women to whom I recommend the CA-125 test are those who have already had ovarian cancer, who carry a mutated BRCA gene, or who have a family history of ovarian cancer. They should have the test annually.

CIRCULATING LYSOPHOSPHATIDIC ACID (LPA). Hope is on the horizon that a more reliable screening test will be available in the near future. The best bet right now seems to be a test for circulating lysophosphatidic acid (LPA), a lipid that appears to promote the growth of cancer cells. A recent study that compared LPA and CA-125 in a small group of patients found that LPA identified 9 out of 10 with early-stage ovarian cancer, whereas CA-125 identified only 2 out of 9. LPA also correctly identified all 24 patients with cancer in the later stages, whereas CA-125 only detected 14 of the 24.

Protecting Yourself Against Ovarian Cancer

So how do you reduce your risk of ovarian cancer? The number-one way is to *see your gynaecologist regularly.* The only reliable way to detect

RISK FACTORS FOR OVARIAN CANCER

What causes ovarian cancer? Many of the same things that cause uterine and breast cancer because, like them, ovarian cancer is an oestrogen-dependent malignancy. Because none of the symptoms, such as pelvic pain or gastrointestinal discomfort, shouts ovarian cancer, your doctor ought to do a complete physical exam to rule out other potential causes. She or he should also take a thorough medical history to assess your risk of having the disease.

FEW OR NO CHILDREN. Each pregnancy protects you from excessive oestrogen exposure because you don't ovulate for nine months. A combined analysis of twelve studies found that one full-term pregnancy lowered the risk of ovarian cancer by 40 percent and each subsequent pregnancy lowered the risk by an additional 14 percent.

NOT BREASTFEEDING. Breastfeeding prolongs the period of anovulation for several more months, providing further protection against ovarian cancer.

OBESITY. Fat cells produce oestrogen. Therefore obesity increases your risk of ovarian cancer, just as it does for breast, uterine, and colon cancer.

POLYCYSTIC OVARIES. As I explained in my discussion of uterine cancer, women with polycystic ovaries are at an increased risk of developing oestrogen-dependent cancers.

INFERTILITY. There has been some concern that fertility drugs may cause ovarian cancer. The fact is, no association between fertility drugs and ovarian cancer has been identified; it's the infertility itself that's the problem. Women who can't get pregnant often experience ovulatory abnormalities that may

ovarian cancer at an early, treatable stage is for your doctor to feel an abnormality during a pelvic exam. I happen to have a high level of suspicion, and it has always served me well. Even though ovarian cancer is less common in younger women, I've picked it up in two different 23-year-olds during my career—neither one with a family history of breast or ovarian cancer—just by performing a routine pelvic exam. The number-two way is to *keep your weight down!* Other ways to reduce your risk include having lots of children and breastfeeding them, and taking oral contraceptives.

predispose their ovaries to becoming cancerous. Women who cannot get pregnant even after using fertility drugs are at an especially high risk.

FAMILY HISTORY. Women with one first-degree relative with ovarian cancer have a 5 percent lifetime risk of developing the disease; women with two or more first-degree relatives have a 7 percent risk.

BREAST CANCER GENES. Women who have multiple relatives with breast and/or ovarian cancer should be offered genetic counseling about the breast cancer genes, BRCA1 and BRCA2 (see page 258). A woman who has the BRCA1 mutation has a 55 percent chance of developing ovarian cancer by age 80; a woman who has the BRCA2 mutation has a 28 percent chance. If you carry one of these genes, you might consider a prophylactic oophorectomy once you've finished having children. You should also have a CA-125 blood test and transvaginal ultrasound annually, and a pelvic exam every six months.

BREAST CANCER BEFORE AGE 50. Because of the strong link between breast cancer and ovarian cancer, women diagnosed with breast cancer at an early age have a greater chance of developing ovarian cancer than do women in the general population.

AGE. Because of the cumulative effect of carcinogens and the increased likelihood that a cell will mutate as it gets older, the chance of an ovarian growth being cancerous increases from 13 percent in premenopausal women to 45 percent in postmenopausal women.

When you're on birth control pills, your ovaries are in a state of suspended animation—they don't ovulate and they produce only low levels of oestrogen. Basically, they just sit quietly in your pelvis. Women who have been on the Pill at any time in their lives have a 30 percent reduction of risk, whereas women who have taken the Pill for five years have a 50 percent reduction of risk. And the benefit lasts at least ten years after you stop. Even women with mutations in either BRCA gene can benefit: up to three years on the Pill can cut their risk by 20 percent; six or more years on the Pill can cut their risk by

60 percent. Women who have suffered infertility should also consider taking birth control pills for a few years, not to prevent pregnancy but to reduce their elevated risk of ovarian cancer.

An interesting article from a 1993 issue of the *Journal of the American Medical Association* reported that according to the Harvard University Nurses' Health Study, tubal ligation reduces the risk of ovarian cancer up to 80 percent. So does hysterectomy that preserves the ovaries, although not to such a great extent—only about 33 percent. It's not totally clear why these surgical procedures have such a benefit. One hypothesis is that surgery compromises the blood flow through the ovarian branches of the uterine arteries, resulting in decreased ovarian hormone production. Another is that blocking or removing the Fallopian tubes prevents potentially carcinogenic material from flowing up through the vagina and uterus, out the tubes to the ovaries.

A fascinating recent study suggests that among its many benefits, good old aspirin may also help prevent ovarian cancer. Taking aspirin at least 3 times a week for 6 months reduces your risk of ovarian cancer by 40 percent, and taking it at least 4 times a week for 5 years reduces your risk by 50 percent. Why? Probably because aspirin suppresses the inflammatory response, which may be a trigger for cancer.

Because ovarian cancer is so serious, it is treated extremely aggressively. This means total hysterectomy—ovaries, uterus, and Fallopian tubes all removed—and chemotherapy in all but the most localized cases. The benefits of radiotherapy are debatable. Even if cancer is present in only one ovary, I like to remove both because in 5 percent of cases there is cancer hidden in the other one. The only exception is in a young woman, in which case I try to salvage the uterus and, if possible, one ovary so she can still have a baby. One of the 23-year-olds I diagnosed, now age 29, recently underwent fertility treatments and is now pregnant with twins.

Although you shouldn't stay up nights worrying about ovarian cancer, in your perimenopausal years your risk does begin to increase, so you should do whatever you can to protect yourself. Make sure to have regular gynaecologic exams and *tell your doctor immediately if you experience any pelvic pain, persistent gastrointestinal symptoms, or unusual bleeding.* Until there's a reliable screening test available, we have to rely on the low-tech, old-fashioned method of catching this devilish disease: hands-on medical care and doctor-patient communication.

CERVICAL CANCER

Cervical cancer is not oestrogen related, and its incidence does not increase with age. It results from a sexually transmitted disease whose incidence peaks in women in their late teens and twenties. So why am I mentioning it here? Because *perimenopausal women who are not monogamous are at just as great a risk as young women.*

Cervical cancer is caused by human papillomavirus (HPV), also known as condyloma or venereal warts—a virus that you can catch at any time in your life. A virus of the lower genital tract, it is implicated in causing not only cervical cancer but vaginal, vulvar, and anal cancer as well. The fact of the matter is that as long as you have a cervix, you are at risk for cervical cancer. And if you have had multiple sex partners, began having sex at an early age, smoke, or have a history of herpes, your risk is increased.

HPV is the most common sexually transmitted viral infection in the United States, infecting 40 to 80 percent of adults and an estimated two-thirds of college women. So why don't more women have cervical cancer? Because the majority of women are able to mount an immune reaction strong enough to eradicate the infection. But in a small percentage of women in whom the infection does not regress, the disease can go on to cause *cervical dysplasia,* or precancer of the cervix. If you are over age 40 and test positive for HPV, it is likely that you have been harboring it for a long time without being able to fight it off, putting you at increased risk for cervical cancer.

Over seventy types of HPV exist, and some are more aggressive than others. Women who carry subtypes 6 and 11, for example, are likely to develop genital warts. Those who carry subtypes 16, 18, 31, and 45 are at especially high risk for cervical cancer.

Even though there is evidence that the incidence of cervical cancer is increasing, the death rate has plummeted over the past thirty years. Credit goes to the smear test, a widely used and effective screening tool, which has reduced cervical cancer deaths by 70 percent. Although a single smear test is far from 100 percent accurate—some estimate that it shows false-negative results 20 to 50 percent of the time—if you have it done annually, as all women over the age of 18 should, the cumulative result over several years is quite reliable.

In the traditional smear test, a long Q-tip–like stick is swabbed along the outside and inside of your cervix to pick up loose cells, which are then placed on a slide and sent to a laboratory for examination. The technicians who read the smears are trained to detect abnormal cells that might indicate cervical dysplasia. They can differentiate between low-grade or slow-progressing abnormalities and high-grade or aggressive ones, which are caused by different viral strains.

A new procedure called the ViroPap identifies the various types of HPV in order to help determine the risk of developing cervical cancer. It has been suggested that the ViroPap test be available to all women age 40 and up because of their increased risk of cervical cancer if they test positive for HPV.

The biggest news on the smear front is the development of a new-and-improved smear called ThinPrep. In one recent comparison, the regular smear, in which the cells from the swab are wiped directly onto a slide, where they can bunch up on top of each other, had a false-negative rate of 5.6 percent, meaning it misses abnormalities in 1 out of 18 cases. The ThinPrep, in which cells collected by a spiral swab and a plastic spatula are swirled in a liquid and then applied to a slide in a thin layer, had a false-negative rate of only 2.2 percent. In another, the conventional smear test detected only 77.8 percent of high-grade squamous intraepithelial lesions (HSIL)—the worst kind of cancer— and 90.9 percent of carcinomas, whereas the ThinPrep detected 92.9 percent of HSIL and 100 percent of carcinomas.

Once you've been exposed to HPV, no matter what age you are, you should have smear tests religiously every six months for the rest of your life. And if you've been fortunate enough not to contract HPV, continue to have yearly smear tests. To avoid future infection, use condoms with a spermicide containing nonoxyl-9, but realize that this does not provide complete protection.

COLON CANCER

I've been repeatedly shocked by how uninformed my perimenopausal patients are about colon cancer, and I am now on a personal campaign to bring it to their awareness. After lung and breast cancer, colon cancer is the third leading cause of cancer deaths among women in the United States, causing approximately 30,000 deaths annually. Although

ANAEMIA—AN OFTEN OVERLOOKED SIGN

All too frequently, anaemia in perimenopausal women is automatically chalked up to excessive menstrual bleeding. But it could very well be caused by a gastrointestinal problem—an ulcer, tumor, polyp, or haemorrhoids. I routinely send any patient over age 40 with a haemoglobin count under 10 or with any other abdominal symptoms for a full gastrointestinal evaluation.

its incidence increases significantly after menopause, it's important to learn the symptoms, begin regular screening, and modify your risk factors in your perimenopausal years, because the earlier you catch colon cancer, the better your chances of survival.

People often get into trouble with colon cancer because they either haven't paid attention to the symptoms or are too shy to talk about them with their doctor. The warning signs include blood in the stool—either bright red blood coming out of the rectum, or blackened stool when you're not taking iron or Pepto-Bismol—gradually worsening constipation or alternating constipation and diarrhoea, feeling that your bowel is never completely empty, lower abdominal pain, and fatigue. Understandably, these complaints can easily be mistaken for haemorrhoids or a passing digestive problem. *If you are experiencing any of these symptoms for more than a week or two, see your doctor immediately,* because colon cancer often doesn't cause discomfort until it's very advanced.

Colon cancer usually develops slowly when a polyp—a normally benign growth that looks much like a skin tag—transforms into a malignancy over five to ten years. This gives us a large window in which to catch and excise any suspicious growths. Fortunately, colon cancer can be cured in 92 percent of cases if it is diagnosed early. Unfortunately, if colon cancer isn't detected until it is advanced, the five-year survival rate is only 8 percent. For this reason, it's crucial that you be screened on a regular basis.

There are five major screening tools for colon cancer, and together they provide a highly effective means of detecting the disease in its early stage.

RISK FACTORS FOR COLON CANCER

Although everyone is at risk for colon cancer, certain medical, genetic, and lifestyle conditions up the ante.

PERSONAL OR FAMILY HISTORY OF POLYPS. There's a 30 to 50 percent chance that if you have one polyp, you will have multiple polyps. Because there's a 5 percent chance that each polyp can become malignant, if you have a personal history of polyps, your risk could be significantly increased. Women who have a hereditary condition called *inherited polyposis syndrome* make lots of polyps and are at especially high risk.

CHRONIC INFLAMMATORY BOWEL DISEASE. Ulcerative colitis or Crohn's disease put you at a higher risk of colon cancer. Be sure to mention any current or past bowel problems you might have to your doctor.

PERSONAL OR FAMILY HISTORY OF BREAST, OVARIAN, OR UTERINE CANCER. Breast, ovarian, uterine, and colon cancer are all hormonally sensitive, meaning that if your tissues are hyperresponsive to oestrogen stimulation, either because of genetics or because they became sensitized in utero, you are at risk for developing all four types of cancer. Four hereditary nonpolyposis colorectal cancer (HNPCC) genes have been identified: hMSH2, hMLH1, PMS1, and PMS2. Women who have mutations in any of these genes have a 68 to 75 percent lifetime risk of colon cancer, a 30 to 39 percent risk of endometrial cancer, and a 10 percent risk of ovarian cancer. Women who carry a mutated copy of the breast cancer gene BRCA2 (see page 258) are at high risk of developing not only breast cancer but pancreatic and colon cancer as well.

FAECAL OCCULT BLOOD TEST. This is a simple test to detect the presence of blood in the stool. Whenever I perform a pelvic exam on a patient age 40 or older, I wipe a small stool sample on a card and put a chemical on it to test for blood. This could indicate the presence of a polyp or tumor, or even something as benign as a haemorrhoid. If the sample tests positive, I send my patient home with a kit containing a more accurate follow-up screen. The nice part about this is that you can do it in the privacy of your own home. The not-so-nice part is that it entails collecting small samples of stool from three different bowel movements, smearing them onto a special card, then popping it

HIGH-FAT, LOW-FIBER DIET. Living on junk food is not a good idea in general, but especially not when your colon's health is concerned. A high-fat, low-fiber diet makes your intestine sluggish. Without regular bowel movements, potential carcinogens sit in your intestines longer, giving them a greater opportunity to cause mutations that may initiate cancer. Also, to break down fat, your gallbladder releases bile acids, which in excessive amounts can damage the lining of your intestines. Red meat particularly increases your risk of colon cancer: the long-term Harvard University Nurses' Health Study in the United States found that women who ate red meat had a 249 percent greater risk of developing colon cancer than women who ate fish or skinless chicken.

OBESITY. Women who are obese are at a higher risk of colon cancer for two reasons. One is that their fat cells produce excess oestrogen, which puts them at risk for hormonally sensitive cancers. The other is they are probably eating lots of fat and not exercising, both of which increase the chances of developing the disease.

SEDENTARY LIFESTYLE. Exercise reduces the risk of colon cancer by several means. It enhances gut motility, moves food through the system rapidly so carcinogens don't sit around too long, and decreases the gut's concentration of bile acid, which contributes to colon cancer.

SMOKING. Talk about carcinogens! Cigarette smoke is full of them, and once they're in your bloodstream they can affect all the tissues in your body, including your intestines.

in the post to your doctor. For two days before the test, you need to avoid red meat, raw fruits and vegetables, vitamin C, aspirin, and other nonsteroidal anti-inflammatory drugs, such as ibuprofen and aspirin, as any of these can cause a false-positive reading.

If the home test reveals blood in your stool, you need to have a full gastrointestinal workup, as the blood could be caused by anything from polyps and tumors to ulcers or haemorrhoids. Beginning at age 40, or age 30 if you have a family history of colon cancer, you should have a faecal occult blood test every year. Annual faecal occult blood testing has decreased the mortality from colon cancer by up to 33 percent.

DIGITAL RECTAL EXAMINATION. This procedure, in which your doctor feels for any polyps, tumors, or haemorrhoids in the lower three to four inches of your rectum and anus with a gloved and well-lubricated finger, should be done as part of your routine pelvic exam.

FLEXIBLE SIGMOIDOSCOPY. Whenever a patient age 50 or older comes to see me, I always ask her whether she's had her sig-moidoscopy yet. Nine times out of ten I get a blank look. Flexible sig-moidoscopy is an excellent screening test, reducing the death rate from colon cancer by 60 to 70 percent. It's imperative that you have one beginning at age 50 (or age 35 if you have a family history of colon polyps or cancer) and every 10 years thereafter, alternating with colonoscopy (so you're checked every five years).

The test entails having a thin lighted flexible scope, about the di-ameter of your little finger, inserted into your rectum, enabling your doctor to examine the lower two feet of your colon. If your doctor spies polyps or other growths, he or she can take samples or even re-move them altogether during the procedure. You'll need to take a lax-ative the night prior to the test and an enema right before it begins, but you won't need any anaesthetic—it's about as uncomfortable as a pelvic exam.

DOUBLE-CONTRAST BARIUM ENEMA. In this test your colon is filled with barium and air and then x-rayed, illuminating the walls of the rectum and entire colon. It requires no anaesthesia, although, as you can imagine, it causes some discomfort. The double-contrast bar-ium enema detects 72 percent of tumors larger than 1 centimeter. If your doctor finds a suspicious growth, he or she will recommend colonoscopy to verify and biopsy it.

COLONOSCOPY. If your sigmoidoscopy or double-contrast barium enema shows an abnormal growth or if you are at high risk for colon cancer, you'll need to have a colonoscopy. Basically this is the same type of procedure as the flexible sigmoidoscopy, except the scope is about three times as long, enabling your doctor to examine your en-tire large intestine. Colonoscopy not only detects cancer but also picks up polyps, which can be removed at the time of the test. For this one you'll have to take a mild sedative. If you have a first-degree relative who had colon cancer before the age of 55, you should have colonoscopy beginning at age 35. Otherwise, beginning at age 50 have colonscopy every ten years, alternating with flexible sigmoidoscopy (so you're checked every five years).

Reducing Your Risk

How can you protect yourself against colon cancer? Make sure you are screened regularly, stop smoking, and eat a well-balanced low-fat, high-fiber diet. Folate, selenium, mixed carotenes, vitamin E, calcium, and vitamin D have all been shown to reduce the risk of colon cancer. Patients who have taken multivitamin supplements for fifteen years or more have been shown to have a 75 percent decreased risk of colon cancer. But even more effective than taking supplements is getting those vitamins and minerals by eating lots of fruits and vegetables, which provide essential fiber as well. Exercise regularly, as it will help keep you regular and also keep your weight under control.

Multiple studies have shown that exogenous oestrogen (from outside your body) reduces the risk of colon cancer. Why? Because oestrogen reduces bile acid production, and excess bile acid damages the intestinal lining. Oestrogen has also been shown to suppress tumor growth in cultured colon cancer cells. So during perimenopause, consider oral contraceptives, as they can not only reduce your symptoms and provide birth control but also lower your risk of colon cancer by about 35 percent.

You also may want to think about going on hormone replacement therapy, which can reduce your chance of developing the disease by up to 25 percent. It can also protect you from growing polyps, the precursor to colon cancer. Studies have not yet been done to assess whether all types of hormone replacement therapy are equally effective. (I'd be interested to see whether the transdermal oestradiol patch has any effect at all on colon cancer, as the oestrogen it delivers never reaches the gastrointestinal tract.) Although prevention of colon cancer is not a reason in and of itself to choose hormone replacement therapy, you should consider it along with the other pros and cons when you're making your decision, and give it special weight if you are at high risk for this disease.

Not all gastrointestinal changes in perimenopause mean cancer. Many women between the ages of 40 and 49 complain of various symptoms: constipation, heartburn, gas, bloating, reflux. The connection

ASPIRIN—A MIRACLE DRUG

As with heart disease, an aspirin a day has been shown to reduce the incidence of colon cancer. A decade-long study of more than 660,000 men and women by the American Cancer Society revealed that those who took aspirin sixteen or more times a month were half as likely to die of colon cancer as were nonusers. Ask your doctor if he or she recommends taking a daily baby aspirin to ward off colon cancer. But if you have a bleeding disorder or gastric ulcers, this therapy is not for you.

seems to be that decreasing oestrogen levels affect the levels of catecholamines—neurotransmitters that control, among other functions, the motor and sensory action of the bowel. A patient recently came in with several perimenopausal symptoms, but the worst by far was her bowel dysfunction. She was bloated and had horrendous gas. "This is all brand new and came on along with my other symptoms, so I'm convinced it's related to menopause," she told me. After sending her for a thorough gastrointestinal workup, which showed nothing physically wrong, I prescribed low-dose oestrogen and recommended she increase her intake of omega-3 fatty acids by eating more fatty fish, and she has been improving on all fronts.

CHAPTER 12

Eve's Apple:
Your Thyroid Gland

Let's say you come to me with the following symptoms: weight gain, menstrual changes, fertility problems, thinning hair, dry skin, palpitations, insomnia, fatigue, sweating, disturbed concentration, memory loss, depressed mood, and decreased sexual desire. After reading the previous eleven chapters, the answer seems pretty obvious—perimenopause, right? Not necessarily. Those very same symptoms could also indicate thyroid disease.

As a case in point, consider my mother. In her early fifties my mom started having irregular periods. She felt hot all the time and even developed claustrophobia—she always had to sit next to the door when she and my dad went to a restaurant. She had heart palpitations and couldn't sit still. "I felt like I was jumping out of my skin!" Her nails became brittle and she started losing her hair.

On numerous occasions she complained of these symptoms to her doctor, but each time he said, "Don't worry, it's just your changes." Eventually, things got so bad that she couldn't carry the clean clothes up from the basement because of the terrible pain in her lower back and weakness in her legs. The last straw was when she could no longer write her name on a straight line because her hands shook so much.

"I knew something was wrong, but my doctor wouldn't take me seriously," she said. "I began to think I was losing my mind!" Then one day she was looking in the mirror and noticed a huge goiter on her neck. She also realized that her eyes had begun to pop out. At the time, I was in medical school. She called me up and related her symptoms.

"Ma," I said, "you've got a classic case of hyperthyroidism!"

Armed with my diagnosis, she went back to her doctor and demanded a blood test. When the results came in he told her she had the highest free T_4 count he had ever seen. "You have Graves' disease," he said and recommended surgery to remove her overactive thyroid gland.

Just thinking about this story makes me so mad—here my mother was sick as a dog and no one thought to do a simple thyroid test! If her condition hadn't been treated she would have gone into thyroid storm, a very serious condition that can lead to heart arrhythmia, heart failure, and liver disease. Fortunately, she was cured and now, twenty-five years later, is enjoying a wonderfully active, healthy life.

Like my mother, many women develop thyroid disease in their perimenopausal years. Why? Because there is a link between thyroid function and the female sex hormones. Oestrogen and progesterone receptors are found on the thyroid gland, and thyroid hormone receptors are found on the ovaries. So when your oestrogen levels begin to wax and wane, and eventually drop off in perimenopause, you are more likely to experience changes in your thyroid function. It's not surprising, therefore, that women suffer thyroid problems far more frequently than men and that the incidence of thyroid disease in women peaks in their forties and continues into old age. In addition to perimenopause, thyroid disease frequently shows up in puberty, pregnancy, and after menopause—all times in your life characterized by vast hormonal changes.

Like oestrogen, there are receptors for thyroid hormone in virtually every tissue of your body. That's why your symptoms might be extremely diverse and masquerade as other problems, such as depression, stress, or perimenopause. As a standard practice, I test the thyroid hormone levels of all my patients who complain of perimenopausal symptoms. If the levels indicate hypothyroidism (an underactive gland), which affects 10 percent of women by age 50, or hyperthyroidism (an overactive gland), which affects 2 percent of women by age 50, I immediately refer them to an endocrinologist for treatment.

More difficult to diagnose are women who suffer subclinical hyper- or hypothyroidism. These borderline conditions may show up in a blood test, but sometimes they are so subtle that the blood levels appear normal. You may have one or more symptoms of thyroid disease—lingering black mood or fatigue, bouts of anxiety, inexplicable aches and pains, a general "run-down" feeling—or you may have no symptoms at all. The key to getting treatment is to be scrupulous about reporting any and all symptoms to your doctor; make sure you have your thyroid hormone levels checked; and if the levels are normal but you still don't feel right, suggest to your doctor the possibility of subclinical thyroid disease.

Catching thyroid disease in perimenopause is essential because it adversely affects so many other systems that are vulnerable at this time of your life, including your bones, your heart, your reproductive organs, and your brain. It is shocking that more than half the people suffering a thyroid imbalance are undiagnosed or misdiagnosed. Identifying and treating thyroid disease promptly is, to my mind, one of the biggest responsibilities of any women's healthcare provider.

WHAT IS THE THYROID AND HOW DOES IT WORK?

The thyroid is a small butterfly-shaped gland that wraps around the windpipe between the voice box and collarbone at the base of the neck. Although no bigger than a couple of dates, it has an enormous effect on the rest of the body because it controls metabolism. While most of us equate metabolism with weight, as in "I've always had trouble losing weight because I have a slow metabolism" or "She must have a high metabolism—she eats like a pig but never gains an ounce," metabolism really refers to how the body uses energy on a cellular level. That's why, in addition to weight loss or gain, symptoms of thyroid disease include temperature changes, insomnia or exhaustion, bone loss, even children's growth rate.

We've now discovered that the thyroid also influences neurotransmitter levels in the brain. Specifically, thyroid hormones regulate levels of serotonin, noradrenaline, and GABA, which explains why mental symptoms such as moodiness, lack of libido, memory problems, and difficulty concentrating can also signal thyroid problems.

The thyroid regulates your metabolism by producing two hormones that circulate through your bloodstream, T_3 and T_4 (so called because they contain three and four atoms of iodine, respectively). Your thyroid gland produces ten times more T_4 than T_3, but T_4 is converted to T_3 once it's in circulation. Every single cell needs thyroid hormone in order to perform its most basic functions. Think of it as the gas that keeps your engine running. Without enough, you drag along. With too much, you're racing.

The hypothalamus and pituitary glands in the brain monitor and control the amount of thyroid hormone in the body through a negative feedback loop. In general, the hypothalamus secretes thyrotropin-releasing hormone (TRH), which stimulates the pituitary to release thyroid-stimulating hormone (TSH), which in turn stimulates the thyroid to produce T_3 and T_4. High levels of circulating thyroid hormone (T_3 and T_4) inhibit the hypothalamus from secreting TRH and make the pituitary much less sensitive to TRH. The pituitary then produces less TSH, causing the thyroid to slow down production of T_3 and T_4.

Because your ovaries have receptors for thyroid hormones and your thyroid has receptors for oestrogen and progesterone, the two glands are in constant communication. Like your thyroid gland, your ovaries are also controlled by the hypothalamus and pituitary glands in the brain. Under certain conditions, your ovaries and thyroid gland are stimulated simultaneously when your pituitary gland releases TSH, LH, and FSH all at once.

A DELICATE BALANCE

The thyroid and reproductive systems communicate through interlinked feedback loops.

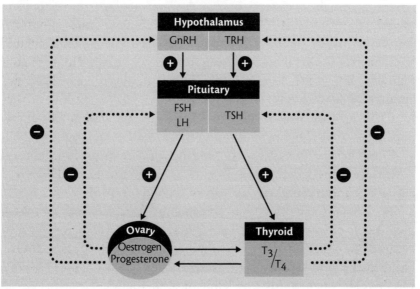

Most T_3 and T_4 travels through the bloodstream bound to a protein called, appropriately, thyroxine-binding globulin (TBG). This inactivates the hormones. To determine how much active thyroid hormone you have in circulation, therefore, it is important to check your blood levels of *free*, or unbound, T_3 and T_4.

THE IMPORTANCE OF SCREENING

As part of the routine series of questions I ask in taking a medical history, I always find out whether there is any kind of thyroid disease in my patient's immediate family. Thyroid disease is hereditary, so "yes" means we have a red flag. My own family is typical: my mother had hyperthyroidism, and my brother and both my grandmothers had thyroid disease. Having a relative with thyroid disease increases your chance of developing it by four times.

Even if the answer is "no," I still check the thyroid gland both visually and through palpation at every visit because thyroid disease is so very common in women. If a goiter can be seen with the naked eye, the disease is already advanced. Less prominent swelling or nodules that can be felt but not seen may indicate either a less severe imbalance or, in very rare cases, cancer of the thyroid.

With patients who are 45 years of age or are experiencing menstrual irregularities (whichever comes first), I always run a blood test to check TSH levels. The normal range is between 1 and 5 mU/l. If TSH is high, then the thyroid is underactive; if TSH is low, the thyroid is overactive. Remember, TSH stimulates the thyroid gland, so if your thyroid is sluggish it will take extra TSH to help it produce a normal amount of thyroid hormone (hypothyroidism). Similarly, if your thyroid is overactive it is in very little need of stimulation (hyperthyroidism).

In addition to TSH, I check circulating levels of free T_4, which indicate how hard the thyroid is working. (In cases where TSH is low, I also check free T_3, as there are two types of hyperthyroidism: high T_3 and high T_4.) If your T_4 count is normal (between 0.7 and 1.5 mU/l) but your TSH level is either high or low, you have what we call subclinical hypo- or hyperthyroidism. When you have your thyroid level checked, make sure your doctor is testing both your TSH and free T_4. Otherwise, he or she may miss subclinical thyroid disease.

WHAT DO THE NUMBERS MEAN?		
Very high TSH (over 10 mU/l)	Low T_4	Hypothyroidism
High TSH (5–10 mU/l)	Normal T_4	Subclinical hypothyroidism
Low TSH (under 1 mU/l)	High T_4 or T_3	Hyperthyroidism
Low TSH (under 1 mU/l)	Normal T_4	Subclinical hyperthyroidism

HYPOTHYROIDISM

When the thyroid gland produces too little thyroid hormone, all the systems in your body slow down, from your brain to your bowel. In addition, because your metabolism is reduced, your body can't generate enough heat to keep you warm. Following is a chart of the most common symptoms of hypothyroidism. Any one of them merits discussion with your doctor.

Ninety percent of all hypothyroid cases are caused by an autoimmune reaction, which occurs when your immune cells attack your own thyroid gland, causing inflammation. This attack causes your body to make antibodies, which can be measured in the blood as a way of diagnosing hypothyroidism. The damaged tissue produces less thyroid hormone, so your T_4 level decreases. Sensing this lack of T_4, your pituitary and hypothalamus try to get your thyroid gland working again by pumping out TSH and TRH, respectively. In response, your thyroid cells multiply, causing the gland to swell. If a goiter becomes apparent, the condition is called Hashimoto's thyroiditis.

No one is completely sure what causes autoimmune hypothyroidism. It often accompanies other autoimmune conditions such as diabetes, rheumatoid arthritis, and lupus (SLE). Oestrogen is most likely a factor in all these autoimmune diseases, as women are three times as likely as men to develop them. Women with early onset of periods and late menopause are at greater risk of developing hypothyroidism,

SYMPTOMS OF HYPOTHYROIDISM

- cold intolerance
- low body temperature
- delayed reflexes
- water retention
- dry skin and hair
- hair loss
- constipation
- weight gain
- lethargy
- fatigue
- mental slowness
- depression

- memory lapses
- slowed speech
- low-pitched or hoarse voice
- hearing loss
- impaired night vision
- carpal tunnel syndrome
- muscle cramps
- aches and stiffness of joints
- hypertension
- irregular periods
- anaemia
- elevated LDL cholesterol

which suggests that overexposure to oestrogen may be a trigger, although no specific mechanism has been identified. There is some speculation that a virus may be involved in initiating the condition; heredity and environment may also play a role.

I have several cases in my practice of patients who came to me with terrible depression, exhaustion, and an inability to lose their pregnancy weight after having a baby. Lo and behold, when I checked their thyroid glands both manually and through blood testing, I found they were in flagrant hypothyroidism. Immediately postpartum, women frequently develop autoimmune hypothyroidism. Basically what's happening is that the immune system, which is suppressed by high levels of progesterone during pregnancy (otherwise the foetus would be rejected as a foreign body), comes back too strongly after the baby is born and begins attacking your own thyroid tissue. This is a permanent condition and requires lifelong thyroid hormone supplementation.

Autoimmune hypothyroidism can be confirmed by a blood test for antithyroid antibodies. If your condition is not autoimmune, it may be caused by one of several other factors. Hypothyroidism can result from an unformed thyroid gland at birth; when the neck has been irradiated for some reason, such as to treat acne (a common practice in the

---

TRANSIENT POSTPARTUM HYPOTHYROIDISM

There is a situation in which women develop *hyper*thyroidism late in pregnancy or right after delivery, and then end up *hypo*thyroidal six weeks or more after childbirth. Blood tests of these women may show the presence of autoantibodies. The condition usually reverts to normal within a year; until it does, patients may need to take thyroid hormone. In some cases, no medication may be necessary.

1960s); or from taking certain drugs such as potassium iodide or lithium.

Whatever the cause, hypothyroidism is treated with some form of thyroid hormone. The most commonly prescribed is synthetic T_4, known as Synthroid. Discovered over a century ago, it has proven extremely safe, even when taken for decades. The dose must be carefully calibrated according to your weight and the severity of your condition, as overtreatment can result in osteoporosis (see Chapter 8). It must be taken in the morning on an empty stomach, half an hour before breakfast with water only. Treatment is lifelong, although your dose may change as your hormones fluctuate. For example, in perimenopause you may need less Synthroid. If you are being treated for hypothyroidism, have your TSH and free T_4 levels checked annually.

A more natural alternative, called Armour thyroid, is extracted from cows and pigs. Unlike Synthroid, which is pure T_4, Armour thyroid contains both T_3 and T_4. For most people, it makes absolutely no difference which is taken, because the body converts T_4 to T_3 anyway. A very small portion of patients do feel better on Armour; however, the reason for this is unclear.

SUBCLINICAL HYPOTHYROIDISM

Geneen, age 50, was a new patient who came to me complaining of infrequent periods, hot flushes, insomnia, fatigue, memory loss, depression, mood swings, and breast soreness. She had no family history of thyroid disease, and upon exam her thyroid gland felt perfectly

THE CHOLESTEROL CLUE

One of the symptoms of hypothyroidism is high LDL ("bad") cholesterol. This is because thyroid hormone is necessary to activate the LDL receptors on cell membranes. If the receptors aren't working, cholesterol cannot be absorbed from the bloodstream into cells and instead builds up in the bloodstream.

Whenever a patient's cholesterol test shows high LDL levels, I immediately order a thyroid test to see if hypothyroidism is also a factor. If it is, treatment with thyroxine may reduce the cholesterol level by an average of 8 percent.

normal. As part of my perimenopausal workup, I sent off her blood samples for hormone studies, cholesterol, triglycerides, cardiac profile, and thyroid studies. Her hormones came back in the menopausal range, which didn't surprise me, and her lipid profile looked good: total cholesterol under 200, high HDLs, and low LDLs. But she also had an elevated TSH of 8, normal free T_4, and negative thyroid antibodies, signaling subclinical hypothyroidism.

The question then became, how to treat her? Her symptoms could just as easily have been caused by her perimenopausal status as by her thyroid condition. We had a long discussion, weighing the pros and cons of hormone replacement versus thyroid medication, and ultimately decided to start her on hormone replacement therapy.

Three months later Geneen returned. "So, how are you feeling?" I asked.

"My physical symptoms are much better—I still get the occasional period, my breasts aren't sore anymore, and I haven't had a hot flush since I saw you last. But emotionally I'm still not myself. I'm weepy and exhausted, and I spend most of my day in a fog."

"Sounds like those symptoms may be from the hypothyroidism rather than the perimenopause," I told her and explained how the two conditions could be very hard to distinguish. "I think it's time you saw a specialist about your thyroid problem." I referred her to an endocrinologist, who put her on a low dose of Thyroxine.

Within four weeks Geneen called me back. "I definitely feel an improvement. My mood has lifted and I have more energy."

"Report back to me in two months," I said, "and we'll evaluate how both treatments are working for you."

Although 10 percent of women will develop clinical hypothyroidism at some point during their lives, another 10 percent will develop subclinical hypothyroidism between ages 40 and 60, the years when it's easiest to confuse with perimenopause. Many will experience one or more symptoms, but others may have none at all. All require monitoring, however, as one-quarter of these cases will eventually become full-blown hypothyroidism.

There is a debate in the medical community about whether or not to treat subclinical hypothyroidism. Some say that treatment is not needed until symptoms appear; others believe that early treatment can forestall the progression to overt hypothyroidism. My belief is that if you're suffering, you should be treated. If your complaints coincide with perimenopausal changes, it's up to you and your doctor whether you try hormone replacement therapy or thyroid medication first. You may find that one approach or the other exclusively improves your symptoms: or as in Geneen's case, you may end up on a combination of the two.

Even if you don't have symptoms, if your blood tests show high LDL cholesterol, antithyroid antibodies, or a rising TSH level, you should start taking thyroid hormone, as these are all indicators that your subclinical condition may progress. But if your lipid profile is good, you don't have antithyroid antibodies, and you aren't experiencing any symptoms, I don't think it's necessary to go on medication. In this case, I'd prefer to watch and wait, following you closely with yearly TSH/free T_4 tests.

HYPERTHYROIDISM

Hyperthyroidism speeds up your metabolism, burning up your energy stores and leading to a host of symptoms in all parts of your body. It is far less common than hypothyroidism, affecting 2 percent of women, usually in their thirties or forties.

The most common cause of hyperthyroidism, accounting for 85 percent of all cases, is Graves' disease, an autoimmune condition that

SYMPTOMS OF HYPERTHYROIDISM

- heat intolerance
- elevated body temperature
- strong reflex response
- excessive perspiration
- warm, moist skin
- fine, soft hair and hair loss
- separation of nail plate from nail bed
- frequent and/or loose bowel movements
- frequent urination
- increased appetite
- weight loss
- fatigue
- insomnia

- nervousness
- irritability
- increased heart rate
- heart palpitations
- shortness of breath
- tremor
- weakness in extremities
- bone loss
- bulging, staring eyes
- irregular periods
- anaemia
- low LDL cholesterol
- goiter

affects women five times more often than men. For some reason—hormonal, environmental, genetic, or infectious—the body begins to make antibodies to the thyroid gland. One of these antibodies, called thyroid-stimulating immunoglobulin (TSI), mimics TSH, plugging into the TSH receptors on your thyroid gland and thereby stimulating thyroid hormone production. With high levels of circulating thyroid hormone, actual TSH levels decline until they are ultimately undetectable.

Graves' disease can be confirmed by a blood test that detects thyroid-stimulating antibodies (TSI) as well as elevated free T_4/T_3 and low TSH levels. It can also be diagnosed by the presence of a "diffuse goiter," which makes you look as if you swallowed a rolled-up sock. The goiter is caused by the overstimulation of the thyroid gland, which makes the cells enlarge and multiply.

Another dead giveaway is a peculiar change that occurs in the eyes of a very small percentage of Graves' patients, called *exophthalmos*. To put it simply, patients become bug-eyed—their eyes pop out, their eyelids retract, they blink less and look as if they're staring all the time. Why this eye problem should be connected to the thyroid gland is a bit of a mystery. The most popular hypothesis is that the autoantibodies that attack the thyroid gland also attack the tissue behind the eye,

YET ANOTHER REASON NOT TO SMOKE

Just in case you still aren't persuaded of the evils of smoking, here's another unpleasant condition it can cause: goiter. Nicotine and benzpyrene, both components of cigarette smoke, increase thyroid hormone synthesis. The thyroid gland expands in response to this stimulation, causing a goiter.

Because of this, one might expect smokers to have extremely elevated T_3 and T_4 levels. Yet they don't—their thyroid hormone levels are only slightly higher than normal. This is because another product of cigarette smoking called thiocyanate (a derivative of cyanide) builds up in their bloodstream. Thiocyanate inhibits overproduction of thyroid hormone. It does not, however, reduce the goiter that forms in response to the gland's overstimulation.

causing the eye muscles first to become inflamed and then to degenerate. Smokers with Graves' disease are more likely to have eye involvement than are nonsmokers.

Most non-Graves' hyperthyroidism occurs as a result of a toxic nodule goiter, in which certain "hot" spots on the thyroid gland pump out lots of extra thyroid hormone. Known as Plummer's disease, it mainly affects older women. Other causes of hyperthyroidism include TSH-producing tumors on the pituitary gland; radiation of the neck; viruses such as mumps, Coxsackie, and influenza; and eating a diet low in iodine.

There are several options for treating hyperthyroidism. We usually begin with antithyroid medication such as propylthiouracil (PTU—100 to 600 mg per day) or methimazole (Tapazole—10 to 40 mg per day), both of which inhibit thyroid hormone synthesis. If you don't go into remission within six to twelve months, we move on to either radioactive iodine therapy to destroy the thyroid (taken orally as long as you are not pregnant or planning a pregnancy) or surgical removal of almost all of the gland. If you're treated with radioactive iodine or surgery, you'll have to take thyroid hormone supplements for the rest of your life.

SUBCLINICAL HYPERTHYROIDISM

You have subclinical hyperthyroidism when your blood test shows low TSH but normal free T_4. No good studies have been done to prove that treatment is universally recommended for this condition. I do monitor patients closely who have subclinical hyperthyroidism, however, because in certain cases treatment may be warranted. In particular, if you show signs of bone loss from excess thyroid hormone exposure or are over age 55 and have cardiac disease that might be exacerbated by hyperthyroid-induced heart palpitations, I think it's important to take action.

If you have subclinical hyperthyroidism, you should have your TSH and free T_4 levels checked annually. If your T_4 level begins to rise, you may be on the way to developing overt hyperthyroidism. In that case, treatment is a good idea to prevent development of a goiter or of Graves' ophthalmopathy.

THYROID NODULES

"Bumps and lumps" in the thyroid gland are extremely common. While they are diagnosed in 5 percent of women, it is believed that as many as 25 percent of all Americans have them. The vast majority of these nodules are benign: they don't affect thyroid function but occasionally may produce symptoms of hoarseness or pressure on the throat. Those that are associated with hypothyroidism or hyperthyroidism may shrink when the condition is treated.

A typical case of a patient with benign thyroid nodules is Alicia, a 46-year-old who came in for a routine exam. Five years earlier I had put her on oral contraceptives to control her irregular bleeding and perimenopausal symptoms including insomnia, anxiety, and memory loss. As I was feeling her thyroid as part of her check-up I noticed that she had two nodules on the left side of her gland.

"Have you ever had anything wrong with your thyroid before?" I asked. "And does anyone in your family have any kind of thyroid disease?"

"No," she replied.

"I'm going to run some blood tests to check out your thyroid function. In the meantime, I'd like you to see an endocrinologist who may want you to have a thyroid scan."

Alicia's TSH, free T_3, and free T_4 levels were all perfectly normal. But when the endocrinologist did a sonogram of her thyroid gland, he confirmed the nodules on her left side. He then performed a fine-needle aspiration, sampling tissue from each of the nodules. The cells were sent to pathology and found to be benign. He decided to continue following her thyroid nodules without any treatment because all her tests were in the normal range and she was feeling fine.

I commonly find thyroid nodules when I'm examining patients, but it is extremely rare for any of them to turn out to be cancerous. Thyroid cancer affects only 1 in 10,000 people. If you happen to be that one and your nodules are malignant, you need to have your entire thyroid gland removed. After surgery, you must take radioactive iodine to kill off any cancer cells that may have spread and to destroy any remaining thyroid tissue.

BE GOOD TO YOUR THYROID

Unfortunately, there's little you can do to decrease your risk of thyroid cancer besides watching your weight in perimenopause and taking a multivitamin and natural vitamin E supplement. Early detection is the key. So make sure your doctor feels your thyroid gland on a yearly basis when he or she carries out your smear test.

As far as other thyroid disorders are concerned, don't overlook symptoms that you may be having or automatically chalk them up to aging, stress, or hormone changes. Have your TSH and free T_4 levels checked every five years after age 45, and report any unusual symptoms to your doctor.

RISK FACTORS FOR THYROID CANCER

Like cancers of the breast, uterus, ovaries, and colon, thyroid cancer is an oestrogen-responsive tumor. Therefore, any situation that raises your exposure to unopposed oestrogen can increase your risk, including:

FEMALE SEX

EARLY MENARCHE AND LATE MENOPAUSE

INFERTILITY (because infertility is frequently caused by anovulation)

SURGICAL MENOPAUSE (because surgery is commonly related to fibroids and endometriosis, which are oestrogen-dominated diseases)

PREGNANCY

OBESITY

NOT SMOKING (smoking *decreases* your risk of thyroid cancer because it reduces both your circulating oestrogen levels and your body weight)

Other, non–oestrogen-related risk factors are:

GENETICS

IRRADIATION OF THE NECK (about 10 percent of people who received neck irradiation to treat acne, eczema, and tonsillitis will develop thyroid cancer, and three times that many will have some form of thyroid abnormality)

CHAPTER 13

Dr. Corio's Prescription for a Healthy Perimenopause

If you've ever needed motivation to make changes in your lifestyle, perimenopause is a great opportunity. Adopting a healthy diet and exercise plan that helps you keep your weight under control, your muscles and bones toned, and your body fed with beneficial nutrients can not only help control the symptoms you may be experiencing but also decrease your risk of developing a host of health problems such as diabetes, osteoporosis, heart disease, and cancer later in life.

What constitutes a healthy diet and exercise plan? Every year it seems there's a new "best" way to control your weight. At first carbohydrates were good and protein was bad; now carbs are the villain and protein is the hero. And what about fat? The "experts" recommend that anywhere from 10 to 40 percent of your calories should come from fat—that's a big spread. And are some fats better than others?

Exercise can be just as confusing. Is aerobic exercise better than strength training? Could swimming really be good for your heart but not for your bones? Is it better to exercise an hour a day or ten minutes three times a day? And who even has ten minutes three times a day? If you hate gyms or simply don't have time for them, rest assured, there are plenty of other ways to get fit. It does take a little determination to get in the swing, but once you begin to see and feel the effects you'll likely as not wish you'd started exercising years ago.

Vitamins and minerals play an important role in keeping us at our peak. Ideally, we'd get all our nutrients from the foods we eat. But in today's world, that just isn't practical. For that reason, it's wise to take a multivitamin as well as calcium/magnesium and natural vitamin E supplements daily, plus any other vitamins and minerals you may want to try to address specific health issues. Herbs may also enter the picture in perimenopause, if they haven't already. At this stage in the game you and your doctor should also begin discussing hormone replacement therapy. To prepare for this conversation, you need to be as knowledgeable as possible about the ever-increasing number of options out there. At the end of this chapter you'll find lots of information on both natural and synthetic formulations to help you make this important decision.

THE MEDITERRANEAN DIET

My grandma Noni died at 98 of pure old age—no cancer, no heart disease, nothing. Her entire life she ate a traditional Sicilian diet: tons of vegetables, fruit, nuts, olive oil, and garlic; small portions of meat, fish, eggs, and pasta; few sweets, lots of homemade bread, and a little glass of red wine every night. My other grandmother, also from Sicily, lived to age 94. Up until her dying day she was making homemade pasta, which she would lay out all over the beds and chairs to dry so that there was no place to sit down when you went to visit. There was always salami and provolone cheese in her fridge to munch on, as well as bowls of nuts and fruit. She cooked with lots of garlic and onions, especially in her delicious homemade tomato sauce. She and my grandfather grew grapes in the garden, and he made red wine in the cellar.

I was raised in a close Sicilian family, with both sets of grandparents living right up the street. My brothers and sisters and I would always be in and out of their homes sharing their meals and listening to their stories. My parents continue to eat in the traditional way—there's always a bowl of nuts out, and every night after dinner my father ritually cuts a plate of fruit for dessert. In the autumn we gorge on figs from the tree in the garden, and year-round we indulge in my mother's amazing homemade pasta. We always have fish once a week and at least once a week eat homemade soup—pea soup, lentil soup, or an incredible fourteen bean soup. The olive oil flows liberally—on salad, on bread, on pasta—as does the red wine.

Now you may think I'm pushing the Mediterranean diet—the traditional diet of Crete, Greece, and southern Italy—because it's the diet I was brought up on and, goodness knows, it's delicious. But the fact of the matter is that numerous scientific studies have shown it to be one of the most healthful ways to eat. In Italy, patients who'd had heart attacks in the past and who followed a Mediterranean diet for 6 years reduced their mortality rate by 40 percent. Heart disease and cancer rates in these areas are extremely low (although they're on the rise now that modern conveniences such as prepared and fast food are making inroads), and people enjoy an excellent quality of life well into old age.

Why? Because the Mediterranean diet includes ideal proportions of protein, carbohydrates, and fat as well as lots of fresh fruits, vegetables, legumes, and whole grains that are rich in nutrients and protective antioxidants. Refined sugar was, until recently, a rarity—growing up we didn't know from cake, candies, or ice cream. The only thing we might on occasion have for dessert besides fruit was gelato, a frozen dessert that doesn't have nearly the fat content of ice cream.

Just as important as its health benefits, researchers have found that the Mediterranean diet is satisfying—an important criterion if you're planning to make a lifelong change. The problem with so many fad diets is that they're unrealistically stringent or fussy, making them impossible or even hazardous to follow long-term. By contrast, the Mediterranean diet is all about enjoying and appreciating food.

It is not, however, about losing weight—be forewarned. Rather, by presenting this diet I'd like to teach you a new way to eat to decrease your risk of certain medical diseases. If you wish to make modifications in order to shed a few pounds, remember that to lose weight you need to cut calories, pure and simple. You also need to exercise—something you should be doing anyway, as I'll explain shortly. Once you get in the habit of eating modest portions of wholesome food, you'll probably find your weight begins to stabilize, which is much healthier than constantly gaining and losing the same five, ten, or fifteen pounds anyhow.

So what exactly is the Mediterranean diet? While it's based on a foundation of carbohydrates, it doesn't mean plopping down to eat a huge plate of ravioli every night. The fact is there are many different kinds of carbohydrates, just as there are different kinds of fats and proteins. Ideally, you should get almost equal amounts of calories from each group daily—30 to 40 percent from protein, 30 to 40 percent from carbohydrates, and 30 percent from fat. The trick is to learn to distinguish the "good" carbohydrates, fats, and proteins from the "bad" ones. That will help you make sensible choices, so that when you do sit down for pasta dinner you know that linguini with seafood in a sauce of olive oil and garlic is a better pick than spaghetti carbonara, which is loaded with bacon, eggs, cream, and cheese.

CARBOHYDRATES

Also known by my patients as "the white stuff," carbohydrates include simple starches such as pasta, bread, potatoes, and rice. But they also include fruits and vegetables, cereals, whole grains, and dairy products. These complex carbohydrates are loaded with vitamins, minerals, fiber, and phytochemicals essential to maintaining a healthy body and mind.

Regardless of whether they're simple or complex, all carbohydrates are broken down into the same end product: sugar. That's why diets that recommend gorging on carbohydrates don't help you lose weight—they may actually cause you to put on pounds. It's like eating straight sugar, which, even if you are restricting your fat intake, will make you fat.

Nevertheless, we do need a certain amount of carbohydrates in our diet to provide us with the energy to fuel our daily metabolism and, especially, to feed our brains, which use more than two-thirds of our circulating carbohydrates while we're at rest. Those carbohydrates that aren't used to maintain our bodily functions are stored as glycogen in the liver and muscles. When we eat too many carbohydrates, those repositories become full and the excess is converted to fat and stored in our adipose tissue. As you learned in Chapter 6, insulin is the hormone responsible for fat storage. It is also responsible for mopping up excess sugar from the bloodstream when we eat a high-carb snack and our blood sugar spikes. Too many carbohydrates can lead to insulin resistance, which puts us at risk for a host of health problems mentioned throughout the previous chapters.

So in addition to watching the amount of carbohydrates you eat, it's important to know when to eat them and which ones are preferable. Because of the rise in blood sugar they may cause, carbohydrates should be eaten at regular intervals throughout the day, not in huge quantities all at once. Also, if you are going to indulge in carbohydrates, complex ones are a better choice than simple ones. Complex carbohydrates contain lots of fiber, which slows down the digestion

GLYCEMIC INDEX OF CARBOHYDRATE FOODS

GRAINS, BREADS, AND CEREALS			
White bread	95	Spaghetti	60
Instant rice	90	Couscous	60
Rice cake	80	Pita bread	55
Rice Krispies	80	Wild rice and brown rice	55
French bread	75	Oatmeal	55
Digestive biscuits	75	Special K	55
Regular crackers	75	Oat and bran bread	50
White bagel	75	Sponge cake	45
Cheerios, white flour	75	All-Bran, no sugar added	45
Total cereal	75		
Puffed wheat	75	**FRUITS**	
Corn flakes	70–75	Watermelon	70
Corn, corn chips	70	Pineapple	65
White rice	70	Raisins	65
Taco shells	70	Ripe bananas	60
Croissant	70	Mango	50
Cream of Wheat	70	Kiwi	50
Shredded wheat	70	Grapes, wine	50
Grape-Nuts	65	Pears	45
Whole wheat crackers	65	Peaches	40
		Plums	40

process, allowing vitamins and minerals to be absorbed and protecting you from a sudden blip in blood sugar that can lead to insulin resistance. They also keep you full longer, so you end up eating less and not feeling hungry an hour after you get up from the table.

Ideally, carbohydrates should always be paired with protein, as protein moderates insulin release. So a piece of bread with a slice of Edam cheese is actually better for you than a plain piece of bread. Similarly, spaghetti with a few meatballs is preferable to spaghetti with plain tomato sauce.

One way of differentiating among carbohydrates in terms of which ones are better for you than others is the glycemic index. Carbohydrates with a low glycemic index are preferable, because they are absorbed more slowly and stimulate less insulin secretion than those

Apples	40	Soybeans	15
Oranges	40	Green and yellow vegetables	0–15
Dried apricots	30		
Grapefruit	25	**DAIRY PRODUCTS**	
Tomatoes	15	Ice cream, premium	60
Fresh apricots	10	Yogurt with fruit	35
		Whole milk	30+
VEGETABLES		Skim milk	30–
Baked potatoes	95	Plain yogurt, no sugar	15
Parsnips	95		
Carrots	85	**MISCELLANEOUS**	
French fries	80	Maltose (as in beer)	105
Beets	75	Glucose	100
Sweet potatoes	55	Pretzels	80
Yams	50	Honey	75
Green peas	45	Refined sugar	75
Black-eyed peas	40	Popcorn	55
Pinto and green beans	40	Nuts	15–30
Chickpeas	35		
Lima and black beans	30		
Kidney and butter beans	30		

with a high glycemic index. Fiber-rich complex carbohydrates such as whole grains tend to have a lower glycemic index than simple ones such as white rice. And within the complex category, brightly colored fruits and vegetables have lower glycemic indexes than "brown" foods such as whole grains, beans, potatoes, and root vegetables.

Knowing the glycemic index of a number of foods will help you make healthful substitutions: a handful of nuts rather than a handful of pretzels, an apple instead of a banana, a sweet potato instead of a white one. Of course, sometimes you just can't help eating a high-glycemic carbohydrate. For example, I think whole wheat pasta is revolting and would rather have a smaller portion of the real stuff. Just remember to indulge selectively and try to get most of your carbohydrates from foods on the low end of the scale.

PROTEIN

Over the past couple of decades, protein phobia has affected many people, particularly women. For some reason, many of my patients believe protein is bad for them and avoid it like the plague. Some are probably still suffering aftereffects of the low-protein high-carbohydrate diet wave. Others have cut back gradually, eating less red meat without substituting adequate protein-rich vegetables and legumes. Still others tell me they "read somewhere" that too much protein leaches calcium from their bones, so they're not eating protein to protect themselves from osteoporosis. My answer is that you'd have to be eating far more protein than most of us could stomach to have an adverse effect on your bone density; and if you're getting enough calcium in your diet and taking a calcium/magnesium supplement, you shouldn't have to worry as much. In most cases eating too little protein is far more dangerous to your health than eating too much.

Protein is, apart from water, the most common substance in our bodies, accounting for up to half of our dry body weight. It is an essential building block of all cells, and it is a key ingredient in hormones, enzymes, neurotransmitters, and antibodies that make our bodies work and help us fight disease. Skin, hair, and nails are made up of protein, which is why in Chapter 6 I mentioned that a low-protein diet could be a culprit if yours are dry or brittle. Protein also builds muscle, which is critical in perimenopause when our muscle mass is beginning to decline. Muscle mass causes your metabolism to speed up, so if you're skimping on protein to lose weight, you may find yourself actually losing muscle mass and slowing down your metabolism, making weight loss even harder to achieve. Protein also helps flush excess water from our bodies, so a low-protein diet can lead to bloating and weight gain by causing you to retain fluid.

In addition to weight gain and deteriorating skin, hair, and nails, protein deficiency can cause loss of concentration, fatigue, irritability, food cravings, and lack of sex drive—all problems you may be facing anyway because of your perimenopausal hormone fluctuations. To keep your symptoms under control, it's important that you consume adequate protein. The recommended amount is 0.8 g per kg (2.2 pounds) of body weight—that's 49 grams a day for a 135-pound woman.

Proteins are made up of building blocks called amino acids. When we eat protein, it gets broken down into its component amino acids.

These are then reassembled into the proteins our body needs. Of the twenty amino acids necessary for human life, half can be produced by our own bodies. The other half, called essential amino acids, must be ingested. The most efficient source of essential amino acids is animal protein. Plant proteins are incomplete, meaning they don't provide a full complement of essential amino acids. This is why vegetarians must be careful to pair certain foods, such as corn and beans, to make sure they get adequate amounts of all the essential amino acids. Tofu, another good non-meat protein source, is also full of phytoestrogens, which can be extremely beneficial to perimenopausal women (see page 364).

As with carbohydrates, all proteins are not created equal. Eggs are the most complete, so unless you are on a cholesterol-restricted diet, it's wise to eat three to four eggs a week. Fish is a great source of protein, especially salmon, tuna, and other fatty fish that are high in omega-3 fatty acids, which have numerous healthful properties (see page 345). Poultry and meat are also good sources, but unfortunately most of what's available in supermarkets has been pumped up with growth hormones. In perimenopause, this can be a problem, as some of these hormones have oestrogenic properties that can put you at risk for certain cancers or exacerbate conditions such as endometriosis and fibroids. If at all possible, buy organic.

As with dairy—another good protein source—red meat does have the drawback of being high in fat. That's why it's best to eat it sparingly—once a week, for example—and to choose lean cuts. Excessive consumption of red meat also increases your homocysteine level, which can put you at risk for heart disease. On the other hand, if you're experiencing excess bleeding, I recommend you indulge in the occasional steak, as red meat is an excellent source of iron.

In the best of all possible worlds, we'd eat a little protein at every meal, as it helps fill us up and keep our blood sugar even. That could mean a poached egg with whole wheat toast for breakfast, a nice tossed salad with a scoop of tuna salad for lunch, a handful of peanuts and a piece of fruit as a snack, and some roast chicken with couscous and vegetables for dinner. Or, you could do what I do: have a tuna sandwich for breakfast, and have a bowl of bran cereal with 1 percent milk as a late-night snack. Do whatever works for you, but make sure to get the protein—you'll feel much better, I guarantee it.

How Much Protein Is in the Food You Eat?

When I say "Eat 49 grams of protein a day," that doesn't mean that you should weigh the egg you eat for breakfast. Different foods contain different amounts of protein. Here's a U.S. Department of Agriculture list of some common protein sources. Note that some of the serving sizes, such as 3 or 3.5 ounces of fish, chicken, and other meats, are smaller than typical portions.

PROTEIN FOOD AND SERVING SIZE	GRAMS OF PROTEIN
DAIRY PRODUCTS	
Buttermilk, 1 cup	8
Cheese, 1 oz., cheddar	7
Cottage cheese (1/2 cup, low-fat)	15.5
Cream cheese, 1 oz.	7
Milk, 1 cup, whole/low-fat/skim	8
Soy milk (nonfat), 1 cup	6
Yogurt, 8 oz., low-fat, plain	12
Yogurt, 8 oz., low-fat, fruit	6
SEAFOOD	
Bluefish, 3.5 oz., baked/broiled	26
Flounder, 3.5 oz., baked	30
Halibut, 3.5 oz., broiled	21
Mackerel, 3.5 oz., broiled	22
Salmon, 3.5 oz., baked/broiled	27
Scallops, 3.5 oz., steamed	18
Swordfish, 3.5 oz., broiled	28
Tuna, 3.5 oz., canned in water	26

FAT

The other day I had lunch with a friend. We both ordered salad appetizers with oil and vinegar on the side. While I proceeded to douse my salad with olive oil and sprinkle on the vinegar, she didn't touch the oil. "How can you have just vinegar?" I asked, my mouth puckering at the mere thought.

PROTEIN FOOD AND SERVING SIZE	GRAMS OF PROTEIN
POULTRY	
Capon, 3.5 oz., roasted	29
Chicken, 3.5 oz., roasted	27
Turkey, 3.5 oz., roasted	28
FRESH MEATS	
Beef, ground, 3 oz., broiled	21
Beef, bottom round, 3 oz., broiled	25
Beef tenderloin, 3 oz., broiled	21
Ham, 3 oz., roasted	18
Veal, 3 oz., round, broiled	23
PROCESSED MEATS	
Beef bologna, 1 oz.	3
Beef frankfurter, 1	6
Chicken roll, 1 oz.	6
Ham, sliced, 1 oz.	5
Turkey bologna, 1 oz.	4
MISCELLANEOUS	
Tofu, 4 oz.	10
Eggs, 1 large, boiled	6
Peanuts, 1 oz.	7
Soy nuts, 1 oz.	12

"Oil is too fattening," she replied virtuously.

"You're wrong there," I replied and proceeded to explain to her why certain fats are in fact not fattening but can actually help you lose weight.

When you eat, say, a piece of bread dipped in olive oil, the fat slows down the absorption of the carbohydrates. With a more gradual influx of carbohydrates, your blood sugar doesn't spike and your pancreas doesn't need to release a jolt of insulin to control it. The fat therefore helps protect you against insulin resistance.

Fat also stimulates the stomach lining to release a hormone called *cholecystokinin,* which travels to the brain and tells it that you're full and that you should stop eating. If you don't eat enough fat, you'll always be hungry and end up grabbing high-carb snacks that will really put on the pounds.

Besides aiding weight control, fat is an important part of the diet for a number of other reasons. For one thing, without fat you can't absorb the fat-soluble vitamins A, D, E, and K. For another, fats are the raw material from which hormones such as oestrogen, progesterone, testosterone, and DHEA are formed. Fats such as myelin form a protective sheath around nerve cells; fat also stabilizes neurotransmitters, especially serotonin. People eating an extremely low-fat diet are susceptible to mood disorders and depression. In addition, fat is a critical component of cell membranes, keeping them flexible and permeable.

The confusion about fats stems in part from the fact that there are many different kinds of fats, and some are definitely not good for you, whereas others can actually improve your health. Fat naturally occurs in three forms: saturated, monounsaturated, and polyunsaturated. The food we eat generally contains all three types, but in various proportions, so that a particular food is classified according to which of the three it contains more of. In addition, there are man-made trans-fatty acids and cholesterol, which is found in food we eat but is also manufactured by our own bodies.

SATURATED FATS. Saturated fats include butter, cheese, and animal fat, which are hard at room temperature, as well as other dairy fat and tropical oils such as coconut and palm oil. These "bad" fats are associated with high levels of LDL cholesterol, atherosclerosis, and heart disease. Indeed, the Harvard University Nurses' Health Study found that each 5 percent increase in calories from saturated fats raised the women's risk of coronary disease by 17 percent. Saturated fats should be less than 10 percent of your daily caloric intake.

MONO- AND POLYUNSATURATED FATS. While some consumption of saturated fats is inevitable, especially if you eat meat, wherever possible try substituting mono- or polyunsaturated fats, which are actually good for you and should be consumed regularly. Monounsaturated fats, such as fat found in olives, avocados, and of course olive oil, increase HDL levels, lower triglycerides, moderate insulin levels, and act as antioxidants, protecting against heart disease and cancer. Polyunsaturated fats such as those found in nuts; in corn, safflower, peanut, sesame, soybean, cottonseed, flaxseed, and canola oil; as well as in fatty fish, also benefit the heart and have antioxidant qualities.

ESSENTIAL FATTY ACIDS. As with proteins, there are two polyunsaturated fats known as essential fatty acids that the body requires but cannot produce on its own. Both of these essential fatty acids, alpha-linolenic acid (omega-3) and linoleic acid (omega-6), can be obtained in varying proportions from meats, fish, vegetables, grains, and nuts. Fatty fish and flaxseed oil, for example, are particularly rich in omega-3 fatty acids, whereas other vegetable oils are good sources of omega-6 fatty acids. Among participants in the Harvard University Nurses' Health Study, those who consumed the most omega-3 fatty acids had up to a 50 percent decrease in their risk of fatal heart attacks as opposed to those who ate the least.

TRANS–FATTY ACIDS. One of the reasons the incidence of heart disease rose so dramatically during the twentieth century is the introduction of fats that have been chemically altered from their natural state. These hydrogenated oils, also known as trans-fatty acids, occur when hydrogen atoms are added to the unsaturated bonds in poly- and monounsaturated fats to stabilize them and make them solid at room temperature. Trans-fatty acids are serious bad news for the heart. The Harvard study found that each 2 percent increase in calories from trans-fatty acids raised the participants' risk of heart disease by 93 percent! Hydrogenated fats increase LDL cholesterol and triglyceride levels while lowering HDL levels. Trans-fatty acids have also been associated with increased breast cancer risk. Make it a habit to read the labels when you go food shopping—especially on margarine—and avoid hydrogenated oils like the plague.

CHOLESTEROL. Finally, a word on cholesterol. For years we've been told to watch our dietary cholesterol intake if we want to protect ourselves against heart disease. And while high blood levels of cholesterol are associated with increased risk of coronary disease, recent research has revealed that there's surprisingly little correlation between how much cholesterol we eat and how high our circulating levels are. Eighty percent of the cholesterol in our bloodstream is manufactured by our livers; only 20 percent comes from outside sources. In fact, if you don't eat enough cholesterol, your body will begin to overproduce it, increasing insulin production in order to free up the carbohydrates it needs as raw material.

So why not go out and eat a diet rich in cholesterol? Because cholesterol-rich foods such as high-fat dairy products and meats (especially organ meats such as liver and kidney) are full of other kinds of fats you should be avoiding. On the other hand, many people have for years been unnecessarily depriving themselves of eggs and either using the horrible substitutes or eating egg-white omelets for fear of cholesterol. It turns out that three or four eggs a week will not adversely affect your cholesterol; I recommend eggs as a great low-calorie source of protein.

DAIRY

As with protein, a lot of my patients are shunning dairy products these days—and often compromising their health in the process. Dairy products are an excellent source of carbohydrates, protein, and calcium, three critical elements in a balanced diet for perimenopausal women.

While some people legitimately cannot digest dairy products, those who can (and who aren't vegan) should make them a part of their daily diet. "But dairy products are full of fat!" protest my weight-watching patients. True, and it's saturated fat, which isn't great for your health. But how about skim milk? Lowfat cheese? Nonfat yogurt? All these products have just as much protein as their full-fat counterparts. The cheeses common in the traditional Mediterranean diet such as ricotta and mozzarella were originally made from goat's milk, which is much lower in fat than cow's milk. Feta, common in Greek cuisine, is another good—but salty—low-fat cheese, and although Parmesan is fatty, it is usually used sparingly as a condiment.

A patient recently told me she is not eating dairy because she's afraid that the hormones pumped into cows will increase her risk of breast cancer. If this is your concern, it's not reason enough to forego the benefits of dairy. Organic milk, cheese, and yogurt made from non–hormone-treated cow's milk is available practically everywhere now. It costs a little more, but if it gets you back to eating dairy, it's well worth the added expense.

FOOD AND DRINK

In presenting the benefits of the Mediterranean diet, I discussed the healthful properties of a number of foods. Here are some specifics on several additional foods and beverages that have been studied extensively and proven to have positive effects on the body.

Garlic

Amount   1 to 2 cloves daily

Benefits • decreases cholesterol   • decreases blood pressure
            • decreases risk of blood clots

Warning   Do not take with bloodthinners.

Omega-3 Fatty Acids

Amount   2 to 3 servings fatty fish per week, or up to six 1,000 mg
              fish oil capsules daily
            1 to 2 teaspoons flaxseed oil daily, or 3 to 5 tablespoons
              freshly ground flaxseed

Benefits • relieves PMS symptoms   • decreases heart arrhythmias
            • decreases risk of depression • decreases blood pressure
            • decreases risk of heart   • inhibits tumor growth
                attack   • decreases risk of breast
            • decreases cholesterol   cancer
            • decreases risk of blood clots • improves mental function
            • may protect against   • improves irritable bowel
                Alzheimer's Disease   syndrome

Nuts

Amount   ½ cup five or more times a week (unsalted peanuts are
              particularly healthful)

Benefits	• antioxidant	• lowers blood pressure
	• lowers LDL cholesterol	• relaxes blood vessels
	• lowers triglycerides	• lowers homocysteine

Red Wine or Purple Grape Juice

Amount	One glass per day with food	
Benefits	• antioxidant	• decreases risk of stroke
	• decreases LDL cholesterol	• decreases risk of heart
	• increases HDL cholesterol	attack

Tea (Black or Green, Not Herbal)

Amount	One or more cups a day (caffeinated is more beneficial than decaffeinated)	
Benefits	• antioxidant	• decreases risk of stroke
	• decreases LDL cholesterol	• protects against cancer
	• decreases risk of heart attack	

HOW DO I KNOW IF I NEED TO LOSE WEIGHT?

Simple question, right? Not really: weight is an extremely subjective issue. Different cultures and different parts of the country have different standards. Moreover, every woman brings her own load of body image issues with her every time she steps on the scale, often distorting what the numbers really mean. I have patients who can't even pinch an inch but who are constantly dieting to try to look like some of the unhealthily thin models and actresses they see in the media. Other patients who are seriously overweight shrug their shoulders when I tell them to try to slim down, saying, "It's no use, it's genetic. My whole family is fat."

Although it's true that heredity does play a role in body size, there is a range of healthy weights within which most people should try to fall. It's based on your body mass index (BMI), a measurement representing the relationship between your height and weight. The Department of Health and Human Services in the United States recommends maintaining a BMI of between 19 and 25. But these guidelines apply to men, who naturally have more muscle mass, as well as to women, who naturally have more body fat. A more realistic goal for women should be between 22 and 25. Lower than 22 puts you at risk for osteoporosis (see Chapter 8), whereas higher than 25 puts you at risk for heart disease, diabetes, oestrogen-dependent tumors, and a host of other obesity-related diseases.

Consult the chart on page 350 to determine your BMI. Even if your BMI is within the healthy range, it's preferable not to have gained more than 10 pounds since age 18 (unless you were underweight), as such an increase poses independent health risks.

If your body mass index is greater than 25, you are considered overweight and should immediately take action. That *doesn't* mean jumping on the latest weight-loss bandwagon, which now happens to be high-protein low-carbohydrate diets. Eating excessive protein (substantially more than the 0.8 g per 2.2 pounds body weight recommended earlier in this chapter) and inadequate carbohydrates can lead to bone loss and a condition called ketosis. Even though there are some diet gurus who think ketosis is the ultimate weight-control strategy, the fact of the matter is that it's extremely dangerous longterm. Ketosis stresses the liver and kidneys to the point at which your kidneys could actually fail, and it also can cause nausea, fatigue, headaches, and potentially even brain damage. Any weight loss on an extremely high-protein, low-carbohydrate diet is due to loss of muscle mass and water weight, not fat. Indeed, when you go off the diet, you're likely to put back the weight you lost from muscles as fat, setting you back even further in your efforts. The best way to lose weight is to commit to a low-fat, moderate-carbohydrate, reduced-calorie eating plan you can live with long-term and begin a regular exercise program, which I'll describe shortly.

Another measurement you should keep your eye on is your waisthip ratio (WHR), which shouldn't exceed 0.80. To calculate your WHR, simply divide your waist measurement by your hip measurement: if your waist is 33 inches and your hips are 45 inches, your WHR is 0.73. As I've explained, abdominal fat accumulation is extremely dangerous for women, as it puts us at risk for heart disease, diabetes, and cancer. In fact, a waistline of greater than 35 inches has been shown to increase health problems for women regardless of hip size. So if you find yourself repeatedly letting out your skirts, take out

Body Mass Index Chart

Height (Feet and Inches)

Weight (Pounds)	5'0"	5'1"	5'2"	5'3"	5'4"	5'5"	5'6"	5'7"	5'8"	5'9"	5'10"	5'11"	6'0"	6'1"	6'2"	6'3"	6'4"
100	20	19	18	18	17	17	16	16	15	15	14	14	14	13	13	12	12
105	21	20	19	19	18	17	17	16	16	16	15	15	14	14	13	13	13
110	21	21	20	19	19	18	18	17	17	16	16	15	15	15	14	14	13
115	22	22	21	20	20	19	19	18	17	17	17	16	16	15	15	14	14
120	23	23	22	21	21	20	19	19	18	18	17	17	16	16	15	15	15
125	24	24	23	22	21	21	20	20	19	18	18	17	17	16	16	16	15
130	25	25	24	23	22	22	21	20	20	19	19	18	18	17	17	16	16
135	26	26	25	24	23	22	22	21	21	20	19	19	18	18	17	17	16
140	27	26	26	25	24	23	23	22	21	21	20	20	19	18	18	17	17
145	28	27	27	26	25	24	23	23	22	21	21	20	20	19	19	18	18
150	29	28	27	27	26	25	24	23	23	22	22	21	20	20	19	19	18
155	30	29	28	27	27	26	25	24	24	23	22	22	21	20	20	19	19
160	31	30	29	28	27	27	26	25	24	24	23	22	22	21	21	20	19
165	32	31	30	29	28	27	27	26	25	24	24	23	22	22	21	21	20
170	33	32	31	30	29	28	27	27	26	25	24	24	23	22	22	21	21
175	34	33	32	31	30	29	28	27	27	26	25	24	24	23	22	22	21
180	35	34	33	32	31	30	29	28	27	27	26	25	24	24	23	22	22
185	36	35	34	33	32	31	30	29	28	27	27	26	25	24	24	23	23
190	37	36	35	34	33	32	31	30	29	28	27	26	26	25	24	24	23
195	38	37	36	35	33	32	31	31	30	29	28	27	26	26	25	24	24
200	39	38	37	35	34	33	32	31	30	30	29	28	27	26	26	25	24
205	40	39	37	36	35	34	33	32	31	30	29	29	28	27	26	26	25
210	41	40	38	37	36	35	34	33	32	31	30	29	28	28	27	26	26
215	42	41	39	38	37	36	35	34	33	32	31	30	29	28	28	27	26
220	43	42	40	39	38	37	36	34	33	32	32	31	30	29	28	27	27
225	44	43	41	40	39	37	36	35	34	33	32	31	31	30	29	28	27
230	45	43	42	41	39	38	37	36	35	34	33	32	31	30	30	29	28
235	46	44	43	42	40	39	38	37	36	35	34	33	32	31	30	29	29
240	47	45	44	43	41	40	39	38	36	35	34	33	33	32	31	30	29
245	48	46	45	43	42	41	40	38	37	36	35	34	33	32	31	31	30
250	49	47	46	44	43	42	40	39	38	37	36	35	34	33	32	31	30

☐ Underweight   ☐ Weight Appropriate   ☐ Overweight   ☐ Obese the tape measure and check to see whether you're letting your belly get the best of you.

EXERCISE

You've heard it a thousand times before. Make this number one-thousand-and-one: exercise is critical for weight control and health. And it's never too late to start. It is shocking that only 20 percent of American adults get regular moderate exercise, meaning the other 80 percent qualify as "sedentary" and are at risk for innumerable diseases and a shortened life expectancy. Part of the problem is that we live in a convenience-oriented society—you can do your banking or buy a burger without leaving the comfort of your car, and thanks to the Internet you can now shop for everything from groceries to gardening tools without leaving the comfort of your living room. The result of this cushy lifestyle is that we're getting fatter and fatter and, in spite of modern medical advances, more and more susceptible to heart attacks, stroke, diabetes, hypertension, and certain types of cancer.

Now I'm not saying you should turn in your Toyota for a horse and buggy. I am saying, however, that because it's so easy not to be physically active in our society, you'll have to make an extra effort to get the kind of exercise you need to protect your health. And how much is that? *At least 30 minutes of weight-bearing aerobic exercise three times a week, and at least 30 minutes of strength training twice a week.*

"Hey—wait a minute," you may be thinking. "That sounds complicated. I have to do two different kinds of exercise? Why can't I just find one thing I can tolerate and do it five times a week?" For several reasons. First, it will get boring, and if you're bored, your motivation will decline. Second, there is no perfect exercise that works out every muscle in your body: jogging, for example, is great for the heart, the buttocks, and the legs (except the knees) but does little for your arms or your back. And finally, although aerobic exercise is great for your cardiovascular health, strength training exercise is essential for your muscles and bones.

What's the difference? Aerobic exercise is any exercise that raises your heart rate. Ideally, you should aim to get your pulse up to between 60 and 80 percent of your maximum heart rate for at least

30 minutes three times a week. Your maximum heart rate is 220 minus your age; that means if you're 45, your maximum heart rate is 175. Sixty to 80 percent of 175 is between 105 and 140 beats per minute.

Even though jogging, biking, swimming, playing tennis, rowing, dancing, StairMastering, and NordicTracking are all great ways to get aerobic exercise, simple walking can also do the trick. Many women enjoy walking because apart from a comfortable pair of supportive shoes, it doesn't involve a big investment; it can be done anytime, anywhere; and it can be done with a friend. Indeed, enlisting a buddy to exercise with you—no matter what you choose to do—is a great way to make the activity more fun and help you stick to your commitment.

When I say walking, however, I don't mean window shopping. To get an aerobic workout, you need to walk fast enough to reach your target heart rate. That means getting out of breath—although not so out of breath that you can't speak. At first you may find you get sufficient exercise by walking a 20-minute mile. After a while, as you get in better shape, you'll need to pick up the pace to achieve the same aerobic benefit.

Those of you who don't have a half-hour break will be glad to know that studies have shown that three 10-minute aerobic exercise sessions a day yield just as great a benefit as one 30-minute session. Quickie sessions are easy to incorporate into your everyday routine: bike to the post office instead of driving, vigorously weed the garden, climb up and down the stairs, scrub the bathtub, vacuum the house. Just make sure to work hard enough to get your heart rate up and sustain the activity for the full 10 minutes.

Whereas aerobic exercise improves the health of your heart, strength training exercise is essential for the health of your muscles and bones. Why? Because putting pressure on your bones promotes increased density; also, when your muscles pull on your bones they increase the bones' strength. Actual weight-lifting is one way to achieve this effect, but other exercises can also help you build bone. Basically, any exercise that involves fighting gravity—jumping rope, jogging, aerobic dancing, hiking, tennis, volleyball, skiing, walking—is considered weight-bearing. Any exercise in which you do not have to support your own weight—swimming, water aerobics, and bicycling—is non–weight-bearing and will not benefit your bones significantly.

But what if your doctor has told you to swim for your arthritis or your bad back? Fine (it counts for your aerobic workout)—but also lift weights twice a week. If you bicycle five times a week, cut back to three and play tennis on the other two days. If you're a walker, a runner, or an aerobics fiend, you still may want to do some additional weight-lifting because those activities benefit your hip and spine bones, but not your shoulders, arms, or wrists. The bonus to doing weight-bearing exercise is that it also increases muscle mass. Because muscle burns more calories than fat, it'll help you keep your weight down in the long term.

"But I take calcium supplements," you may say. "Won't that keep my bones in shape?" In a word, no. Without calcium, your bones will definitely deteriorate, but taking calcium alone without exercise will not increase your bone density. The flip side is also true: doing weight-bearing exercise without getting adequate calcium won't increase your bone density, either. Weight-bearing exercise promotes bone remodeling, which as you'll recall from Chapter 8 occurs when osteoclasts break down bone and osteoblasts rebuild it. If you don't have enough calcium in your system, the osteoblasts won't have any raw material with which to manufacture new bone. Similarly, even if you have plenty of calcium, if your bones aren't actively turning over (being broken down and rebuilt), the calcium won't be incorporated into them and will simply remain in circulation. By the same token, oestrogen replacement therapy is not a substitute for exercise, either—in terms of both bone and cardiovascular health.

As far as exercise is concerned, I have to confess that I haven't always practiced what I preach. For years I was so crazed and sleep-deprived working around the clock and raising two children that I didn't have time to blink, much less work out. Moreover, the prospect of joining a gym and spending a half-hour a day in a stuffy room packed with sweaty bodies was not exactly a turn-on. Eventually, however, I admitted that I had to start taking better care of myself. Being on my feet all day, I wasn't worried about weight-bearing exercise, but I knew I needed to do something aerobic.

After a while I began to ask my patients what they were doing to keep fit, and their answers made me think about exercise in a whole new way. Sure, some were going to gyms, but others were ballroom dancing, kick-boxing, doing yoga, and horseback riding. One of my 70-year-old patients was ice-skating! I realized that the reason these women were able to stick to their exercise commitments was because *they chose activities they loved to do and would do anyway, regardless of the health benefits.*

So I asked myself what I like to do in my spare time—being outdoors, enjoying beautiful scenery, exploring different neighborhoods, admiring people's gardens and homes—and decided to try bicycling. Now, whenever I have a day off or if I get home before dark, I jump into a pair of shorts, put on a helmet, and take a half-hour spin. Not only do I feel more awake and alive and relaxed, but I also find it easier to control my weight. My only regret is that I spent so many years depriving myself of this wonderfully healthful indulgence.

VITAMIN AND MINERAL SUPPLEMENTS

Even though a balanced Mediterranean-style diet will provide you with an excellent array of nutrients, perimenopausal women often need to supplement their diets in order to achieve the amounts they need to moderate their symptoms and protect themselves against disease.

Across the board I recommend that at the very least my perimenopausal patients take a good multivitamin as well as calcium/ magnesium and natural vitamin E supplements daily. In addition, you may wish to add one or more of the following to your regimen *if your multivitamin does not already contain the recommended dose.* All the following recommendations have been described in more detail in individual chapters throughout the book.

Don't forget to inform your doctor before you begin taking any dietary supplements—there may be interactions with drugs you are already taking or health reasons you should not take a particular product.

Vitamin A

Dose   5,000 IU daily

Benefits   • acts as antioxidant   • regulates bone remodeling
            • improves skin health

Vitamins B₆, B₁₂, and Folic Acid

Dose B_6: 50 to 100 mg daily *but no more than* 200 mg daily
B_{12}: 50 to 100 mcg daily
Folic acid: 400 mcg daily

Benefits
- relieves PMS symptoms
- relieves hot flushes
- enhances mood
- decreases risk of depression
- improves memory
- produces hydrochloric acid necessary for absorption of calcium
- lowers homocysteine levels
- decreases risk of atherosclerosis
- relieves fibrocystic breasts
- decreases risk of colon cancer

Vitamin C

Dose 500 mg twice a day of ester vitamin C

Benefits
- acts as antioxidant
- improves memory
- decreases incidence of urinary tract infections
- increases collagen in skin
- increases collagen in bone
- decreases risk of stroke
- decreases risk of atherosclerosis

Vitamin D

Dose 400 IU daily

Benefits
- enhances calcium absorption from intestines
- increases bone strength

Natural Vitamin E

Dose 400 to 800 IU daily

Benefits
- acts as antioxidant
- relieves hot flushes
- improves memory
- slows progression of Alzheimer's disease
- reduces wrinkles
- decreases risk of stroke
- decreases risk of atherosclerosis
- protects against cancer

• relieves fibrocystic breasts	• decreases risk of colon cancer

Warning   Do not take with bloodthinners.

Vitamin K

Dose   100 mcg daily

Benefits   • increases osteocalcin and improves bone density

Warnings   Do not take with bloodthinners.
                Do not take if you are pregnant.

Boron

Dose   3 mg daily

Benefit   • helps vitamin D stimulate intestinal absorption
                 of calcium

Calcium

Dose   1,200 mg daily taken in two 600 mg doses with food, preferably at the end of the day (e.g., one pill with dinner and another at bedtime with a light snack)

Benefits

• relieves PMS symptoms	• decreases risk of stroke
• builds bone	• decreases risk of colon cancer
• decreases heart palpitations	
• decreases blood pressure	

Mixed Carotenes

Dose   3 to 6 mg daily

Benefits

• acts as antioxidant	• protects against cancer
• improves memory	• decreases risk of colon cancer
• decreases risk of heart disease	

Coenzyme Q10

Dose   50 mg daily or 100 mg daily if you are at risk for heart
              disease

Benefits   • relieves angina   • decreases heart palpitations
              • decreases blood pressure   • decreases risk of breast
                                                 cancer

Iron

Dose   28 mg ferrous sulphate taken on an empty stomach with
              vitamin C (your body will absorb what it needs and
              excrete any excess in your stool)

Benefit   • prevents and treats iron-deficiency anaemia

Magnesium

Dose   600 mg daily taken with calcium in divided doses with
              food at the end of the day

Benefits   • relieves PMS symptoms   • builds bone
              • reduces fatigue   • decreases blood pressure
              • improves feelings of   • relieves angina
                well-being   • decreases heart palpitations
              • may prevent migraine
                headaches

Phosphatidyl Serine (PS) and Acetyl-L-Carnitine (ALC)

Dose   100 to 300 mg PS daily
              500 to 2,000 mg ALC daily

Benefits   • increases attention   • improves judgment
              • improves concentration   • relieves depression (PS)
              • improves short- and
                long-term memory

Selenium

Dose   200 mcg daily taken with vitamin E

Benefit   • decreases risk of colon cancer

Herbs

One of the treatment options my perimenopausal patients are most grateful to hear about—especially if they're reluctant to go on hormones or medications—is herbs. Although herbs are not for everyone, many women find that herbs can be enough to carry them through part if not all of their perimenopause.

More than 70 million Americans are currently taking herbal products in the belief that these natural remedies will improve their health. Unfortunately, they may be doing themselves more harm than good. Although the active ingredients in herbs are often identical to those in conventional medications, because herbs are classified as dietary supplements and not as drugs they are not regulated. This leaves some unscrupulous manufacturers free to dilute the active ingredients or misrepresent the health benefits of their products. Herbs can also have serious side effects if taken in combination with certain other herbs or medications.

As a physician, I am comfortable prescribing the herbs listed in this appendix because I have seen them work in my patients. Nevertheless, it is your responsibility to educate yourself about the herbs you are interested in—their effects and side effects, drug interactions, and contraindications—because everyone's response to herbs is different. *To protect yourself, take these precautions:* (1) always tell your doctor before beginning an herbal regimen; (2) ask your doctor or pharmacist to recommend reliable brands; (3) check the amount of active ingredient in the product; (4) check the expiration date; (5) do not exceed the

> ### *Beware of Blue Cohosh*
>
> Also known as blueberry root, papoose root, and squawroot, blue cohosh is not the same as black cohosh and should not be taken to treat menstrual or menopausal symptoms. Traditionally used to induce labor, it has been shown to cause severe birth defects in rats that were given it during the early stages of pregnancy. I do not recommend it under any circumstances.

recommended dosage; (6) do not take if pregnant or breastfeeding; and (7) if side effects occur, stop immediately and consult your doctor.

Black Cohosh (Remifemin)

Dose One Remifemin pill in morning, one pill in evening

Benefits
- improves irregular bleeding
- relieves painful periods
- relieves PMS symptoms
- relieves hot flushes
- relieves insomnia
- relieves heart palpitations
- improves mood
- relieves anxiety
- decreases incidence of migraine headaches

Chamomile

Dose Tea or 300 to 400 mg dried chamomile daily before bed-time

Benefit
- relieves insomnia

Chasteberry (Vitex)

Dose 10 mg chasteberry seeds three times a day

Benefits
- improves irregular bleeding
- relieves amenorrhoea
- increases LH, thereby increasing progesterone and protecting against unopposed oestrogen
- relieves fibrocystic breasts

Evening Primrose Oil

Dose   1,000 to 3,000 mg daily

Benefits   • relieves menstrual   • relieves anxiety
           problems   • improves mood
          • relieves hot flushes   • relieves fibrocystic breasts

Feverfew

Dose   125 mg daily

Benefit   • decreases incidence of migraine headaches

Warning   Do not take with bloodthinners or within two to three weeks of surgery because it can cause problems with blood pressure and bleeding.

Ginkgo Biloba

Dose   30 to 50 mg three times a day

Benefits   • acts as antioxidant   • improves concentration
          • improves mood   • acts as antidepressant
          • improves short–term   • stimulates libido
           memory

Warning   Do not take with bloodthinners or within two to three weeks of surgery because it can cause problems with blood pressure and bleeding.

Hawthorn

Dose   100 to 250 mg three times a day

Benefits   • relieves angina
          • decreases heart palpitations
          • decreases blood pressure

Kava Kava

Dose   60 to 120 mg daily

Benefits
- relieves insomnia
- reduces anxiety
- improves mood
- reduces irritability and stress

Warnings Do not take with benzodiazepines (Nitrazepam, Valium, Temazepam).
Do not use with alcohol or with other antidepressants.

Liquorice (DGL)

Dose   500 mg daily

Benefits
- acts as anti-inflammatory
- reduces heavy bleeding
- has mild phytoestrogenic properties

Saint John's Wort

Dose   Start with one 300 to 500 mg tablet daily with breakfast and, if necessary, work up to three pills a day with meals (takes six to eight weeks to be effective).

Benefits
- relieves insomnia
- relieves depression
- reduces anxiety
- stimulates libido

Warnings Consult your physician before taking Saint John's wort if you are on any prescription medication. Saint John's wort has been shown to interact with the following drugs:
- oral contraceptives
- statins (Lipitor, Lipobay)
- beta-blockers (Inderal, Tenormin)
- calcium channel blockers (Adalat, Cardene, Tildiem, Verelan, Plendil)
- digitalis (Digoxin)
- theophylline (Nuelin, Theo-Dur)
- warfarin (Adenocoumarol)
- certain antibiotics (Biaxin, E-Mycin)
- SSRI antidepressants (Prozac, Lustral)
- MAO inhibitors
- drugs that cause sun sensitivity (Isotretinoin, tetracycline, doxycycline)

Uva Ursi

Dose   250 to 500 mg three times a day for four days

Benefits   • prevents urinary tract infections
             • has antiviral, antibacterial, and antifungal properties

Warning   Uva Ursi is not effective if your urine is acidic, so avoid vitamin C and cranberry juice if you are taking it.

Valerian

Dose   150 to 300 mg a half hour before bedtime

Benefit   • relieves insomnia

Warning   Do not take with barbiturates (Phenobarbital, Primidone) or benzodiazepines (Nitrazepam, Valium, Temazepam).

Phytoestrogens

Throughout this book I've been touting the benefits of phytoestrogens for relief of perimenopausal symptoms. Foods are much more effective sources of phytoestrogens than supplements. In particular, I do not recommend soy powders or pills because they lack the soy protein needed to activate the soy isoflavones. Eating a diet rich in fruits, vegetables, legumes, and whole grains will provide a good distribution of phytoestrogens, but if you want a special boost, incorporate soy products and flaxseed into your diet.

Soy

Dose   Up to 50 mg soy isoflavones incorporating between 10 and 30 g soy protein daily through food sources

Benefits
- acts as antioxidant
- relieves menstrual cramping
- regulates periods
- relieves hot flushes
- relieves insomnia
- decreases heart palpitations
- improves mood
- decreases incidence of migraine headaches
- improves memory
- increases bone density
- increases HDL cholesterol
- decreases lipoprotein (a)
- lowers blood pressure
- decreases risk of stroke
- decreases risk of heart attack
- decreases risk of breast cancer
- decreases risk of ovarian cancer
- decreases risk of uterine cancer

• decreases LDH cholesterol, triglycerides, and total cholesterol

Warning   May exacerbate fibroids and endometriosis.

SOURCES OF SOY ISOFLAVONES

SOY FOOD	SOY PROTEIN	CALORIES	CALCIUM	ISOFLAVONES
Tofu (4 ounces)	10 g	120	120–300 mg	30 mg
Textured vegetable protein—cooked (1/2 cup)	12 g	60	85 mg	35 mg
Soy flour (1/2 cup)	23 g	163	200 mg	55–90 mg
Tempeh (1/2 cup)	16 g	204	80 mg	40–50 mg
Soybeans—(edamame beans) cooked (1/2 cup)	14 g	149	88 mg	55–90 mg
Soy milk—nonfat (1 cup)	6 g	80	200–300 mg	25 mg
Soy protein (1–2 tbsp)	15–30 g	50–100	50 mg	60–120 mg
Roasted soy nuts (1 ounce)	12 g	120	48 mg	78 mg

Flaxseed

Dose   3 to 5 tablespoons (25 to 50 g) daily freshly ground flaxseed or 1 to 2 teaspoons flaxseed oil (2 to 9 g)

Benefits
• acts as antioxidant
• relieves PMS symptoms
• relieves menstrual cramps
• relieves hot flushes
• improves mood
• relieves anxiety
• relieves depression
• improves memory
• decreases blood pressure
• decreases risk of atherosclerosis
• decreases LDL cholesterol
• protects against cancer
• decreases risk of breast cancer
• inhibits tumor growth

TOO MUCH OF A GOOD THING

Often when I ask a perimenopausal patient whether she's taking anything to relieve her symptoms, she'll reply, "Oh, yes! I picked up these great supplements at the health food store, made just for women, that contain lots of phytoestrogens, plus I'm drinking soy shakes, eating tofu, and sprinkling soy powder on my cereal every morning."

Although phytoestrogens can help equilibrate your hormone levels during perimenopause, too many can tip the balance in a potentially dangerous direction. Overstimulating your oestrogen receptors can lead to excessive bleeding, which sets the stage for precancer of the uterus. So it's important to monitor your phytoestrogen intake and not exceed the recommended dose.

In addition, be wary of the plethora of over-the-counter "For Women Only" formulations. These supplements are not regulated, so there's no guarantee that they contain what they say they do in the doses they say they have. Plus, they may include ingredients—such as megadoses of phytoestrogens—that could do you more harm than good.

Hormones in Perimenopause

Every day there are more options for perimenopausal women who need or want to take hormones to regulate their symptoms. Treatment has to be individualized: some women need more hormonal support; others experience side effects from stronger products and will benefit from a lower dose. Oral contraceptives contain three times the amount of oestrogen as standard hormone replacement therapy and six times the amount as low-dose oestrogen replacement therapy. Morever, as your perimenopause progresses, you may need to adjust your regimen. When I prescribe hormones to a patient, I see her or have her report to me by phone every two months until we are both pleased with the results.

ORAL CONTRACEPTIVES

Many women still fear the Pill because they recall the sometimes serious side effects that were occasionally associated with oral contraceptives in the early days. Today, those high-dose pills are virtually off the market; all I ever prescribe are low-dose oral contraceptives that have minimal side effects. If you do find you're experiencing bloating or mood swings, ask your doctor to prescribe a different brand—there are a zillion out there to choose from.

One kind of birth control pill I do not recommend for perimenopausal women is Micronor, the progestogen-only mini-Pill. This drug can affect your bleeding pattern, which is the last thing you want to do in perimenopause.

Dose   20 to 35 mcg oestrogen plus progestogen

Benefits
- regulates periods and menstrual blood flow
- reduces risk of iron-deficiency anaemia
- reduces painful periods
- relieves hot flushes
- relieves insomnia
- relieves vaginal dryness
- decreases risk of urinary tract infections
- decreases risk of pelvic inflammatory disease
- controls unwanted hair growth
- reduces acne
- protects against pregnancy
- reduces incidence of ectopic pregnancy
- increases bone density
- may lower risk of stroke and heart attack
- decreases symptoms of fibrocystic breasts
- decreases incidence of ovarian cysts
- decreases symptoms of fibroids
- decreases symptoms of endometriosis
- decreases risk of ovarian cancer
- decreases risk of endometrial cancer
- decreases risk of colon cancer

Warnings   Do not take if you are over age 35 and smoke.
Do not take if you have a history of thrombophlebitis or any other clotting disorder.

HORMONE REPLACEMENT THERAPY

As with birth control pills, many women shy away from hormone replacement therapy because of stories they've heard about the early days when women suffered side effects from high doses or developed uterine cancer as a result of the original practice of prescribing unopposed oestrogen. Nowadays we always prescribe progestogens to counterbalance the oestrogen except when a woman has had a hysterectomy. Also, the standard dose of hormone replacement therapy is only one-third that of a low-dose birth control pill.

"But I don't want to get my period for the rest of my life—that's the one thing I've been looking forward to about menopause," patients often complain. "I mean, it'll be a little embarrassing shopping for Tampax when I'm 80." Rest assured, hormone replacement therapy won't make you menstruate indefinitely. Under combined therapy, which means taking both oestrogen and progestogens daily, 95 percent of patients who start hormone replacement therapy with menopause stop bleeding within one year.

All treatment plans for hormone replacement should be determined on a case-by-case basis. Some women find natural products easier to tolerate than synthetics, whereas others find natural products aren't strong enough and require synthetics. Depending on their symptoms, some women may benefit from an added jolt of testosterone. I frequently have to adjust the dose my patients are taking or the type—oral, patch, cream, or gel—several times until we find a level that works for them. And then, as their perimenopause progresses or they cross over into menopause, we often need to change yet again.

To my delight, many of my patients who have been difficult to treat with oral hormone replacement have responded wonderfully to skin-based therapies. For example, I have a perimenopausal patient who was suffering a myriad of symptoms including hot flushes and insomnia. But by far the worst was a "spacy" feeling she described as "like being on Cloud Nine." I put her on Hormonin (oral natural oestrogen) and oral micronized progesterone (OMP), and several months later she reported feeling even worse—emotionally volatile, crying for no reason, forgetting everything, still not sleeping, and feeling "like a zombie." So I switched her to an oral natural oestrogen and Provera. (The OMP sedated her so much she was dragging all day.) Still she complained of hot flushes, insomnia, and memory loss. Finally I put her on a standard-dose natural oestrogen patch with Provera and shortly thereafter she told me her memory was great, she was sleeping, and she felt "like a normal person again." It is interesting that as I reviewed the blood tests in her chart I noticed that while she was on oral oestrogen replacement, her blood levels for oestrogen were only moderate and tended to decline over time. But when I put her on the patch her blood levels were excellent and remained elevated, indicating that her body absorbed oestrogen much better through the skin than the gut.

If you do decide to go on hormone replacement therapy, the key to having a successful experience is to be entirely frank with your doctor about your concerns and, once you are on hormones, about how they are making you feel. If you don't tell your doctor, for example, that your hot flushes are actually worse or that you still have no sex drive, he or she won't be able to make the adjustments necessary to provide you with relief. My patients who report the most satisfaction with their hormone replacement therapy are often the ones with whom I've spent the most time fine-tuning their treatment.

OESTROGEN

When most people talk about hormone replacement therapy, what they're really thinking about is oestrogen. It's our declining endogenous oestrogen levels, after all, that are responsible for our perimenopausal symptoms, and it's oestrogen's protective effect on virtually every system of the body that we lose after menopause.

Oestrogen supplements are available in five forms: standard pills, low-dose pills, transdermal patches and gels, and vaginal creams. The standard treatment provides the greatest benefits, but for various reasons you and your doctor may decide that low-dose pills, transdermal products, or vaginal cream is best for you. Low-dose formulations are indicated by an asterisk on the product charts that begin on page 378.

Standard Oestrogen Replacement Therapy

Benefits

- acts as antioxidant
- acts as anti-inflammatory
- reduces hot flushes
- relieves insomnia
- decreases heart palpitations
- improves memory
- improves cognitive function
- improves concentration
- reduces anxiety and irritability
- improves mood
- may decreases risk of Alzheimer's disease
- decreases vaginal atrophy
- relieves painful intercourse
- increases vaginal moisture
- decreases incidence of vaginitis
- relieves itchy skin
- increases skin collagen
- increases sebum production and skin moisture
- decreases wrinkles
- increases lean body mass
- decreases waist-hip ratio
- improves bone density
- relieves joint pain
- decreases total and LDL cholesterol
- increases HDL cholesterol and triglycerides
- decreases blood pressure
- decreases lipoprotein (a)
- decreases risk of heart disease by 50 percent

- decreases incidence of urinary tract infections
- relieves incontinence
- decreases risk of colon cancer
- relieves irritable bowel syndrome

Warnings Do not take if you have a history of blood clots.

If you have had breast cancer or are at high risk, consult your doctor.

Side effects include increased bleeding, breast tenderness, and bloating.

Low-Dose Oestrogen Replacement Therapy

Many of my patients who resist standard oestrogen replacement therapy are willing to try low-dose oestrogen because it is safer and has fewer side effects: less bleeding, less breast tenderness, less bloating, possibly less risk of thrombophlebitis (blood clots) and possibly no risk of breast cancer. Because of the low dose, this form of oestrogen may be taken without a progestogen; however, I still like to prescribe a continuous low dose of natural progesterone or synthetic progestogen as well. If you don't take a progestogen daily, at least every three to four months you should take one for 10 to 14 days to decrease your risk of uterine cancer.

Benefits
- relieves hot flushes
- relieves insomnia
- improves memory
- improves cognitive function
- improves mood
- improves bone density
- decreases risk of heart disease by 20 to 30 percent

Transdermal Oestrogen (Patches) and Percutaneous Gels

I've become a convert to transdermal delivery of oestrogen in recent years, as I've seen both low-dose and standard oestrogen patches and gels work wonderfully on my patients. The absorption of hormones through the skin is often superior to absorption through the gut, and blood levels stay constant. If you are on oral hormone replacement therapy and still don't feel great, ask your doctor about the possibility of changing over to a transdermal product.

Benefits   • all the benefits of oestrogen (see page 370) plus . . .
- decreases incidence of   • is the preferred option
  migrane headaches   for smokers
- lowers triglyceride levels

Warning   The patch or gel will lower your total and LDL cholesterol but will not raise your HDL cholesterol, so if
your HDLs are below 35, you would gain more benefit from oral oestrogen than from the patch.

Vaginal Oestrogen

If your symptoms are localized to your vagina and bladder, the most
effective treatment is oestrogen applied directly to the vagina.

Benefits   • relieves vaginal atrophy   • decreases incidence of
- relieves painful intercourse   urinary tract infections
- increases vaginal lubrication   • relieves incontinence
- decreases incidence of
  vaginitis

PROGESTOGEN SUPPLEMENTS

Thanks to progestogen supplements, the incidence of uterine cancer
has dropped significantly. Not only do I prescribe progestogens with
oestrogens as part of hormone replacement therapy, but I often prescribe progestogens alone for women whose endogenous oestrogen
levels are elevated or who do not wish to take oestrogen supplements.
My preference is for natural progesterone, since it has favorable effects
on both heart and bone without causing unpleasant side effects.
Synthetic progestogens have more adverse side effects than natural
progesterone, but some women cannot take the natural because they
are allergic to peanuts (peanut oil being one of the main ingredients of
natural progesterone) or because it makes them too drowsy. For them,
synthetic progestogens are an alternative.

Progestogens

Benefits   • counterbalances excess   • controls growth of
  oestrogen   fibroids
- relieves hot flushes   • controls endometriosis

Warnings   Side effects include fluid retention, breast tenderness, weight gain, depression, and migraine headaches.

Progestogens increase LDL and total cholesterol levels, and they decrease HDL cholesterol levels, negating the positive effects of oestrogen.

Progestogens increase the risk of coronary artery vasospasm.

Oral Progesterone

Benefits
- relieves PMS symptoms
- relieves painful periods
- controls abnormal bleeding
- decreases hot flushes
- relieves insomnia
- relieves depression
- relieves anxiety
- builds bone
- does not negate the positive cardiovascular effects of oestrogen
- controls endometriosis

Warnings   If you are allergic to peanuts, do not take oral micronized progesterone.

Doses of greater than 400 mg may make you drowsy.

Progesterone Cream or Percutaneous Gel

Benefits
- builds bones
- counteracts oestrogen dominance
- controls excessive bleeding
- relieves PMS symptoms
- decreases hot flushes
- relieves endometriosis symptoms

Warnings   Progesterone cream or gel should not be substituted for the progestogen in conventional hormone replacement therapy, as neither is strong enough to counteract oestrogen dominance at the level of the uterus.

TESTOSTERONE

Testosterone has many of the same beneficial effects as oestrogen. And because the ovaries continue to produce testosterone for five years after menopause, we tend not to think about supplementing our declining testosterone levels in perimenopause. In some instances, however, adding testosterone supplements to perimenopausal hormone replacement therapy can have a powerful effect, notably on bone and on cognitive symptoms such as concentration, memory, mood, and libido (remember, the brain is the ultimate erogenous zone).

The reason you may need testosterone replacement if you're taking oestrogen replacement is that oestrogen supplements can actually drag down your testosterone levels. This is because oral oestrogen increases your levels of sex hormone binding globulin (SHBG), which mops up your circulating testosterone, making it unavailable to the brain. When you take oral oestrogen and testosterone, however, your SHBG levels decrease, thereby freeing up more testosterone and oestrogen.

Testosterone is available in several different forms: synthetic and natural pills, sublingual lozenges, ointments, gels, and soon-to-be-approved patches. You and your doctor can decide which form is best for you depending on your individual needs.

Benefits	• relieves hot flushes	• relieves insomnia
	• decreases incidence of migraine headaches	• improves libido
		• improves sexual function
	• improves cognitive function	• improves orgasm
	• improves concentration	• increases lean muscle mass and decreases body fat
	• improves memory	
	• improves mood	
	• decreases anxiety	• builds bone
	• reduces fatigue	• decreases triglyceride and HDL cholesterol levels
	• maintains height	

Warnings   Testosterone supplements can negatively alter your cholesterol profile and adversely affect your liver, so if you are taking them, make sure to have your lipids and liver function tested regularly.

COMBINED PRODUCTS

New products are constantly entering the market. Some of these combine oestrogen and progestogens or oestrogen and testosterone, making life a lot easier because you have fewer pills to take. The problem is that none of the commercially available products is 100 percent natural. Most are totally synthetic.

THE WAVE OF THE FUTURE

It's a great time to be going through perimenopause. The tables in this appendix reflect only the products available today, but wait—there are roughly thirty new hormone preparations in development. Patches offer many potential advantages such as more continuous delivery, making your hormone levels more stable throughout the day and night. Gels are also going to become more popular because they're well absorbed through the skin and easy to use. Europeans are already enjoying many of these new advances. The real breakthrough—which isn't too far in the future—will be when a hormone product, like a custom-made suit, will be tailored just for you.

Transdermal Oestrogen (Patches) Percutaneous Gels and Sprays

BRAND NAME	ACTIVE INGREDIENTS	SOURCE	STRENGTHS (RELEASED PER 24 HOURS)
Patches **Dermestril septem**	Oestradiol	Natural	0.025, 0.05, 0.075, 0.1 mg once weekly
Elleste-Solo MX40	Oestradiol	Natural	0.025, 0.04 mg twice weekly
Elleste-Solo MX80	Oestradiol	Natural	0.05, 0.075, 0.08, 0.1 mg twice weekly
[Also Fematrix (same doses)]			
Estraderm MX	Oestradiol	Natural	0.025, 0.05, 0.075, 0.1 mg twice weekly
Evorel	Oestradiol	Natural	0.025, 0.05, 0.075, 0.1 mg twice weekly
FemSeven	Oestradiol	Natural	0.025, 0.05, 0.075, 0.1 mg once weekly

BRAND NAME	ACTIVE INGREDIENTS	SOURCE	STRENGTHS (RELEASED PER 24 HOURS)
Nuvelle TS twice weekly	Oestradiol and levonorgestrel	Oestradiol: natural Levonorgestrel: synthetic	0.08, 0.05 oestradiol 0.1 mg twice weekly; 0.02 levonorgestrel
Evorel Sequi	Oestradiol and norethisterone acetate	Oestradiol: natural Norethisterone acetate: Synthetic	0.05 mg 17beta-oestradiol and 0.17 mg norethisterone acetate; replaced every 3–4 days over a 28-day cycle
Gels **Oestrogel**	Oestradiol	Natural	0.06%, 1.5 mg* gel once daily
Spray **Aerodiol**	17beta-oestradiol	Natural	300 mcgn nasal spray twice daily

Oral Oestrogen

BRAND NAME	ACTIVE INGREDIENTS	SOURCE	STRENGTHS
Hormonin	Oestriol 0.27 mg, Oestradiol 0.6 mg, Oestrone 1.4 mg	Natural	Tablets: 1 to 2 tablets once daily
Ovestin	Oestriol	Natural	Tablets: 1 mg daily
(non-branded)	Ethinyl oestradiol	Synthetic (Plant sources)	Tablets: 0.01 mg once daily
Harmogen	Oestropipate (oestrone sulphite)	Synthetic	Tablets: 1.5 mg once daily
Premarin	Conjugated equine oestrogens (CEE)	Synthetic (Urine of pregnant mares)	Tablets: 0.625, 1.25 mg daily
Climaval Elleste-Solo Progynova	Oestradiol	Natural	Tablets: 1 mg, 2 mg once daily

Vaginal Oestrogen

BRAND NAME	ACTIVE INGREDIENTS	SOURCE	STRENGTHS
Premarin	Conjugated equine oestrogens (CEE)	Synthetic (Urine of pregnant mares)	Cream: 0.625 mg/1 g base
Estring	Oestradiol	Natural	Ring: 2 mg reservoir, change every 90 days
Vagifem	Oestradiol	Natural	Cream: 1.5 mg/1 g base Vaginal Tablets: 0.025 mg once daily
Ortho-Gynest	Oestriol	Natural	Cream: 0.01%
Ovestin	Oestriol	Natural	Cream: 0.1%

PROGESTOGENS

BRAND NAME	ACTIVE INGREDIENTS	SOURCE	STRENGTHS
Provera	Medroxyprogesterone acetate (MPA)	Synthetic	Tablets: 2.5, 5, and 10 mg
Adgyn Medro	Medroxyprogesterone acetate (MPA)	Synthetic	Tablets: 5 mg
Micronor	Norethisterone	Synthetic	Tablets: 1 mg
[non-branded] Primolut N Utorlan	Norethisterone	Synthetic	Tablets: 5 mg

PROGESTERONE

BRAND NAME	ACTIVE INGREDIENTS	SOURCE	STRENGTHS
Crinone	Micronized progesterone	Natural	Gel: 45 mg
Cyclogest	Progesterone	Natural	Pressaries: 200 and 400 mg
Gestone	Progesterone	Natural	Injection: 25 and 50 mg

Combined Products

BRAND NAME	ACTIVE INGREDIENTS	SOURCE	STRENGTHS
Oestrogen and Progestogens			
Prempak-C	Conjugated equine oestrogens (CEE) and medroxyprogesterone acetate (MPA)	Synthetic	Tablets: 0.625 mg CEE days 1–14; 0.625 mg CEE and 5 mg MPA days 15–28
Premique	Conjugated equine oestrogens (CEE) and medroxyprogesterone acetate (MPA)	Synthetic	Tablets: 0.625 mg CEE and 2.5 mg MPA daily; 0.625 mg CEE and 5 mg MPA daily
Evorel & Sequi	*See Transdermal*	*See Transdermal*	*See Transdermal*
Climagest	Oestradiol and norethisterone	Oestradiol: natural Norethisterone: synthetic	Tablets: oestradiol 1, 2 mg days 1–28; norethisterone 1 mg days 17–28
Cyclo-Progynova	Oestradiol and levonorgestrel	Oestradiol: natural Levonorgestrel: synthetic	Tablets: oestradiol 2 mg days 1–21; levonorgestrel 0.025 mg days 10–21

BRAND NAME	ACTIVE INGREDIENTS	SOURCE	STRENGTHS
Kliofem	Oestradiol and norethisterone acetate	Oestradiol: natural Norethisterone: synthetic	Tablets: 2 mg oestradiol and 1 mg norethisterone acetate
Kliovance	Oestradiol and norethisterone acetate	Oestradiol: natural Norethisterone: synthetic	Tablets: 1 mg oestradiol and 500 mcg norethisterone acetate

TESTOSTERONE

BRAND NAME	ACTIVE INGREDIENTS	SOURCE	STRENGTHS
Testosterone	Testosterone	Synthetic	Implants: 100 and 200 mg

Checklist of Screening Tests

Throughout this book I've recommended a variety of routine screening tests that you should have at certain intervals beginning in your perimenopausal years. Here's a quick summary that you can photocopy and take to your next doctor's appointment.

Test	*When to Have It*
Bloodwork	
Chemistries (including glucose and liver function tests), lipid profile (total cholesterol, HDL, LDL, triglycerides), C-reactive protein, and homocysteine	Every five years if they're in the normal range; if abnormal, they may need to be repeated annually.
FBC (haemoglobin/ haematocrit) and ferritin	Every five years unless you suffer heavy bleeding or anaemia, in which case you need to be followed more closely.
TSH/free T_4	Beginning at age 45 or when your periods become irregular, whichever comes first, you should have your TSH and free T_4 tested every five years. Have these hormone levels checked immediately if you have any of the symptoms of thyroid disease (see pages 325 and 329)

Hormone studies (FSH, LH, oestradiol, progesterone, testosterone)	Periodically from the time you experience your first perimeno-pausal symptoms until you reach menopause.
Bone densitometry (hip, spine, and wrist)	At age 45 or when you have your first hot flush, whichever comes first, you should have a bone densitometry scan. If the results show bone loss, you will need to have a scan every one to two years. If you have a thyroid condition, you should have your bones checked annually.
Mammogram (and breast sonogram if you have dense breasts)	Have a baseline done at age 35 (or age 30 if you have a family history of breast cancer), then screenings every three years beginning at age 50.
Smear test	3 yearly, unless you have had an abnormal one, in which case you should have one every year.
Faecal occult blood test	Annually beginning at age 40 (or age 30 if you have a family history of colon cancer).
Sigmoidoscopy or colonoscopy	Alternate between having sigmoidoscopy and colonoscopy every five years beginning at age 50 (or age 35 if you have a family history of colon cancer).

REFERENCES

CHAPTER 1:
HOW DO I KNOW IF I'M IN PERIMENOPAUSE?

Khandwala, Salil S. "Primary Care of the Perimenopausal Woman." *Primary Care Update Ob/Gyns* 5.1 (1998): 43–49.

London, Steve N., and Charles B. Hammond. "The Climacteric." In *Danforth's Obstetrics and Gynecology*, 6th ed. Philadelphia: J. B. Lippincott, 1990. 857.

Sherman, Barry M., Joanne H. West, and Stanley G. Korenman. "The Menopausal Transition: Analysis of LH, FSH, Oestradiol, and Progesterone Concentrations During Menstrual Cycles of Older Women." *Journal of Clinical Endocrinology and Metabolism* 42 (1976): 629–636.

Speroff, Leon, Robert H. Glass, and Nathan G. Kase. *Clinical Gynecologic Endocrinology and Infertility*, 5th ed. Baltimore: Williams & Wilkins, 1994. 183–230.

University of Medicine and Dentistry of New Jersey—Robert Wood Johnson Medical School Department of Obstetrics, Gynecology, and Reproductive Sciences. *Recognition and Management of the Perimenopausal Patient in Clinical Practice.* Somerville, NJ: EMBRYON, 1998. 3–4.

CHAPTER 2
THE FIRST SIGN: MENSTRUAL IRREGULARITIES

Awwad, Johnny T., Thomas L. Toth, and Isaac Schiff. "Abnormal Uterine Bleeding in the Perimenopause." *International Journal of Fertility* 38 (1993): 261–269.

Bales, Lauren. "Treatment of the Perimenopausal Female." *Primary Care Update Ob/Gyns* 5.2 (1998): 90–94.

Brody, Jane E. "Americans Gamble on Herbs as Medicine." *New York Times*, 9 February 1999, F1, F7.

Cassidy, Aedin, Marion Faughnan, Roisin Hughes, Claire Fraser, Angela Cathcart,

Norman Taylor, Kenneth Setchell, and Sheila Bingham. "Hormonal Effects of Soy." *American Journal of Clinical Nutrition* 68 suppl. (1998): 1531S–1533S.

Firshein, Richard. *The Nutraceutical Revolution.* New York: Riverhead Books, 1998. 144–160.

Nagele, Fritz, Tarina Rubinger, and Adam Magos. "Why Do Women Choose Endometrial Ablation Rather Than Hysterectomy?" *Fertility and Sterility* 69.6 (1998): 1063–1066.

Seltzer, Vicki L., Fred Benjamin, and Stanley Deutsch. "Perimenopausal Bleeding Patterns and Pathologic Findings." *Journal of the American Medical Association* 45 (1990): 132–134.

Shochey, Candace. "Perimenopause and Heavy Menstrual Flow: Standard Treatments and Alternative Treatment Modalities." *Nurse Practitioner* (September 1994): 73–75.

Weber, Asma A. "Effects of Estrogens and Androgens on the Libido of Women Following Surgical and Natural Menopause." *Menopausal Medicine* 7.1 (1999): 5–8.

Weiner, Michael A., and Janet A. Weiner. *Herbs That Heal.* Mill Valley, CA: Quantum Books, 1994. 113–114, 212–213.

Worcester, Sharon. "New Progesterones Offer Good Alternatives." *Ob. Gyn. News*, 1 July 1999, 11.

CHAPTER 3
CAN SOMEBODY OPEN A WINDOW? HOT FLUSHES, INSOMNIA, AND OTHER JOYS

Albertazzi, Paola, Francesco Pansini, Gloria Bonaccorsi, Laura Zanotti, Elena Forini, and Domenico de Aloysio. "The Effect of Dietary Soy Supplementation on Hot Flushes." *Obstetrics & Gynecology* 91.1 (1998): 6–11.

Altman, Lawrence K. "Antidepressants Ease Hot Flashes, Cancer Study Shows." *New York Times*, 23 May 2000, A23.

Asplund, R., and H. Aberg. "Nocturnal Micturition, Sleep and Well-Being in Women of Ages 40–64 Years." *Maturitas* 24 (1996): 73–81.

Bachman, David L. "Sleep Disorders With Aging: Evaluation and Treatment." *Geriatrics* 47.9 (1992): 53–61.

Bachmann, Gloria A. et al. "Role of Androgens in the Menopause." *OBG Management* suppl. 10.7 (1998): 16–18.

Bales, Lauren. "Treatment of the Perimenopausal Female." *Primary Care Update Ob/Gyns* 5.2 (1998): 90–94.

Begley, Sharon. "Understanding Perimenopause." *Newsweek Special Edition* (Spring/Summer 1999): 34.

Boschert, Sherry. "Progesterone Cream Soothes Vasomotor Ills." *Ob. Gyn. News*, 1 January 1999, 11.

Brody, Jane E. "Americans Gamble on Herbs as Medicine." *New York Times*, 9 February 1999, F1, F7.

Casper, R. F., S. S. C. Yen, and M. M. Wilkes. "Menopausal Flushes: A Neuroendocrine Link With Pulsatile Luteinizing Hormone Secretion." *Science* 205 (1979): 823–825.

Cheng, Guang-Shing. "Paroxetine Relieves Hot Flashes in Breast Cancer Survivors." *Ob. Gyn News*, 1 May 2000, 5.

Clark, Ann J., Juanzetta Flowers, Larry Boots, and Shashidhar Shettar. "Sleep Disturbance in Mid-Life Women." *Journal of Advanced Nursing* 22 (1995): 562–568.

Coope, Jean. "Hormonal and Non-Hormonal Interventions for Menopausal Symptoms." *Maturitas* 23 (1996): 159–168.

Erlik, Yohanan, Ivanna V. Tataryn, David R. Meldrum, Peter Lomax, Joseph G. Bojorek, and Howard L. Judd. "Association of Waking Episodes With Menopausal Hot Flushes." *Journal of the American Medical Association* 245.17 (1981): 1741–1744.

Firshein, Richard. *The Nutraceutical Revolution.* New York: Riverhead Books, 1998. 242–254.

Foster, Steven. "Seven Herbs to See You Through Winter." *Herbs for Health* (January/February 1999): 58–60.

Gannon, Linda. "The Potential Role of Exercise in the Alleviation of Menstrual Disorders and Menopausal Symptoms: A Theoretical Synthesis of Recent Research." *Women & Health* 14.2 (1988): 105–127.

Greendale, Gail A., and MaryFran Sowers. "The Menopause Transition." *Endocrinology and Metabolism Clinics of North America* 26.2 (1997): 261–276.

Hahn, Philip M., Jacqueline Wong, and Robert L. Reid. "Menopausal-Like Hot Flashes Reported in Women of Reproductive Age." *Fertility and Sterility* 70.5 (1998): 913–918.

Hendrix, Susan L. "Nonestrogen Management of Menopausal Symptoms." *Endocrinology and Metabolism Clinics of North America* 26.2 (1997): 379–390.

"HRT vs. Remifemin in Menopause." *American Journal of Natural Medicine* 3.4 (1996): 7–10.

"Insomnia: Remedies for the Sleep Impaired." *Mayo Clinic Women's HealthSource* 2.3 (1998): 1–2.

Kass-Annese, Barbara. "Alternative Therapies for Menopause." *Clinical Obstetrics and Gynecology* 43.1 (2000): 162–183.

Klinkenborg, Verlyn. "Awakening to Sleep." *New York Times Magazine,* 5 January 1997, 26–56.

LeBoeuf, Faye J., and Stefanie G. Carter. "Discomforts of the Perimenopause." *JOGNN* 25.2 (1996): 173–180.

Lee, Lauri. "The 'Change' in How Women View Menopause." *Women's Health Connections* 5.4 (1997): 1–5.

London, Steve N., and Charles B. Hammond. "The Climacteric." In *Danforth's Obstetrics and Gynecology,* 6th ed. Philadelphia: J. B. Lippincott, 1990. 857–859.

Lourwood, David L. "Guide to Hormone Replacement Therapy." *Ob/Gyn Special Edition* (Spring 1999): 15–20.

Menopause Guidebook. Cleveland, OH: The North American Menopause Society, 1999. 10.

Mindell, Earl. *Earl Mindell's Supplement Bible.* New York: Fireside Books, 1998, 203–204.

Mohyi, Darush, Khosrow Tabassi, and James Simon. "Differential Diagnosis of Hot Flashes." *Maturitas* 27 (1997): 203–214.

"Palpitations: Be Still My Heart." *Mayo Clinic Women's HealthSource* 2.3 (1998): 6.

Rosano, Giuseppe M. C., Mariano Rillo, Filippo Leonardo, Carlo Pappone, and Sergio L. Chierchia. "Palpitations: What Is the Mechanism, and When Should We Treat Them?" *International Journal of Fertility* 42.2 (1997): 94–100.

Shaver, Joan, Elizabeth Giblin, Martha Lentz, and Kathryn Lee. "Sleep Patterns and Stability in Perimenopausal Women." *Sleep* 11.6 (1988): 556–561.

Slaven, Lorraine, and Christina Lee. "Mood and Symptom Reporting Among Middle-Aged Women: The Relationship Between Menopausal Status, Hormone Replacement Therapy, and Exercise Participation." *Health Psychology* 16.3 (1997): 203–208.

Spiegel, Karine, Rachel Leproult, and Eve Van Cauter. "Impact of Sleep Debt in Metabolic and Endocrine Function." *Lancet* 354 (1999): 1435–1439.

Taylor, Maida. "Alternatives to Conventional HRT: Phytoestrogens and Botanicals." *Contemporary Ob/Gyn* (June 1999): 27–50.

University of Medicine and Dentistry of New Jersey—Robert Wood Johnson Medical School Department of Obstetrics, Gynecology, and Reproductive Sciences. *Recognition and Management of the Perimenopausal Patient in Clinical Practice.* Somerville, NJ: EMBRYON, 1998. 12.

"Women May Prefer Natural Progesterone Over Synthetic." *Mayo Clinic Women's HealthSource* 3.8 (1999): 3.

Chapter 4
I'm Losing My Mind! Oestrogen and the Brain

Arpels, John C. "The Female Brain Hypoestrogenic Continuum From the Premenstrual Syndrome to Menopause." *The Journal of Reproductive Medicine* 41.9 (1996): 633–639.

Baker, Barbara. "Tamoxifen May Reduce the Risk of Alzheimer's." *Ob.Gyn. News,* 15 June 1998, 16.

Begley, Sharon. "Understanding Perimenopause." *Newsweek Special Edition* (Spring/Summer 1999): 34.

Berger, Alisha. "When 'Silent Strokes' Evoke Depression." *New York Times,* 5 October 1999, F8.

"Blueberries May Reduce Effects of Aging." *New York Times,* 21 September 1999, F8.

Blum, Deborah. *Sex on the Brain.* New York: Viking, 1997.

Brinton, Roberta Diaz, Julie Tran, Pam Proffitt, and Maria Montoya. "17 B-Oestradiol Enhances the Outgrowth and Survival of Neocortical Neurons in Culture." *Neurochemical Research* 22.11 (1997): 1339–1351.

Brody, Jane E. "Americans Gamble on Herbs as Medicine." *New York Times,* 9 February 1999, F1, F7.

Carroll, Linda. "Is Memory Loss Inevitable? Maybe Not." *New York Times,* 1 February 2000, F7, F12.

Diagnostic and Statistical Manual of Mental Disorders, 4th ed. Washington, DC: American Psychiatric Association, 1994. 317, 327, 350.

"Extinguishing Alzheimer's." *New York Times,* 23 June 1998, F7.

Firshein, Richard. *The Nutraceutical Revolution.* New York: Riverhead Books, 1998. 18–32, 255–270.

Foster, Steven. "Seven Herbs to See You Through Winter." *Herbs for Health* (January/February 1999): 58–60.

Hammond, Charles B. *Therapeutic Options for Menopausal Health*. Durham, NC: Duke University Medical Center, 1998. 25–26.

Harlow, Bernard L., Daniel W. Cramer, and Kathryn M. Annis. "Association of Medically Treated Depression and Age at Natural Menopause." *American Journal of Epidemiology* 141.12 (1995): 1170–1176.

Harlow, Bernard L., Lee S. Cohen, Michael W. Otto, Donna Spiegelman, and Daniel W. Cramer. "Prevalence and Predictors of Depressive Symptoms in Older Premenopausal Women." *Archives of General Psychiatry* 56 (1999): 418–424.

Henderson, Victor W. "Oestrogen, Cognition, and a Woman's Risk of Alzheimer's Disease." *The American Journal of Medicine* 103 (1997): 11S–18S.

"HRT vs. Remifemin in Menopause." *American Journal of Natural Medicine* 3.4 (1996): 7–10.

Jackson, Nancy Beth. "When the Brain's Mailbox Is Full." *New York Times*, 27 July 1999, F6.

Legato, Marianne J. *Gender-Specific Aspects of Human Biology for the Practicing Physician*. Armonk, NY: Futura, 1997. 22.

MacGregor, E. Anne. "Menstruation, Sex, Hormones, and Migraine." *Neurologic Clinics* 15.1 (1997): 125–141.

McBee, Wendy L., Margaret E. Dailey, Elizabeth Dugan, and Sally A. Shumaker. "Hormone Replacement Therapy and Other Potential Treatments for Dementia." *Endocrinology and Metabolism Clinics of North America* 26.2 (1997): 329–345.

Mindell, Earl. *Earl Mindell's Supplement Bible*. New York: Fireside Books, 1998. 120–121, 141–142.

Neri, I. F. Granella, R. Nappi, G. C. Manzoni, F. Facchinetti, and A. R. Genazzani. "Characteristics of Headache at Menopause: A Clinico-Epidemiologic Study." *Maturitas* 17 (1993): 31–37.

Newman, Lawrence C., and Christine L. Lay. *Menstruation-Associated Migraine*. Bala Cynwyd, PA: Meniscus Educational Institute, 1994.

Pearlstein, Teri. "Hormones and Depression: What Are the Facts About Premenstrual Syndrome, Menopause, and Hormone Replacement Therapy?" *American Journal of Obstetrics and Gynecology* 173.2 (1995): 646–653.

Pearlstein, Teri, Karen Rosen, and Andrea B. Stone. "Mood Disorders and Menopause." *Endocrinology and Metabolism Clinics of North America* 26.2 (1997): 279–294.

Rearley, Nicola. *The New Encyclopedia of Vitamins, Minerals, Supplements, and Herbs*. New York: M. Evans, 1998. 348–349.

Scharbo-DeHaan, Marianne. "Maintaining Brain Health As We Age." *Menopausal Issues for Nursing Professionals*. Barrington, IL: The Willow Group, 1998. 12–15.

Schmidt, Peter J., Catherine A. Roca, Miki Bloch, and David R. Rubinow. "The Perimenopause and Affective Disorders." *Seminars in Reproductive Endocrinology* 15.1 (1997): 91–100.

Sherwin, Barbara B. "Oestrogen Effects on Cognition in Menopausal Women." *Neurology* 48.suppl. 7 (1997): S21–S26.

Simon, James A. "Effects of Progestins and Progesterone on CNS Function." *Menopausal Medicine* 6.4 (1998): 8–12.

Slaven, Lorraine, and Christina Lee. "Mood and Symptom Reporting Among

Middle-Aged Women: The Relationship Between Menopausal Status, Hormone Replacement Therapy, and Exercise Participation." *Health Psychology* 16.3 (1997): 203–208.

Stark, Stuart. "Migraine in Women." *The Female Patient* 24 (1999): 53–69.

"Staying Mentally Sharp." *Mayo Clinic Women's HealthSource* 3.10 (October 1999): 1–2.

University of Medicine and Dentistry of New Jersey—Robert Wood Johnson Medical School Department of Obstetrics, Gynecology, and Reproductive Sciences. *Recognition and Management of the Perimenopausal Patient in Clinical Practice.* Somerville, NJ: EMBRYON, 1998. 12.

Van Duijn, C. M. "Menopause and the Brain." *Journal of Psychosomatic Obstetrics and Gynecology* 18 (1997): 121–125.

Washburn, Scott A. "Oestradiol and Progesterone Effects on the Central Nervous System." *Menopausal Medicine* 5.4 (1997): 5–8.

Willoughby, John, and Chris Schlesinger. "Dark-Fleshed Fish: A Taste Worth Acquiring." *New York Times*, 15 September 1999, F3.

CHAPTER 5
NOT TONIGHT, HONEY: SEXUAL CHANGES AND OTHER EMBARRASSMENTS

Bachmann, Gloria A. "Sexual Function in the Perimenopause." *Obstetrics and Gynecology Clinics of North America* 20.2 (1993): 379–389.

Bachmann, Gloria A. et al. "Female Sexuality During the Menopause." *OBG Management* suppl. 11.5 (1999).

Baker, Barbara. "Progestin Plus Conjugated Estrogen Treats Dyspareunia." *Ob. Gyn. News*, 15 November 1999, 11.

Bales, Lauren. "Treatment of the Perimenopausal Female." *Primary Care Update Ob/Gyns* 5.2 (1998): 90–94.

Brody, Jane E. "A Tad of Testosterone Adds Zest to Menopause." *New York Times*, 24 February 1998, F7.

Coope, Jean. "Hormonal and Non-Hormonal Interventions for Menopausal Symptoms." *Maturitas* 23 (1996): 159–168.

Dennerstein, L., A. M. A. Smith, C. A. Morse, and H. G. Burger. "Sexuality and the Menopause." *Journal of Psychosomatic Gynecology* 15 (1994): 59–66.

Douglass, Marcia, and Lisa Douglass. *Are We Having Fun Yet?* New York: Hyperion, 1997.

Fantl, J. Andrew. "The Lower Urinary Tract in Women—Effect of Aging and Menopause on Continence." *Experimental Gerontology* 29.3/4 (1994): 417–422.

Fourcroy, Jean L. "Diagnosis and Treatment of Urinary Incontinence." *Ob/Gyn Special Edition* 2 (1999): 43–46.

Goldberg, Burton. *Alternative Medicine Guide to Women's Health*, vol. 1. Tiburon, CA: Future Medicine Publishing, 1998. 220–221.

Gonzales, Michael, and Mark Zetin. "Sexual Dysfunction in Women." *Ob/Gyn Special Edition* 2 (1999): 63–66.

Greendale, Gail A., and MaryFran Sowers. "The Menopause Transition." *Endocrinology and Metabolism Clinics of North America* 26.2 (1997): 261–276.

Griebling, Tomas L., and Ingrid E. Nygaard. "The Role of Estrogen Replacement

Therapy in the Management of Urinary Incontinence and Urinary Tract Infection in Postmenopausal Women." *Endocrinology and Metabolism Clinics of North America* 26.2 (1997): 347–359.

Kaunitz, Andrew M. "The Role of Androgens in Menopausal Hormone Replacement." *Endocrinology and Metabolism Clinics of North America* 26.2 (1997): 391–397.

Khandwala, Salil S. "Primary Care of the Perimenopausal Woman." *Primary Care Update Ob/Gyns* 5.1 (1998): 43–49.

Kirchengast, Sylvia, Beda Hartmann, Doris Gruber, and Johannes Huber. "Decreased Sexual Interest and Its Relationship to Body Build in Postmenopausal Women." *Maturitas* 23 (1996): 63–71.

Klutke, John J., and Arieh Bergman. "Hormonal Influences on the Urinary Tract." *Urologic Clinics of North America* 22.3 (1995): 629–639.

LeBoeuf, Faye J., and Stefanie G. Carter. "Discomforts of the Perimenopause." *JOGNN* 25.2 (1996): 173–180.

Lee, Lauri. "The 'Change' in How Women View Menopause." *Women's Health Connections* 5.4 (1997): 1–5.

London, Steve N., and Charles B. Hammond. "The Climacteric." In *Danforth's Obstetrics and Gynecology*, 6th ed. Philadelphia: J. B. Lippincott, 1990. 859–860.

"Midlife Sexuality and Women." *Mayo Clinic HealthOasis.* www.mayohealth.org/mayo/9711/html/midlife.htm, 3 November 1997.

Pandit, Lotika, and Joseph G. Ouslander. "Postmenopausal Vaginal Atrophy and Atrophic Vaginitis." *The American Journal of the Medical Sciences* 314.4 (1997): 228–231.

Reichman, Judith. *I'm Not in the Mood.* New York: William Morrow, 1998. 121–123, 137.

Sampselle, Carolyn M., Molly C. Dougherty, Diane Kaschak Newman, and Jean F. Wyman. "Continence for Women: Evidence-Based Practice." *JOGNN* (July/August 1997): 375–385.

"Sexuality: 12 Ways to Turn Up the Heat at Midlife." *Mayo Clinic Women's Health-Source* (January 1998): 4–5.

Sherwin, Barbara. "Sex Hormones and Psychological Functioning in Postmenopausal Women." *Experimental Gerontology* 29.3/4 (1994): 423–430.

Taylor, Maida. "Alternatives to Conventional HRT: Phytoestrogens and Botanicals." *Contemporary Ob/Gyn* (June 1999): 27–50.

Tyler, Aubin. "Bladder Control: There's No Need to Suffer in Silence." *The Female Patient* S16 (1999): 27–31.

Weber, Asma A. "Effects of Estrogens and Androgens on the Libido of Women Following Surgical and Natural Menopause." *Menopausal Medicine* 7.1 (1999): 5–8.

Speroff, Leon et al. "Your Menopausal Patient: Individualizing Management." *Contemporary Ob/Gyn* suppl. (June 1998): 4–25.

CHAPTER 6
MIRROR, MIRROR, ON THE WALL: VISIBLE SIGNS OF PERIMENOPAUSE

Aronne, Louis J. "Weight Gain During the Perimenopause." *Menopause Management* (November/December 1999): 6–11.

Bjorkelund, C., L. Lissner, S. Andersson, L. Lapidus, and C. Bengtsson. "Reproductive History in Relation to Relative Weight and Fat Distribution." *International Journal of Obesity* 20 (1996): 213–219.

Bjorntorp, P. "The Regulation of Adipose Tissue Distribution in Humans." *International Journal of Obesity* 20 (1996): 291–302.

Brody, Jane E. "In a Culture of Sunbathers, Tips for Shielding the Skin." *New York Times*, 15 June 1999, F7.

Callens, A., L. Vaillant, P. Lecomte, M. Berson, Y. Gall, and G. Lorette. "Does Hormonal Skin Aging Exist?" *Dermatology* 193 (1996): 289–294.

Castelo-Branco, C., M. Duran, and J. Gonzalez-Merlo. "Skin Collagen Changes Related to Age and Hormone Replacement Therapy." *Maturitas* 15 (1992): 113–119.

Castelo-Branco, Camil, Francesca Pons, Eduard Gratacos, Albert Fortuny, Juan Antonio Vanrell, and Jesus Gonzalez-Merlo. "Relationship Between Skin Collagen and Bone Changes During Aging." *Maturitas* 18 (1994): 199–206.

Chalmers, Debra A. "Rosacea: Recognition and Management for the Primary Care Provider." *The Nurse Practitioner* 22.10 (1997): 18, 23–24, 26–28, 30.

Chappard, D., Ch. Alexandre, J.-M. Robert, and G. Riffat. "Relationships Between Bone and Skin Atrophies During Aging." *Acta Anatomica* 141 (1991): 239–244.

Clarkson, Thomas B. "The Effects of Hormone Replacement Therapy on Key Risk Factors for Cardiovascular Disease." *HRT Casebook I: Hormone Replacement Therapy Cardiovascular Health*. Fairlawn, NJ: MPE Communications, 2000.

Dunn, Laura B., Mark Damesyn, Alison A. Moore, David B. Reuben, and Gail A. Greendale. "Does Estrogen Prevent Skin Aging?" *Archives of Dermatology* 133 (1997): 339–342.

Epstein, Debbie. "Your Skin: The Great Cover-Up." *The Female Patient* S12 (1998): 5–9.

Fritsch, Jane. "The Secret Loss That Women Try to Keep Under Their Hats." *New York Times*, 21 June 1998, WH19.

Gavin, James. "Diabetes and Menopause." *Menopause Management* (July/August 1998): 10–12.

Goldman, Erik L. "Syndrome W: Weight Gain, White-Coat HT." *Ob. Gyn. News,* 15 (July 1999): 6–7.

Haarbo, Jens, Ulla Marslew, Anders Gotfredsen, and Claus Christiansen. "Postmenopausal Hormone Replacement Therapy Prevents Central Distribution of Body Fat After Menopause." *Metabolism* 40.12 (1991): 1323–1326.

"Hair Loss in Women." *Mayo Clinic Health Letter*, February 1997.

Heymsfield, Steven B., Dympna Gallagher, Eric T. Poehlman, Carla Wolper, Kathy Nonas, Dorothy Nelson, and Zi-Mian Wang. "Menopausal Changes in Body Composition and Energy Expenditure." *Experimental Gerontology* 29.3/4 (1994): 377–389.

Jensen, Jytte, Claus Christiansen, and Paul Rodbro. "Oestrogen-Progesterone Replacement Therapy Changes Body Composition in Early Post-Menopausal Women." *Maturitas* 8 (1986): 209–216.

Kazuaki, Kotani, Katsuto Tonkunaga, Shigenori Fujioka, Takashi Kobatake, Yoshiaki Keno, Shingo Yoshida, Iichiro Shimomura, Seiichiro Tarui, and Yuji Matsuzawa. "Sexual Dimorphism of Age-Related Changes in Whole-Body Fat Distribution in the Obese." *International Journal of Obesity and Related Metabolic Disorders* 18.4 (1994): 207–212.

Kirchengast, S., D. Gruber, M. Sator, B. Hartmann, W. Knogler, and J. Huber. "Menopause-Associated Differences in Female Fat Patterning Estimated by Dual-Energy X-Ray Absorpitometry." *Annals of Human Biology* 24.1 (1997): 45–54.

Kirchengast, S., D. Gruber, M. Sator, W. Knogler, and J. Huber. "The Impact of Nutritional Status on Body Fat Distribution Patterns in Pre- and Postmenopausal Females." *Journal of Biosocial Science* 30 (1998): 145–154.

Lee, Lauri. "Syndrome X." *Women's Health Connections* 6.3 (1998): 1–4.

Mindell, Earl. *Earl Mindell's Supplement Bible*. New York: Fireside Books, 1998. 244–252.

Muti, Paola, Maurizio Trevisan, Salvatore Panico, Andrea Micheli, Egidio Celentano, Jo L. Freudenheim, and Franco Berrino. "Body Fat Distribution, Peripheral Indicators of Androgenic Activity, and Blood Pressure in Women." *Annals of Epidemiology* 6.3 (1996): 181–187.

Otomo-Corgel, Joan. "Periodontal Disease in the Midlife Woman," *Menopause Management* (March/April 2000): 14–18.

Panotopoulos, Georges, Jean-Charles Ruiz, Jocelyne Raison, Bernard Guy-Grand, and Arnaud Basdevant. "Menopause, Fat and Lean Distribution in Obese Women." *Maturitas* 25 (1996): 11–19.

Pierard, Gerald E., Caroline Letawe, Afshin Dowlati, and Claudine Pierard-Franchimont. "Effect of Hormone Replacement Therapy for Menopause on the Mechanical Properties of Skin." *Journal of the American Geriatrics Society* 43 (1995): 662–665.

Schmidt, J. B., M. Binder, W. Macheiner, Ch. Kainz, G. Gitsch, and Ch. Bieglmayer. "Treatment of Skin Ageing Symptoms in Perimenopausal Females With Estrogen Compounds: A Pilot Study." *Maturitas* 20 (1994): 25–30.

Sears, Barry, with Bill Lawren. *Enter the Zone*. New York: HarperCollins, 1995. 9–31, 135–147.

Speroff, Leon, Robert H. Glass, and Nathan G. Kase. *Clinical Gynecologic Endocrinology and Infertility*, 5th ed. Baltimore: Williams & Wilkins, 1994. 589–590.

Spindler, James R., and Joann L. Data. "Female Androgenetic Alopecia: A Review." *Dermatology Nursing* 4.2 (1992): 93–99.

CHAPTER 7
MY BIOLOGICAL CLOCK IS TICKING: CHANGES IN FERTILITY

"Age and Fertility." *Mayo Clinic Women's HealthSource* 2.6 (1998): 1–2.

Bandler, Michael J. "A Prescription for Pregnancy?" *American Baby* (November 1998): 55–61.

Bates, G. William. "Body Weight and Reproduction." In *Infertility*, 2nd ed., Machelle M. Seibel, ed. New York: Prentice Hall, 1997. 409–415.

Blake, Emily J., Tovaghgol Adel, and Nanette Santoro. "Relationships Between Insulin-Like Growth Hormone Factor-1 and Oestradiol in Reproductive Aging." *Fertility and Sterility* 67.4 (1997): 697–701.

Bopp, Bradford L., and David B. Seifer. "Oocyte Loss and the Perimenopause." *Clinical Obstetrics and Gynecology* 41.4 (1998): 898–911.

Boschert, Sherry. "Check Tubes in Infertility Work-Up." *Ob.Gyn. News*, 1 January 1999, 15.

Bovo, Mary Jane. *Contraceptive Guide.* www.mjbovo.com/contracep.htm., 18 August 1997.

Chamoun, Diran, Howard D. McClamrock, and Eli Y. Adashi. "Ovulation Initiation With Clomiphene Citrate." In *Infertility*, 2nd ed., Machelle M. Seibel, ed. New York: Prentice Hall, 1997. 495–506.

Cohen, Matthew A., and Mark V. Sauer. "Fertility in Perimenopausal Women." *Clinical Obstetrics and Gynecology* 41.4 (1998): 958–963.

Damario, Mark A., and Zev Rosenwaks. "Ovum Donation." In *Infertility*, 2nd ed., Machelle M. Seibel, ed. New York: Prentice Hall, 1997. 773–792.

Ekblad, U., and T. Vilpa. "Pregnancy in Women Over Forty." *Annales Chirurgiae et Gynaecologiae* 83 (1994): 68–71.

Epigee Birth Control Guide. www.epigee.org/guide, 18 August 1997.

Gilbert, William M., Thomas S. Nesbitt, and Beate Danielsen. "Childbearing Beyond Age 40: Pregnancy Outcome in 24,032 Cases." *Obstetrics & Gynecology* 93.1 (1999): 9–14.

Gindoff, Paul R., Peter J. Schmidt, and David R. Rubinow. "Response to Clomiphene Citrate Challenge Test in Normal Women Through Perimenopause." *Gynecologic and Obstetric Investigation* 43 (1997): 186–191.

Hillard, Paula J. Adams, Daniel R. Jishell Jr., and Lee P. Shulman. *Combined Hormonal Injectable Contraceptive.* Houston, TX: MedPro Communications, 1999.

Holland, Eileen G. "Guide to Oral Contraception Management." *Ob/Gyn Special Edition* 2 (1999): 57–62.

Hummel, William P., and L. Michael Kettel. "Assisted Reproductive Technology: The State of the ART." *Annals of Medicine* 29 (1997): 207–214.

Jancin, Bruce. "Optimize Emergency Contraceptive Use." *Ob. Gyn. News*, 15 December 1998, 9.

———. "Tubal Ligation Underused to Cut Ovarian Ca Risk." *Ob.Gyn. News*, 15 January 1999, 14.

Jimenez, Sherry L. M. "Rethinking Birth Control." *American Baby* (September 1998): 49–55.

Johnson, Kate. "Explain Pregnancy Risks to Women Over Age 40." *Ob.Gyn. News*, 1 September 1998, 40.

———. "Finding Pathology in 'Normal' Infertility Patients." *Ob.Gyn. News*, 1 March 2000, 18.

———. "Laparoscopy Can Wait in Infertility Investigation." *Ob.Gyn. News*, 1 October 1998, 22.

———. "Tell Women Over Age 40 That Their Fertility Drops." *Ob.Gyn. News*, 1 August 1998, 26.

Klein, Nancy A., and Michael R. Soules. "Endocrine Changes of the Perimenopause." *Clinical Obstetrics and Gynecology* 41.4 (1998): 912–920.

Kolata, Gina. "Scientists Face New Ethical Quandaries in Baby-Making." *New York Times*, 19 August 1997, C1, C8.

LaValle, James B. "Guide to Herb, Vitamin, and Mineral Use in Pregnancy." *Ob/Gyn Special Edition* 2 (1999): 51–55.

References · 397

Lobo, Rogerio A. "The Perimenopause." *Clinical Obstetrics and Gynecology* 41.4 (1998): 895–897.

Lunenfeld, Bruno, and Eitan Lunenfeld. "Ovulation Induction With Human Menopausal Gonadotropin." In *Infertility*, 2nd ed., Machelle M. Seibel, ed. New York: Prentice Hall, 1997. 507–523.

Maroulis, George B. "Aging and Reproduction." In *Infertility*, 2nd ed., Machelle M. Seibel, ed. New York: Prentice Hall, 1997. 435–443.

Moon, Mary Ann. "Low-Dose OCs Don't Raise Heart Attack Risk." *Ob. Gyn. News*, 1 January 1999, 10.

Nachtigall, Lila E. "The Symptoms of Perimenopause." *Clinical Obstetrics and Gynecology* 41.4 (1998): 921–927.

Parchment, Winsome J. "Ob/Gyn On Call." *Parents* (August 1998): 59–60.

Pettigrew, R., and D. Hamilton-Fairley. "Obesity and Female Reproductive Function." *British Medical Bulletin* 53.2 (1997): 341–358.

"The Pill Revisited." *Mayo Clinic Women's HealthSource* (August 1998): 4–5.

Ringel, Marcia. "The Pill: It's Not Just for Birth Control Anymore." *The Female Patient* 513 (1998): 5–9.

Sauer, Mark V., Richard J. Paulson, Beth A. Ary, and Rogerio A. Lobo. "Three Hundred Cycles of Oocyte Donation at the University of Southern California: Assessing the Effect of Age and Infertility Diagnosis on Pregnancy and Implantation Rates." *Journal of Assisted Reproduction and Genetics* 11.2 (1994): 92–96.

Schmidt-Sarosi, Cecilia. "Infertility in the Older Woman." *Clinical Obstetrics and Gynecology* 41.4 (1998): 940–950.

Seibel, Machelle M. "Diagnostic Evaluation of an Infertile Couple." In *Infertility*, 2nd ed., Machelle M. Seibel, ed. New York: Prentice Hall, 1997. 3–27.

Shaaban, Mamdouh M. "The Perimenopause and Contraception." *Maturitas* 23 (1996): 181–192.

"Sterilization: Yours? Mine? Ours." *Mayo Clinic Women's HealthSource* (September 1998): 6.

Sweeny, Danielle. "Multiple-Birth Baby Boom." www.babycenter.com, 20 September 1999.

Taechakraichana, Nimit, Kobchitt Limpaphayom, Tanimporn Ninlagarn, Krasean Panyakhamlerd, Sukanya Chaikittisilpa, and Nikorn Dusitsin. "A Randomized Trial of Oral Contraceptive and Hormone Replacement Therapy on Bone Mineral Density and Coronary Heart Disease Risk Factors in Postmenopausal Women." *Obstetrics & Gynecology* 95.1 (2000): 87–94.

"Time Lends Hand to Test-Tube Fertilization." *New York Times*, 27 July 1999, F14.

Tunick, Barbara. "When 1 and 1 Don't Make 3." *The Female Patient* 512 (1998): 17–20.

Westhoff, Carolyn. "Contraception at Age 35 Years and Older." *Clinical Obstetrics and Gynecology* 41.4 (1998): 951–957.

"What Makes Multiples More Likely." *American Baby* (August 1998): 18.

"What Medications Can Affect My Fertility?" www.babycenter.com/expert/6146.html, 6 April 2000.

CHAPTER 8
DON'T CRY OVER SPILLED MILK: YOUR BONES

Arnala, I., J. Saastamoinen, and E. M. Alhava. "Salmon Calcitonin in the Prevention of Bone Loss at Perimenopause." *Bone* 4.6 (1996): 629–632.

Baker, Barbara. "Risedronate Appears Effective for Osteoporosis." *Ob. Gyn. News*, 15 July 1999, 1–2.

Bone, Henry G., Susan L. Greenspan, Clark McKeever, Norman Bell, Michael Davidson, Robert W. Downs, Ronald Emkey, Pierre J. Meunier, Sam S. Miller, Anthony L. Mulloy, Robert R. Recker, Stuart R. Weiss, Norman Heyden, Thomas Musliner, Shailaja Suryawanski, A. John Yates, and Antonio Lombardi. "Alendronate and Estrogen Effects in Postmenopausal Women with Low Bone Mineral Density." *Journal of Clinical Endocrinology and Metabolism* 85.2 (2000): 720–726.

Brody, Jane E. "Finding Calcium Sources Outside the Dairy Case." *New York Times*, 20 October 1998, F7.

Brunk, Doug. "Some Calcium Supplements Aren't Absorbed." *Ob. Gyn. News*, 1 February 2000, 15.

Bykowski, Mike. "Many Women Unaware They Have Osteoporosis." *Ob. Gyn. News*, 15 January 1999, 6.

Chittacharoen, Apichart, Urusa Theppisai, Rojana Sirisriro, and Chalermsri Thanantaseth. "Pattern of Bone Loss in Surgical Menopause: A Preliminary Report." *Journal of the Medical Association of Thailand* (November 1997): 731–736.

"Combating Osteoporosis." *OBG Management* (June 1998): 55–65.

Cosman, F., and R. Lindsay. "Is Parathyroid Hormone a Therapeutic Option for Osteoporosis?" *Calcified Tissue International* 62 (1998): 475–480.

Cummings, Steven R., Lisa Palermo, Warren Browner, Robert Marcus, Robert Wallace, Jim Pearson, Terri Blackwell, Stephen Eckert, and Dennis Black. "Monitoring Osteoporosis Therapy with Bone Densitometry." *Journal of the American Medical Association* 283. 10 (2000): 1318–1321.

Delmas, Pierre D., Nina H. Bjarnason, Bruce H. Mitlak, Anne-Catherine Ravoux, Aarti S. Shah, William J. Huster, Michael Draper, and Claus Christiansen. "Effects of Raloxifene on Bone Mineral Density, Serum Cholesterol Concentrations, and Uterine Endometrium in Postmenopausal Women." *The New England Journal of Medicine* 337.23 (1997): 1641–1687.

Eastell, Richard. "Treatment of Postmenopausal Osteoporosis." *The New England Journal of Medicine* 338.11 (1998): 736–745.

Ebeling, Peter R., Lynne M. Atley, Janet R. Guthrie, Henry G. Burger, Lorraine Dennerstein, John L. Hopper, and John D. Wark. "Bone Turnover Markers and Bone Density Across the Menopausal Transition." *Journal of Clinical Endocrinology and Metabolism* 81.9 (1996): 3366–3371.

"Emerging Role of Estrogen/Androgen Therapy." *Managing the Mid-Life Woman*, 18 June 1998, 2.

Firshein, Richard. *The Nutraceutical Revolution*. New York: Riverhead Books, 1998. 49–67.

Gaby, Alan. "Preventing and Reversing Osteoporosis." *Health Counselor* 7.6: 51–53.

Gambacciani, M., M. Ciaponi, B. Cappagli, L. Piaggesi, and A. R. Genazzani. "Effects of Combined Low Dose of the Isoflavone Derivative Ipriflavone and Estrogen Replacement on Bone Mineral Density and Metabolism in Postmenopausal Women." *Maturitas* 28 (1997): 75–81.

Gambacciani, Marco, Adriana Spinetti, Fabio Taponeco, Barbara Cappagli, Silvia Maffei, Pietro Manetti, Laura Piaggesi, and Piero Fioretti. "Bone Loss in Perimenopausal Women: A Longitudinal Study." *Maturitas* 18 (1994): 191–197.

Genant, Harry K., Johna Lucas, Stuart Weiss, Mark Akin, Ronald Emkey, Heidi McNaney-Flint, Robert Downs, Joseph Mortola, Nelson Watts, Hwa Ming Yang, Niranyan Banav, John J. Brennan, and Joseph C. Nolan. "Low-Dose Esterified Estrogen Therapy." *Archives of Internal Medicine* 157 (1997): 2609–2615.

Goldman, Erik. "Growing Up in the North May Increase Osteoporosis Risk." *Ob. Gyn. News*, 1 December 1999, 5.

Heaney, Robert P., ed. "Calcium: Answers for Lifelong Health." *OBG Management* suppl., October 1998.

Heersche, Johan N. M., Carlton G. Bellows, and Yoichiro Ishida. "The Decrease in Bone Mass Associated With Aging and Menopause." *The Journal of Prosthetic Dentistry* 79.1 (1998): 14–16.

Jackson, Nancy Beth. "New Therapy Builds Bone Without Unpleasant Side Effects." *New York Times*, 1 June 1999, F14.

Jassal, Simerjot K., Elizabeth Barrett-Connor, and Sharon L. Edelstein. "Low Bioavailable Testosterone Levels Predict Future Height Loss in Postmenopausal Women." *Journal of Bone and Mineral Research* 10.4 (1995): 650–654.

Johnson, Kate. "Low BMD Tied to Calcified Arteries." *Ob. Gyn. News*, 15 December 2000, 1–2.

Kass-Annese, Barbara. "Alternative Therapies for Menopause." *Clinical Obstetrics and Gynecology* 43.1 (2000): 162–183.

Keen, Richard, and Paul J. Kelly. "Genetic Factors in Osteoporosis." *Drugs & Aging* 11.5 (1997): 333–337.

Krahe, C., R. Friedman, and J. L. Gross. "Risk Factors for Decreased Bone Density in Premenopausal Women." *Brazilian Journal of Medical and Biological Research* 30 (1997): 1061–1066.

Kulak, Carolina A. Moreira, and John P. Bilezikian. "Osteoporosis: Preventive Strategies." *International Journal of Fertility* 43.2 (1998): 56–64.

Labrie, Fernand, Alain Belanger, Van Luu-The, Claude Labrie, Jacques Simard, Leonello Cusan, Jose-Luis Gomez, and Bernard Candas. "DHEA and the Intracrine Formation of Androgens and Estrogens in Peripheral Layer Tissues." *Steroids* 63 (1998): 322–328.

Labrie, Fernand, Pierre Diamond, Leonello Cusan, Jose-Luis Gomez, Alain Belanger, and Bernard Candas. "Effect of 12-Month Dehydroepiandrosterone Replacement Therapy on Bone, Vagina, and Endometrium in Postmenopausal Women." *Journal of Clinical Endocrinology and Metabolism* 82.10 (1997): 3498–3505.

Lane, Joseph. "Osteoporosis: Etiology, Diagnosis, Prevention and Treatment." *Ob/Gyn Special Edition* 2 (1999): 21–24.

Leb, G., H. Warnkross, and B. Obermayer-Pietsch. "Thyroid Hormone Excess and Osteoporosis." *Acta Medica Austriaca* 21 (1994): 65–67.

Lee, Lauri. "Boning Up on Osteoporosis." *Women's Health Connections* 5.2 (1997): 1–5.

London, Steve N., and Charles B. Hammond. "The Climacteric." In *Danforth's Obstetrics and Gynecology*, 6th ed. Philadelphia: J. B. Lippincott, 1990. 860–864.

McCord, Holly. "4 Surprising Nutrients Your Bones Are Starving For." *Prevention* (May 2000): 148–149.

Mindell, Earl. *Earl Mindell's Supplement Bible*. New York: Fireside Books, 1998. 147–148.

Mundy, G., R. Garrett, S. Harris, J. Chan, D. Chen, G. Rossini, B. Boyce, M. Zhao, and G. Gutierrez. "Stimulation of Bone Formation in Vitro and in Rodents by Statins." *Science* 286 (1999): 1946–1949.

Murray, Michael T. "Keep Bones and Joints Healthy With Boron." *Health Counselor* (June/July 1997): 32–33.

Nelson, Miriam E., with Sarah Wernick. *Strong Women Stay Young*. New York: Bantam Books, 1997.

Notelovitz, Morris. "Oestrogen Therapy and Osteoporosis: Principles & Practice." *The American Journal of the Medical Sciences* 313.1 (1997): 2–10.

Packer, Lester. *The Antioxidant Miracle*. New York: John Wiley & Sons, 1999. 92–102, 133–141.

Pollack, Michael. "High Blood Pressure and Osteoporosis." *New York Times*, 21 September 1999, F8.

Potter, Susan M., JoAnn Baum, Hongyu Teng, Rachel J. Stillman, Neil F. Shay, and John W. Erdman Jr. "Soy Proteins and Isoflavones: Their Effects on Blood Lipids and Bone Density in Postmenopausal Women." *American Journal of Clinical Nutrition* 68 suppl. (1998): 1375S–1379S.

Raggio, Cathleen. "Osteoporosis in Children and Adolescents." *Hospital for Special Surgery Health Connection* 7.2 (1999): 6.

Robinson, Susan. "Teaching Teenage Girls About Osteoporosis." *Hospital for Special Surgery Health Connection* 7.2 (1999): 7.

Rosen, Clifford J., and Cathy R. Kessenich. "The Pathophysiology and Treatment of Postmenopausal Osteoporosis." *Endocrinology and Metabolism Clinics of North America* 26.2 (1997): 295–311.

Shapiro, Lynn. "BMD Screening Advised in White Women Over Age 65." *Ob. Gyn. News*, 15 December 1998, 1, 5.

Siemenda, Charles, Christopher Longcope, Munro Peacock, Siu Hui, and C. Conrad Johnston. "Sex Steroids, Bone Mass, and Bone Loss." *Journal of Clinical Investigation* 97.1 (1998): 14–21.

Solomon, Jacqueline. "Osteoporosis." *Office Nurse* (December 1998): 19–26.

"Statins Decrease the Risk of Fractures Among Older Women." *Ob/Gyn Clinical Alert* 17.4 (August 2000): 25–6.

Trichopoulou, Antonia, Evangelos Georgiou, Yiannis Bassiakos, Loren Lipworth, Pagona Lagiou, Charalambos Proukakis, and Dimitrios Trichopoulos. "Energy Intake and Monounsaturated Fat in Relation to Bone Mineral Density Among Women and Men in Greece." *Preventive Medicine* 26 (1997): 395–400.

Tucker, Miriam E. "Exercise, Calcium, and Drugs Key to Bone Loss." *Ob. Gyn. News*, 15 June 1998, 13.

"Wait to Take This Drug: Raloxifene (Evista) for Osteoporosis." *Worst Pills/Best Pills* (February 1998): 11, 13.

Wasnich, Richard D. "Don't Wait for a Fracture." *The Female Patient* 23 (October 1998): 19–33.

CHAPTER 9
BEATING THE ODDS: YOUR HEART

Anthony, Mary S., Thomas B. Clarkson, and J. Koudy Williams. "Effects of Soy Isoflavones on Atherosclerosis." *American Journal of Clinical Nutrition* 68 suppl. (1998): 1390S–1393S.

Barbieri, Robert L., Joseph Carver, Martha Hill, Robert W. Rebar, and Vicki L. Seltzer, eds. *Cardiovascular Disease in Women.* APGO Educational Series on Women's Health Issues. Golden, CO: Medical Education Collaborative, 1998.

Barbieri, Robert L., Richard S. Legro, Sandra J. Lewis, Brian W. Walsh, and Francine K. Welty, eds. *Managing Hyperlipidemia in Women.* APGO Educational Series on Women's Health Issues. Beachwood, OH: Current Therapeutics, 1999.

Bratman, Steven. *The Alternative Medicine Ratings Guide.* Rocklin, CA: Prima Health, 1998. 77, 156–157.

Brink, Susan. "Unlocking the Heart's Secrets." *U.S. News & World Report* 125.9 (1998): 58–66.

Brody, Jane E. "Calcium Takes Its Place as a Superstar of Nutrients." *New York Times,* 13 October 1998, F1, F9.

———. "Health Sleuths Assess Homocysteine as Culprit." *New York Times,* 13 June 2000, F1, F6.

———. "Paradox or Not, Cholesterol in France Is on the Rise." *New York Times,* 22 June 1999, F1, F6.

———. "Some Ailments Found Guilty of Sex Bias." *New York Times,* 10 November 1998, F12.

———. "Tea: The Latest Health Food (But Hold the Clotted Cream)." *New York Times,* 7 September 1999, F7.

———. "The Fatty Nut Finds Its Place at the Table." *New York Times,* 8 February 2000, F8.

———. *The New York Times Book of Health.* New York: Times Books, 1997. 257–286.

———. "Yet Another Reason to Fight the Fat." *New York Times,* 28 July 1998, F7.

Brown, Donald J. "Protecting Your Heart With Hawthorn, CoQ10, and More." *Herbs for Health* (July/August 1998): 24–28.

"Cardiologists Share the Latest Wisdom." *New York Times,* 16 November 1999, F8.

Carlson, Cornelia. "The Benefits of Flax." *Herbs for Health* (September/October 1998): 63–65.

Carlson, Karen J., Stephanie A. Eisenstat, and Terra Ziporyn. *The Women's Concise Guide to a Healthier Heart.* Cambridge, MA: Harvard University Press, 1997. 68, 74–75.

Cerrato, Paul. "Contrary to Popular Belief, Coronary Artery Disease Kills Almost as Many Women as Men." *Office Nurse* (February 1999): 17–19.

Chang, Kenneth. "Aggressive Approaches Can Bolster Heart Health." *New York Times,* 21 November 2000, F6.

"Chocolate: How to Indulge Your Craving Without Giving In to the Guilt." *Mayo Clinic Women's HealthSource* (February 2000): 7.

Clarkson, Thomas B. "The Effects of Hormone Replacement Therapy on Key Risk Factors for Cardiovascular Disease." *HRT Casebook I: Hormone Replacement Therapy Cardiovascular Health*. Fair Lawn, NJ: MPE Communications, 2000.

Colvin, Perry L., Bruce J. Auerbach, Donald R. Koritnik, William R. Hazzard, and Deborah Applebaum-Bowden. "Differential Effect of Oral Oestrone Versus 17B-Oestradiol on Lipoproteins in Postmenopausal Women." *Journal of Clinical Endocrinology and Metabolism* 70 (1990): 1568–1573.

"Could a Chocolate a Day Keep the Doctor Away?" *Mayo Clinic Women's HealthSource* (December 1999): 3.

DeMott, Kathryn. "No Cardiac Benefit for HRT in Women With Heart Disease." *Ob.Gyn. News*, 15 September 1998, 1, 5.

"Don't Have a Stroke." *Consumer Reports on Health* 10.9 (1998): 1, 3–5.

"Drugs & Herbs." *Consumer Reports on Health* (July 1999): 7.

"Facts on Women and Tobacco." *CDC's TIPS*. www.cdc.gov/tobacco/womenfac/htm, 3 April 1998.

"Fiber Minimizes Low Risk of Heart Disease." *Mayo Clinic Women's HealthSource* (September 1999): 3.

"Fiber: Strands of Protection." *Consumer Reports on Health* (August 1999): 1, 3–5.

Firshein, Richard. *The Nutraceutical Revolution*. New York: Riverhead Books, 1998. 18–22, 79.

Frohlich, M., H. Schunkert, H.-W. Hense, A. Tropitzsch, P. Hendricks, A. Doring, G. A. J. Riegger, and W. Koenig. "Effects of Hormone Replacement Therapies on Fibrinogen and Plasma Viscosity in Postmenopausal Women." *British Journal of Haematology* 100 (1998): 577–581.

"From Cause to Cure: Understanding and Preventing Heart Disease." *A Special Advertising Supplement to the New York Times Magazine*, 27 September 1998, 45–68.

Gazella, Karolyn A. "The Homocysteine Theory of Heart Disease: Interview With Kilmer S. McCully, M.D." *American Journal of Natural Medicine* 5.6 (1998): 22–24.

"Gender Differences in Cardiac Care." *Mayo Clinic Women's HealthSource* 3.1 (1999): 4–5.

Gerhard, Marie, Brian W. Walsh, Ahmed Tawakol, Elizabeth A. Haley, Shelly J. Creager, Ellen W. Seely, Peter Ganz, and Mark A. Creager. "Oestradiol Therapy, Combined With Progesterone and Endothelium-Dependent Vasodilation in Postmenopausal Women." *Circulation* 98 (1998): 1158–1163.

Goldman, Erik L. "Daily Aspirin Urged After Age 50 to Prevent First MI." *Ob.Gyn. News*, 1 January 1999, 1, 4.

Grady, Denise. "As Silent Killer Returns, Doctors Rethink Tactics to Lower Blood Pressure." *New York Times*, 14 July 1998, F1, F5.

———. "Nicotine's Image Takes a Turn for the Worse." *New York Times*, 17 November 1998, F1, F8.

———. "Study Cites Risks for Women Under 50 With Heart Attacks." *New York Times*, 21 July 1999, A10.

Hammond, Charles B. *Therapeutic Options for Menopausal Health*. Durham, NC: Duke University Medical Center, 1998. 25–26.

"Heart Disease Is the Number 1 Killer of Women in the United States." *Heart-Strong Woman*. The American College of Obstetricians and Gynecologists, 1998.

Hochman, Judith S., Jacqueline E. Tamis, Trevor D. Thompson, W. Douglas Weaver, Harvey D. White, Frans Van de Werf, Phil Aylward, Eric J. Topol, and Robert M. Califf. "Sex, Clinical Presentation, and Outcome in Patients With Acute Coronary Syndromes." *The New England Journal of Medicine* 341.4 (1999): 226–232.

Hulley, Stephen, Deborah Grady, Trudy Bush, Curt Furberg, David Herrington, Betty Riggs, and Eric Vittinghoff. "Randomized Trial of Estrogen Plus Progesterone for Secondary Prevention of Coronary Heart Disease in Postmenopausal Women." *Journal of the American Medical Association* 280.7 (1998): 605–613.

"Hypertension: Bringing Your Numbers Down to Size." *Mayo Clinic Women's HealthSource* 1.10 (1997): 1–2.

Johnson, Kate. "Foods Serve as Adjuncts to HRT." *Ob.Gyn. News*, 1 November 1998, 1–2.

MacMahon, Stephen. "Blood Pressure and the Risk of Cardiovascular Disease." *The New England Journal of Medicine* 342.1 (2000): 50–51.

Matthews, Karen A., Rena R. Wing, Lewis H. Kuller, Elaine N. Meilahn, and Pam Plantinga. "Influence of the Perimenopause on Cardiovascular Risk Factors and Symptoms of Middle-Aged Healthy Women." *Archives of Internal Medicine* 154 (1994): 2349–2355.

Meschia, Michele, Fiorenza Bruschi, Maurizio Soma, Fabio Amicarelli, Rodolfo Paoletti, and Piergiorgio Crosignani. "Effects of Oral and Transdermal Hormone Replacement Therapy on Lipoprotein(A) and Lipids." *Menopause* 5.3 (1998): 157–162.

Mindell, Earl. *Earl Mindell's Supplement Bible*. New York: Fireside Books, 1998. 3–4, 81–82.

Nagourney, Eric. "For Hypertension, an Eye on Vitamin C." *New York Times*, 4 January 2000, F8.

Newton, Katherine M., and Andrea Z. LaCroix. "Hormone Replacement Therapy and Tertiary Prevention of Coronary Heart Disease." *Menopausal Medicine* 7.2 (1999): 5–8.

Noble, Holcomb B. "A Handful of Nuts and a Healthier Heart." *New York Times*, 17 November 1998, F10.

———. "Report Links Heart Attacks to Marijuana." *New York Times*, 3 March 2000, A13.

"On Your Mind." *Consumer Reports on Health* (September 1998): 12.

Pansini, Francesco, Gloria Bonaccorsi, Marina Calisesi, Carlo Campobasso, Gian Pietro Franze, Giuseppe Gilli, Giancarlo Locorotondo, and Gioacchino Mollica. "Influence of Spontaneous and Surgical Menopause on Atherogenic Metabolic Risk." *Maturitas* 17 (1993): 181–190.

Perry, Arlette C., Paul C. Miller, Mark D. Allison, M. Loreto Jackson, and E. Brooks Applegate. "Clinical Predictability of the Waist-to-Hip Ratio in Assessment of Cardiovascular Disease Risk Factors in Overweight, Premenopausal Women." *American Journal of Clinical Nutrition* 68 (1998): 1022–1027.

Reavley, Nicola. *The New Encyclopedia of Vitamins, Minerals, Supplements, and Herbs*. New York: M. Evans, 1998. 331–334, 666–667.

Salomaa, V., V. Rasi, J. Pekkanen, E. Vahtera, M. Jauhiainen, E. Vartiainen, C. Ehnholm, J. Tuomilehto, and G. Myllyla. "Association of Hormone Replacement Therapy With Hemostatic and Other Cardiovascular Risk Factors." *Arteriosclerosis, Thrombosis, and Vascular Biology* 15.10 (1995): 1549–1555.

Smith, Kathleen A. "Healthy Lifestyle Choices and Their Impact on the Quality of Life of Women Over Age 40." In *Menopausal Issues for Nursing Professionals: Quality of Life and Menopause.* Barrington, IL: The Willow Group, 1998. 6–11.

Sotelo, Margarita, and Susan R. Johnson. "The Effects of Hormone Replacement Therapy on Coronary Heart Disease." *Endocrinology and Metabolism Clinics of North America* 26.2 (1997): 313–327.

Sowers, MaryFran, and Catherine Sigler. "Complex Relation Between Increasing Fat Mass and Decreasing High Density Lipoprotein Cholesterol Levels." *American Journal of Epidemiology* 149.1 (1999): 47–54.

"Soy's Heart-Healthy Claim." *Ob. Gyn. News*, 1 December 1999, 21.

"Statins Decrease the Risk of Fractures Among Older Women." *Ob/Gyn Clinical Alert* 17.4 (August 2000): 25–6.

Stengler, Mark. "Lowering Cholesterol Naturally." *Nature's Impact* (February/March 1999): 32–33.

"Study Sees Benefits of Fiber for Women." *New York Times*, 2 June 1999, A18.

Sullivan, Jay M. "The Role of Estrogen in Secondary Prevention of Cardiovascular Events." *Menopausal Medicine* 7.2 (1999): 7–11.

Taechakraichana, Nimit, Kobchitt Limpaphayom, Tanimporn Ninlagarn, Krasean Panyakhamlerd, Sukanya Chaikittisilpa, and Nikorn Dusitsin. "A Randomized Trial of Oral Contraceptive and Hormone Replacement Therapy on Bone Mineral Density and Coronary Heart Disease Risk Factors in Postmenopausal Women." *Obstetrics & Gynecology* 95.1 (2000): 87–94.

Tang, Alisa. "Cocaine's Grip on the Blood and the Brain." *New York Times*, 21 September 1999, F8.

Tarkan, Laurie. "Chocolate a Health Food? Maybe, but Keep the Aspirin." *New York Times*, 31 October 2000, F7.

Vaccarino, Viola, Lori Parsons, Nathan R. Every, Hal V. Barron, and Harlan M. Krumholz. "Sex-Based Differences in Early Mortality After Myocardial Infarction." *The New England Journal of Medicine* 341.4 (1999): 217–225.

"Vitamin C: Foods Yes, Pills No." *Consumer Reports on Health* 10.11 (1998): 1, 3–5.

Walsh, B., S. Paul, R. Wild, R. Dean, R. Tracy, D. Cox, and P. Anderson. "The Effects of Hormone Replacement Therapy and Raloxifene on C-Reactive Protein and Homocysteine in Healthy Postmenopausal Women: A Randomized, Controlled Trial." *The Journal of Clinical Endocrinology & Metabolism* 85.1 (2000): 214–218.

Warren, Michelle P., and Jaime Kulak Jr. "Is Estrogen Replacement Indicated in Perimenopausal Women?" *Clinical Obstetrics and Gynecology* 41.4 (1998): 976–987.

Washburn, Gregory L. Burke, Timothy Morgan, and Mary Anthony. "Effect of Soy Protein Supplementation on Serum Lipoproteins, Blood Pressure, and Menopausal Symptoms in Perimenopausal Women." *Menopause* 6.1 (1999): 7–13.

Wassef, Farid. "Cardiovascular Disease: Reading the Correct Road Signs." *American Journal of Natural Medicine* 5.7 (1998): 12–15.

Wexler, Laura F. "Studies of Acute Coronary Syndromes in Women—Lessons for Everyone." *The New England Journal of Medicine* 341.4 (1999): 275–276.

Wild, Robert A. "Review of 'Randomized Trial of Estrogen Plus Progestin for Secondary Prevention of Coronary Heart Disease in Postmenopausal Women.' " Reprints and Reviews Series. Chicago: Pragmaton Office of Medical Education (1999). 1–7.

———. "Risk Factors: Assessment and Preventive Measures." *Clinical Obstetrics and Gynecology* 41.4 (1998): 966–975.

Williams, J. Koudy, Remi Delansorne, and Jaques Paris. "Oestrogens, Progestins, and Coronary Artery Reactivity in Atherosclerotic Monkeys." *Journal of Steroid Biochemistry & Molecular Biology* 65.1–6 (1998): 219–224.

"Women Don't Realize Risk of Heart Attack." *ACOG Today* 43.2 (1999): 1, 9.

Zoler, Mitchel L. "Raloxifene Lowers Serum CV Risk Factors in Women." *Ob. Gyn. News*, 15 December 1998, 1, 4.

———. "Studies Offer More Data on HRT's Heart Benefits." *Ob. Gyn. News*, 15 May 1999, 1, 4.

CHAPTER 10
BOSOM BUDDIES: YOUR BREASTS

Altman, Lawrence K. "Drug Is Found to Fight Return of Breast Cancer." *New York Times*, 15 May 1998, A16.

"Arm Lymphedema." *Mayo Clinic Women's HealthSource* (August 1999): 6.

Baker, Barbara. "Breast Ca Before Age 50 Raises Ovarian Ca Risk." *Ob. Gyn. News*, 1 May 1999, 1, 5.

Barakat, Richard R. "Tamoxifen and Endometrial Neoplasia." *Clinical Obstetrics and Gynecology* 39.3 (1996): 629–640.

Boschert, Sherry. "Tamoxifen Lowers Breast Cancer Rate in High-Risk Groups." *Ob. Gyn. News*, 15 June 1999, 1, 5.

Bratman, Steven. *The Alternative Medicine Ratings Guide.* Roclin, CA: Prima Health, 1998. 123–124.

"Breast Cancer and Diet Fat: No Link Found." *New York Times*, 10 March 1999, A15.

"Breast Cancer: Clearing Up the Confusion." *Consumer Reports on Health* (July 1999): 1, 3–6.

"Breast Reconstruction After Mastectomy." *Mayo Clinic Women's HealthSource* (December 1998): 4–5.

"Breast Removal an Option for High-Risk Women." *Mayo Clinic Women's Health-Source* (May 1999): 3.

"Breast-Ovarian Cancer Screening." *ACOG Committee Opinion* 176 (October 1996): 20–21.

Brody, Jane E. "Another Round in Drink-a-Day Debate." *New York Times*, 2 February 1999, F7.

———. "Living Proof: Mammograms Are Not Always Enough." *New York Times*, 9 March 1999, F6.

———. "Risks for Cancer Can Start in Womb." *New York Times*, 21 December 1999, F1, F6.

Calle, Eugenia E., Heidi L. Miracle-McMahill, Michael J. Thun, and Clark W. Heath Jr. "Cigarette Smoking and Risk of Fatal Breast Cancer." *American Journal of Epidemiology* 139.10 (1994): 1001–1007.

"Carcinoma of the Breast." *ACOG Technical Bulletin* 158 (August 1991): 303–308.

Carlson, Cornelia. "The Benefits of Flax." *Herbs for Health* (September/October 1998): 63–65.

Chalas, Eva, and Fidel Valea. "The Gynecologist and Surgical Procedures for Breast Disease." *Clinical Obstetrics and Gynecology* 37.4 (1994): 948–953.

"Common Questions About Testing for Hereditary Cancer Predisposition." *Contemporary Ob/Gyn* (November 1998): 117–118.

Cummings, S. R., S. Eckert, K. A. Krueger, D. Grady, T. J. Powles, J. A. Cauley, L. Norton, T. Nickelsen, N. H. Bjarnason, M. Morrow, M. E. Lippman, D. Black, J. E. Glusman, A. Costa, and V. C. Jordan. "The Effect of Raloxifene on Risk of Breast Cancer in Postmenopausal Women." *Journal of the American Medical Association* 281.23 (1999): 2189–2197.

Davis, Devra Lee, Deborah Axelrod, Lisa Bailey, Mitchell Gaynor, and Annie J. Sasco. "Rethinking Breast Cancer Risk and the Environment." *Environmental Health Perspectives* 106.9 (1998): 523–529.

Del Giudice, M. Elisabeth, I. George Fantus, Shereen Ezzat, Gail McKeown-Eyssen, David Page, and Pamela J. Goodwin. "Insulin and Related Factors in Premenopausal Breast Cancer Risk." *Breast Cancer Research and Treatment* 47 (1998): 111–120.

DeMarco, Carolyn. "Breast Cancer Treatment Options: Part I." *Health Counselor* (June/July 1997): 18–20.

———. "Breast Cancer Treatment Options: Part II." *Health Counselor* (August/September 1997): 18–19.

DeMott, Kathryn. "New Technology Sharpens Breast Ca Screening." *Ob.Gyn. News*, 15 May 1999, 5.

Donohue, Maureen. "Breast Ca Risk Rises Slightly Among HRT Users." *Ob.Gyn. News*, 1 March 2000, 1–2.

Drukker, Bruce H. "Fibrocystic Change of the Breast." *Clinical Obstetrics and Gynecology* 37.4 (1994): 903–915.

Early Breast Cancer Trialists' Collaborative Group. "Tamoxifen for Early Breast Cancer." *Lancet* 351 (1998): 1451–1465.

Eisenberg, Anne. "Cancer Regimen Found Safe in Pregnancy." *New York Times*, 16 March 1999, F7.

———. "Clearer Mammograms May Be Near." *New York Times*, 1 December 1998, F7.

Ellis, Toya, and Susan A. Davidson. "Hereditary Breast and Ovarian Cancer." *OBG Management* (December 1998): 53–59.

Firshein, Richard. *The Nutraceutical Revolution.* New York: Riverhead Books, 1998. 36.

Fisher, Bernard, Joseph P. Costantino, D. Lawrence Wickerham, Carol K. Redmond, Maureen Kavanah, Walter M. Cronin, Victor Vogel, Andre Robidoux, Nikolay Dimitrov, James Atkins, Mary Daly, Samuel Wieand, Elizabeth Tan-Chiu, Leslie Ford, and Norman Wolmark. "Tamoxifen for Prevention of Breast Cancer." *Journal of the National Cancer Institute* 90.18 (1998): 1371–1388.

FitzGerald, Frances E. "Breast Cancer Treatments: You *Do* Have Choices." *Nature's Impact* (August/September 1998): 36–41.

Furberg, H., B. Newman, P. Moorman, and R. Millikan. "Lactation and Breast Cancer Risk." *International Journal of Epidemiology* 28 (1999): 396–402. (Carolina Breast Cancer Study.)

Grady, Denise. "In Breast Cancer Data, Hope, Fear and Confusion." *New York Times*, 26 January 1999, F1, F4.

———. "Software to Compute Women's Cancer Risk." *New York Times*, 26 January 1999, F4.

"Guide to Breast Care." *Mayo Clinic Women's HealthSource* (1997).

Henson, Donald Earl, and Robert E. Tarone. "Involution and the Etiology of Breast Cancer." *Cancer* 74 (1994): 424–429.

Hirose, Kaoru, Kazuo Tajima, Nobuyuki Hamajima, Toshiro Takezaki, Manami Inoue, Tetsuo Kuroishi, Shigeto Miura, and Shinkan Tokudome. "Effect of Body Size on Breast-Cancer Risk Among Japanese Women." *International Journal of Cancer* 80 (1999): 349–355.

Holmes, Michelle D., David J. Hunter, Graham A. Colditz, Meir J. Stampfer, Susan E. Hankinson, Frank E. Speizer, Bernard Rosner, and Walter C. Willett. "Association of Dietary Intake of Fat and Fatty Acids with Risk of Breast Cancer." *Journal of the American Medical Association* 281.10 (1999): 914–920.

Huelsman, Karen M., Jill Huppert, and James Fiorica. "Screening Your Patients for Inherited Breast and Ovarian Cancer." *Contemporary Ob/Gyn* (November 1998): 107–132.

Hunter, David J., Donna Spiegelman, Hans-Olov Adami, Lawrence Beeson, Piet A. van den Brandt, Aaron R. Folsom, Gary E. Fraser, Alexandra Goldbohm, Saxon Graham, Geoffrey R. Howe, Lawrence H. Kushi, James R. Marshall, Aidan McDermott, Anthony B. Miller, Frank E. Speizer, Alicja Wolk, Shiaw-Shyuan Yaun, and Walter Willett. "Cohort Studies of Fat Intake and the Risk of Breast Cancer." *The New England Journal of Medicine* 334 (1996): 356–361.

Ingram, David, Katherine Sanders, Marlene Kolybaba, and Derrick Lopez. "Case-Control Study of Phyto-Oestrogens and Breast Cancer." *Lancet* 350 (1997): 990–994.

Jackson, Nancy Beth. "Strand of Hair May Point to Who Has Breast Cancer." *New York Times*, 4 March 1999, A16.

Jacobs, Timothy W., Celia Byrne, Graham Colditz, James L. Connolly, and Stuart J. Schnitt. "Radial Scars in Benign Breast-Biopsy Specimens and the Risk of Breast Cancer." *The New England Journal of Medicine* 340 (1999): 430–436.

Jancin, Bruce. "BRCA-Associated Ca Risks Have Been Overstated." *Ob. Gyn. News*, 1 May 1999, 9.

———. "Diet Has No Major Impact on Risk of Breast Ca." *Ob. Gyn. News*, 1 March 2000, 1–2.

———. "Hormones Can Alter Ca Risk Due to BRCA Genes." *Ob. Gyn. News*, 15 April 1999, 25.

———. "MRI: Best for Early Cancer Detection?" *Ob. Gyn. News*, 1 February 2000, 1–2.

———. "New Analysis Shows Raloxifene Prevents Breast Ca." *Ob. Gyn. News*, 15 January 1999, 1–2.

———. "Raloxifene Lowers Breast Cancer Risk by 72%." *Ob. Gyn. News*, 1 February 2001, 1, 3.

———. "Technologies Aim to Improve Mammography." *Ob. Gyn. News*, 15 February 1999, 12.

Jetter, Alexis. "Breast Cancer in Blacks Spurs Hunt for Answers." *New York Times*, 22 February 2000, F7, F12.

Kaaks, Rudolph, Paul A. H. Van Noord, Isolde Den Tonkelaar, Petra H. M. Peeters, Elio Riboli, and Diederick E. Grobbee. "Breast-Cancer Incidence in Relation to Height, Weight and Body-Fat Distribution in the Dutch 'DOM' Cohort." *International Journal of Cancer* 76 (1998): 647–651.

Kolb, Thomas M., Jacob Lichy, and Jeffrey H. Newhouse. "Occult Cancer in Women With Dense Breasts." *Radiology* 207.1 (1998): 191–199.

Lee, Lauri M. "Breast Cancer: Replace Fear With Knowledge." *Women's Health Connections* 1.4b (October/November 1993): 1–3, 5.

Magnusson, Cecilia, John Baron, Ingemar Persson, Alicja Wolk, Reinhold Bergstrom, Dimitrios Trichopoulos, and Hans-Olov Adami. "Body Size in Different Periods of Life and Breast Cancer Risk in Post-Menopausal Women." *International Journal of Cancer* 76 (1998): 29–34.

Magnusson, Cecilia M., Ingemar R. Persson, John A. Baron, Anders Ekbom, Reinhold Bergstrom, and Hans-Olov Adami. "The Role of Reproductive Factors and Use of Oral Contraceptives in the Aetiology of Breast Cancer in Women Aged 50 to 74 Years." *International Journal of Cancer* 80 (1999): 231–236.

Marchant, Douglas J. "The Breast." In *Danforth's Obstetrics and Gynecology*, 6th ed. Philadelphia: J. B. Lippincott, 1990. 1159–1160.

Mayfield, Eleanor. "Finding Breast Cancer Early." *The Female Patient* S/3 (1998): 25–29.

McAuliffe, Kathleen. "Researchers Shine a Night Light on a Possible Link to Cancer." *New York Times*, 13 June 1999, 15. 22.

Mechcatie, Elizabeth. "FDA Advisory Panel Nods Tamoxifen to Cut Breast Cancer Risk." *Ob. Gyn. News*, 1 October 1998, 1, 6.

Michels, Karin B., Dimitrios Trichopoulos, James M. Robins, Bernard A. Rosner, JoAnn E. Manson, David J. Hunter, Graham A. Colditz, Susan E. Hankinson, Frank E. Speizer, and Walter C. Willett. "Birthweight as a Risk Factor for Breast Cancer." *Lancet* 348 (1996): 1542–1546.

Mindell, Earl. *Earl Mindell's Supplement Bible.* New York: Fireside Books, 1998. 150–152, 172–173.

Moon, Mary Ann. "Prophylactic Mastectomy." *Ob. Gyn. News*, 1 March 1999, 11.

Morabia, Alfredo, Martine Bernstein, Juan Ruiz, Stephane Heritier, Sophie Diebold Berger, and Bettina Borisch. "Relation of Smoking to Breast Cancer by Estrogen Receptor Status." *International Journal of Cancer* 75 (1998): 339–342.

Nachtigall, Lila E. "Sex Hormone-Binding Globulin and Breast Cancer Risk." *Primary Care Update for Obstetrician/Gynecologists* 6.2 (1999): 39–45.

Newcomb, Polly A., Barry E. Storer, Matthew P. Longnecker, Robert Mittendorf, E. Robert Greenberg, Richard W. Clapp, Kenneth P. Burke, Walter C. Willett, and Brian MacMahon. "Lactation and a Reduced Risk of Premenopausal Breast Cancer." *The New England Journal of Medicine* 330.2 (1994): 81–87.

Noble, Holcomb B. "Procedure Helps Detect Cancers of Breast." *New York Times*, 20 April 1999, F7.

"Nonmalignant Conditions of the Breast." *ACOG Technical Bulletin* 156 (June 1991): 612–616.

Norris, John D., Lisa A. Paige, Dale J. Christensen, Ching-Yi Chang, Maria R. Huacani, Daju Fan, Paul T. Hamilton, Dana M. Fowlkes, and Donald P. McDonnell. "Peptide Antagonists of the Human Estrogen Receptor." *Science* 285 (30 July 1999): 744–746.

Peck, Peggy. "Laser Lumpectomy Eliminates Deformity." *Ob. Gyn. News*, 1 February 1999, 9.

————. "Mammography Plus US Sharpens Cancer Detection." *Ob.Gyn. News*, 1 February 1999, 8.

Riordan, Teresa. "Patents: Using Sophisticated Laser Light as an Alternative to Potentially Hazardous X-Ray Mammography." *New York Times*, 12 October 1998, C2.

"Role of the Obstetrician-Gynecologist in the Diagnosis and Treatment of Breast Disease." *ACOG Committee Opinion* 186 (September 1997): 198–199.

Schairer, Catherine, Jay Lubin, Rebecca Troisi, Susan Sturgeon, Louise Brinton, and Robert Hoover. "Menopausal Estrogen and Estrogen-Progestin Replacement Therapy and Breast Cancer Risk." *Journal of the American Medical Association* 283.4 (2000): 485–491.

Sesso, Howard D., Ralph S. Paffenbarger Jr., and I-Min Lee. "Physical Activity and Breast Cancer Risk in the College Alumni Health Study (United States)." *Cancer Causes and Control* 9 (1998): 433–439.

Smith-Warner, Stephanie A., Donna Spiegelman, Shiaw-Shyuan Yaun, Piet A. van den Brandt, Aaron R. Folsom, Alexandra Goldbohm, Saxon Graham, Lars Holmberg, Geoffrey R. Howe, James R. Marshall, Anthony B. Miller, John D. Potter, Frank E. Speizer, Walter C. Willett, Alicja Wolk, and David J. Hunter. "Alcohol and Breast Cancer in Women." *Journal of the American Medical Association* 279.7 (1998): 535–540.

Stoll, B. A. "Teenage Obesity in Relation to Breast Cancer Risk." *International Journal of Obesity and Related Metabolic Disorders* 22.11 (1998): 1035–1040.

Stoll, Basil A. "Perimenopausal Weight Gain and Progression of Breast Cancer Precursors." *Cancer Detection and Prevention* 23.1 (1999): 31–36.

"Study Suggests Why a Cancer Fighter Fails." *New York Times*, 30 July 1999, A13.

"Tamoxifen and Endometrial Cancer." *ACOG Committee Opinion* 169 (February 1996): 231–232.

Titus-Ernstoff, Linda, Matthew P. Longnecker, Polly A. Newcomb, Bradley Dain, E. Robert Greenberg, Robert Mittendorf, Meir Stampfer, and Walter Willett. "Menstrual Factors in Relation to Breast Cancer Risk." *Cancer Epidemiology, Biomarkers & Prevention* 7 (1998): 783–789.

"Ultrasound Plus Mammography Better for Dense Breasts." *Mayo Clinic Women's HealthSource* (March 1999): 3.

University of Pennsylvania Cancer Center. "NCI/PDQ Patient Statement: Breast Cancer." OncoLink.com., November 1998.

"Women's Risk of Lung Cancer Far Greater Than Men's." *Mayo Clinic Women's HealthSource* (February 2000): 3.

Worcester, Sharon. "Educate Patients About Mammography." *Ob.Gyn. News*, 1 May 1999.

Zava, David T., and Gail Duwe. "Oestrogenic and Antiproliferative Properties of Genistein and Other Flavonoids in Human Breast Cancer Cells *In Vitro*." *Nutrition and Cancer* 27.1 (1997): 31–40.

Zava, David T., Charles M. Dollbaum, and Marilyn Blen. "Oestrogen and Progestin Bioactivity of Foods, Herbs, and Spices." *Proceedings of the Society for Experimental Biology and Medicine* 217 (1998): 369–378.

Zhang, Yuqing, Bernard E. Kreger, Joanne F. Dorgan, Greta L. Splansky, L. Adrienne Cupples, and R. Curtis Ellison. "Alcohol Consumption and Risk of Breast Cancer." *American Journal of Epidemiology* 149.2 (1999): 93–104.

Zoler, Mitchel L. "Cancer Risk with BRCA Mutations." *Ob.Gyn. News*, 15 December 2000, 3.

CHAPTER 11
BELOW THE BELT: YOUR UTERUS, OVARIES, CERVIX, AND COLON

"Aspirin Use Linked to 40% Reduction in Ovarian Ca Risk." *Ob.Gyn. News*, 15 April 2001.

Barbieri, Robert L. "Primary Gonadotropin-Releasing Hormone Agonist Therapy for Suspected Endometriosis." *The American Journal of Managed Care* 3.2 (1997): 285–290.

Bini, Edmund J., Philip L. Micale, and Elizabeth H. Weinshel. "Evaluation of the Gastrointestinal Tract in Premenopausal Women With Iron Deficiency Anemia." *The American Journal of Medicine* 105 (1998): 281–286.

Blumenfeld, Michael L., and L. Paige Turner. "Role of Transvaginal Sonography in the Evaluation of Endometrial Hyperplasia and Cancer." *Clinical Obstetrics and Gynecology* 39.3 (1996): 629–640.

Braly, Patricia. "HPV Screening and Treatment." *Ob/Gyn Special Edition* 2 (Spring 1999): 11–13.

Brody, Jane E. "Detecting Colon Cancer When It's Curable." *New York Times*, 28 September 1999, F8.

Brooks, Sandra E. "Preoperative Evaluation of Patients With Suspected Ovarian Cancer." *Gynecologic Oncology* 55 (1994): S80–S90.

Claus, Elizabeth B., and Peter E. Schwartz. "Familial Ovarian Cancer." *Cancer* suppl. 76.10 (1995): 1998–2002.

Davies, Anthony, Roger Hart, and Adam L. Magos. "The Excision of Uterine Fibroids by Vaginal Myomectomy." *Fertility and Sterility* 71.5 (1999): 961–964.

DePriest, P. D., and J. R. van Nagell. "Transvaginal Ultrasound Screening for Ovarian Cancer." *Clinical Obstetrics and Gynecology* 35.1 (1992): 40–44.

DiSaia, Philip J. "Ovarian Disorders." In *Danforth's Obstetrics and Gynecology*, 6th ed. Philadelphia: J. B. Lippincott, 1990. 1067–1103.

DiSaia, Philip J., and Adolf Stafl. "Disorders of the Uterine Cervix." In *Danforth's Obstetrics and Gynecology*, 6th ed. Philadelphia: J. B. Lippincott, 1990. 987–1011.

Dragojevic-Dikic, Svetlana, and Miodrag Vucic. "The Application of GnRH Analogues in the Treatment of Uterine Myomas in Perimenopausal Women." *Ginekologica Polska* 69.1 (1998): 28–32.

Drake, Janet. "Diagnosis and Management of the Adnexal Mass." *American Family Physician* 57.10 (1998): 2471–2476.

Englund, Katarina, Agneta Blanck, Inger Gustavsson, Ulrika Lundkvist, Peter Sjoblom, Allan Norgren, and Bo Lindblom. "Sex Steroid Receptors in Human Myometrium and Fibroids: Changes During the Menstrual Cycle and Gonadotropin-Releasing Hormone Treatment." *Journal of Clinical Endocrinology & Metabolism* 83.11 (1998): 4092–4096.

Esposito, Melissa A., Richard W. Tureck, and Luigi Mastroianni Jr. "Understanding Endometriosis: Part 1." *The Female Patient* 24 (June 1999): 79–85.

———. "Understanding Endometriosis: Part 2." *The Female Patient* 24 (July 1999): 23–35.

Fernandez, Esteve, Carlo La Vecchia, Claudia Braga, Renato Talamini, Eva Negri, Fabio Parazzini, and Silvia Franceschi. "Hormone Replacement Therapy and Risk of Colon and Rectal Cancer." *Cancer Epidemiology, Biomarkers & Prevention* 7 (1998): 329–333.

Gilbert, Susan. "A Less Invasive Alternative for Fibroids." *New York Times*, 6 April 1999, F7.

Giovannucci, Edward, Meir J. Stampfer, Graham A. Colditz, David J. Hunter, Charles Fuchs, Bernard A. Rosner, Frank E. Speizer, and Walter C. Willett. "Multivitamin Use, Folate, and Colon Cancer in Women in the Nurses' Health Study." *Annals of Internal Medicine* 129.7 (1998): 517–524.

Goodman, Marc T., Lynne R. Wilkens, Jean H. Hankin, Li-Ching Lyu, Anna H. Wu, and Laurence N. Kolonel. "Association of Soy and Fiber Consumption With the Risk of Endometrial Cancer." *American Journal of Epidemiology* 146.4 (1997): 294–305.

Grabo, Theresa N., Pamela Stewart Fahs, Lindsay G. Nataupsky, and Harry Reich. "Uterine Myomas: Treatment Options." *JOGNN* 28.1 (1999): 23–31.

Grady, Denise. "A Cancer Test Surpasses the Pap One, Studies Find." *New York Times*, 5 January 2000, A18.

Hankison, S. E., D. J. Hunter, G. A. Colditz, W. C. Willett, M. J. Stampfer, B. Rasner, C. H. Hennekens, and F. E. Speizer. "Tubal Ligation, Hysterectomy, and Risk of Ovarian Cancer." *Journal of the American Medical Association* 270 (1993): 2813–2818.

Harden, Tracey. "Diagnosing Fibroids Is Simple; Deciding What to Do Is Hard." *New York Times*, 13 June 1999, 14.

Hebert-Croteau, Nicole. "A Meta-Analysis of Hormone Replacement Therapy and Colon Cancer in Women." *Cancer Epidemiology, Biomarkers & Prevention* 7 (1998): 653–659.

Linder, J. "Recent Advances in Thin-Layer Cytology." *Diagnostic Cytopathology* 18.1 (1998): 24–32.

Linder, J., and D. Zahniser. "ThinPrep Papanicolaou Testing to Reduce False-Negative Cervical Cytology." *Archives of Pathology and Laboratory Medicine* 122.2 (1998): 139–144.

Marshall, Lynn M., Donna Spiegelman, JoAnn E. Manson, Marlene B. Goldman, Robert L. Barbieri, Meir J. Stampfer, Walter C. Willett, and David J. Hunter. "Risk of Uterine Leiomyomata Among Perimenopausal Women in Relation to Body Size and Cigarette Smoking." *Epidemiology* 9.5 (1998): 511–517.

Marshall, Lynn M., Donna Spiegelman, Marlene B. Goldman, JoAnn E. Manson, Graham A. Colditz, Robert L. Barbieri, Meir J. Stampfer, and David J. Hunter. "A Prospective Study of Reproductive Factors and Oral Contraceptive Use in Relation to the Risk of Uterine Leiomyomata." *Fertility and Sterility* 70.3 (1998): 432–439.

Marshall, Lynn M., Donna Spiegelman, Robert L. Barbieri, Marlene B. Goldman, JoAnn E. Manson, Graham A. Colditz, Walter C. Willett, and David J. Hunter. "Variation in the Incidence of Uterine Leiomyoma Among Premenopausal Women by Age and Race." *Obstetrics & Gynecology* 90.6 (1997): 967–973.

Martin, Dan C., Ozgul Muneyyirci-Delale, and Ceana H. Nezhat. "Ending the Cycle of Pain: Diagnosis and Treatment of Endometriosis." *Ob. Gyn. News* suppl. (1999).

Mathias, John R., Robert Franklin, Don C. Quast, Nelda Fraga, Camille A. Loftin, Lori Yates, and Victoria Harrison. "Relation of Endometriosis and Neuromuscular Disease of the Gastrointestinal Tract." *Fertility and Sterility* 70.1 (1998): 81–88.

Merrill, James A., and William T. Creasman. "Disorders of the Uterine Corpus." In

Danforth's Obstetrics and Gynecology, 6th ed. Philadelphia: J. B. Lippincott, 1990. 1023–1054.

Moon, Mary Ann. "Sexual Function Should Improve After Hysterectomy." *Ob.Gyn. News*, 1 February 2000, 15.

"NIH Develops Consensus Statement on Ovarian Cancer." *American Family Physician* 50.1 (1994): 213–216.

"One Lifetime Colonoscopy." *Ob.Gyn. News*, 15 December 1999, 17.

Parazzini, Fabio, Eva Negri, Carlo La Vecchia, Liliane Chatenoud, Elena Ricci, and Paolo Guarnerio. "Reproductive Factors and Risk of Uterine Fibroids." *Epidemiology* 7.4 (1996): 440–442.

Perez-Medina, Tirso, Oscar Martinez, Gonzalo Folgueira, and Jose Bajo. "Which Endometrial Polyps Should Be Resected?" *The Journal of the American Association of Gynecologic Laparoscopists* 6.1 (1999): 71–74.

Rein, Mitchell S., Robert L. Barbieri, and Andrew J. Friedman. "Progesterone: A Critical Role in the Pathogenesis of Uterine Myomas." *American Journal of Obstetrics & Gynecology* 172.1 (1995): 14–18.

Riman, Tomas, Ingemar Persson, and Staffan Nilsson. "Hormonal Aspects of Epithelial Ovarian Cancer." *Clinical Endocrinology* 49 (1998): 695–707.

Robbins, Jim. "Research Suggests Positive Effects from Living off the Fat of the Sea." *New York Times*, 24 April 2001, F7.

Roberts, J. M., J. K. Thurloe, R. C. Bowditch, J. Humcevic, and C. R. Laverty. "Comparison of ThinPrep and Pap Smear in Relation to Prediction of Adenocarcinoma in Situ." *Acta Cytologica* 43.1 (1999): 74–80.

"Routine Cancer Screening." *ACOG Committee Opinion* 185 (1997): 200–204.

Schlaff, William D. "Surgical Treatment of Uterine Myomata." *OBG Management* (April 1999): 50–56.

Schwarzler, P., H. Concin, H. Bosch, A. Berlinger, K. Wohlgenannt, W. P. Collins, and T. H. Bourne. "An Evaluation of Sonohysterography and Diagnostic Hysteroscopy for the Assessment of Intrauterine Pathology." *Ultrasound in Obstetrics and Gynecology* 11 (1998): 337–342.

Stampfer, Meir J., and Francine Grodstein. "Colorectal Cancer: Does Postmenopausal Estrogen Use Reduce the Risk?" *Menopause Management* (March/ April 1999): 8–10.

Sulak, Patricia J. "Endometrial Cancer and Hormone Replacement Therapy." *Endocrinology and Metabolism Clinics of North America* 26.2 (1997): 399–412.

Talamini, R., S. Franceschi, L. Dal Maso, E. Negri, E. Conti, R. Filiberti, M. Montella, O. Nanni, and C. La Vecchia. "The Influence of Reproductive and Hormonal Factors on the Risk of Colon and Rectal Cancer in Women." *European Journal of Cancer* 34.7 (1998): 1070–1076.

Talbert, Luther M., and Scott M. Kauma. "Endometriosis." In *Danforth's Obstetrics and Gynecology*, 6th ed. Philadelphia: J. B. Lippincott, 1990. 845–852.

Triadafilopoulos, George, MaryAnn Finlayson, and Catherine Grellet. "Bowel Dysfunction in Postmenopausal Women." *Women & Health* 27.4 (1998):55–66.

Winkel, Craig A. "Laparoscopy Plus GnRH Analogues." *Contemporary Ob/Gyn* (April 1999): 99–109.

Yamada, S. Diane, and Kathryn F. McGonigle. "Cancer of the Endometrium and Corpus Uteri." *Current Opinion in Obstetrics and Gynecology* 10 (1998): 57–60.

Zoler, Mitchel L. "Annual Ovarian Ca Screening Needed With CA 125." *Ob.Gyn. News*, 1 June 1999, 24.

————. "Cancer Risk with BRCA Mutations." *Ob.Gyn. News*, 15 December 2000, 3.

Zreik, Tony G., Thomas J. Rutherford, Steven F. Palter, Robert N. Troiano, Ena Williams, Janis M. Brown, and David L. Olive. "Cryomyolysis, a New Procedure for the Conservative Treatment of Uterine Fibroids." *The Journal of the American Association of Gynecologic Laparoscopists* 5.1 (1998): 33–38.

CHAPTER 12
EVE'S APPLE: YOUR THYROID GLAND

"A Thyroid Dilemma." *The New England Journal of Medicine HealthNews* (September/October 1998): 3.

Akslen, L. A., S. Nilssen, and G. Kvale. "Reproductive Factors and Risk of Thyroid Cancer." *British Journal of Cancer* 65 (1992): 772–774.

Arem, Ridha. *The Thyroid Solution*. New York: Ballantine, 1999.

Bertelsen, Jette B., and Laszlo Hegedus. "Cigarette Smoking and the Thyroid." *Thyroid* 4.3 (1994): 327–331.

Bratman, Steven. *The Alternative Medicine Ratings Guide*. Roclin, CA: Prima Health, 1998. 165–166.

Cooper, David S. "Subclinical Thyroid Disease: A Clinician's Perspective." *Annals of Internal Medicine* 129.2 (1998): 135–138.

Faughnan, Marie, Raymond Lepage, Pierre Fugere, Francois Bissonnette, Jean-Hugues Brossard, and Pierre D'Amour. "Screening for Thyroid Disease at the Menopausal Clinic." *Clinical Investigative Medicine* 18.1 (1995): 11–18.

"The Forgotten Hormone: The Ups and Downs of Your Thyroid." *Mayo Clinic Women's HealthSource* (August 1999): 4–5.

Franceschi, S., A. Fassina, R. Talamini, A. Mazzolini, S. Vianello, B. Bidoli, G. Cizza, and C. La Vecchia. "The Influence of Reproductive and Hormonal Factors on Thyroid Cancer in Women." *Revue Epidémiologique et Santé Publique* 38 (1990): 27–34.

Galanti, Maria Rosaria, Lisbeth Hansson, Eiliv Lund, Reinhold Bergstrom, Lars Grimelius, Helge Stalsberg, Eivind Carlsen, John A. Baron, Ingemar Persson, and Anders Ekbom. "Reproductive History and Cigarette Smoking as Risk Factors for Thyroid Cancer in Women." *Cancer Epidemiology, Biomarkers & Prevention* 5 (1996): 425–431.

Goodman, M. T., L. N. Kolonel, and L. R. Wilkens. "The Association of Body Size, Reproductive Factors and Thyroid Cancer." *British Journal of Cancer* 66 (1992): 1180–1184.

Helfand, Mark, and Craig C. Redfern. "Screening for Thyroid Disease: An Update." *Annals of Internal Medicine* 129 (1998): 144–158.

Levi, Fabio, Silvia Franceschi, Cristina Gulie, Eva Negriond, and Carlo La Vecchia. "Female Thyroid Cancer." *Oncology* 50 (1993): 309–315.

Nidecker, Anna. "TSH Test Advised for All Women Over Age of 50." *Ob.Gyn. News*, 15 September 1998, 1–2.

Robin, Noel I. *The Clinical Handbook of Endocrinology and Metabolic Disease*. Pearl River, NY: Parthenon Publishing Group, 1996. 69–126.

Samuels, M. H., J. D. Veldhuis, P. Henry, and E. C. Ridgway. "Pathophysiology of Pulsatile and Copulsatile Release of Thyroid-Stimulating Hormone, Luteinizing Hormone, Follicle-Stimulating Hormone, and a-Subunit." *Journal of Clinical Endocrinology and Metabolism* 71.2 (1990): 425–432.

Singer, Peter A., David S. Cooper, Elliot G. Levy, Paul W. Ladenson, Lewis E. Braverman, Gilbert Daniels, Francis S. Greenspan, I. Ross McDougall, and Thomas F. Nikolai. "Treatment Guidelines for Patients with Hyperthyroidism and Hypothyroidism." *Journal of the American Medical Association* 273.10 (1995): 808–812.

Speroff, Leon, Robert H. Glass, and Nathan G. Kase. *Clinical Gynecologic Endocrinology and Infertility*, 5th ed. Baltimore: Williams & Wilkins, 1994. 667–684.

Stall, Glenn M., Susan Harris, Lori J. Sokoll, and Bess Dawson-Hughes. "Accelerated Bone Loss in Hypothyroid Patients Overtreated With L-Thyroxine." *Annals of Internal Medicine* 113 (1990): 265–269.

Tomer, Yaron, and Terry F. Davies. "Infection, Thyroid Disease, and Autoimmunity." *Endocrine Reviews* 14.1 (1993): 107–117.

Winsa, Brita, Hans-Olov Adami, Reinhold Bergstrom, Anders Gamstedt, Per Anders Dahlberg, Ulf Adamson, Rolf Jansson, and Anders Karlsson. "Stressful Life Events and Graves' Disease." *Lancet* 338 (1991): 1475–1479.

CHAPTER 13
DR. CORIO'S PRESCRIPTION FOR A HEALTHY PERIMENOPAUSE

"Benefits of a Mediterranean Diet." *Ob. Gyn. News*, 15 April 2001, 14.

Brody, Jane E. "New Look at Dieting: Fat Can Be a Friend." *New York Times*, 25 May 1999, F1, F9.

———. "Tea: The Latest Health Food (But Hold the Clotted Cream)." *New York Times*, 7 September 1999, F7.

———. "The Fatty Nut Finds Its Place at the Table." *New York Times*, 8 February 2000, F8.

"Disease-Fighting Foods?" *Consumer Reports on Health* (March 1999): 8–19.

"Drugs & Herbs." *Consumer Reports on Health* (June 2000): 6.

Fabricant, Florence. "From Algae, Perhaps a Healthier Egg." *New York Times*, 22 November 2000, F1.

Gazella, Karolyn A. "Menopause: Preparing for a Smooth Transition, Part 1." *Health Counselor* (August/September 1997): 36–40.

———. "Menopause: Preparing for a Smooth Transition, Part 2." *Nature's Impact* (October/November 1997): 34–38.

Goldman, Erik L. "Oestrogen Shouldn't Replace Exercise." *Ob. Gyn. News*, 1 December 1999, 1–2.

"The Great Weight Debate." *Consumer Reports on Health* (January 1999): 4–6.

Greenwood, Sadja. "Fats in the Diet—Helping Midlife Women Make Healthy Choices." *Menopause Management* (May/June 1999): 20–24.

———. "The Mediterranean Diet: Acceptable and Effective for Americans?" *Menopause Management* (January/February 1999): 16–19.

"Health Maintenance for Perimenopausal Women." *ACOG Technical Bulletin* 210 (August 1995): 470–478.

"It's All in the Mix." *Mayo Clinic Women's HealthSource* (September 1998): 1–2, 7.

Keough, Carol. "Got Hot Flashes? Got Night Sweats? Way Too Young for Menopause? Read This!" *Prevention* (May 1999): 110–117, 194.

Lee, Lauri. "The Complex Story of Carbohydrates." *Women's Health Connections* 6.2 (1998): 1–5.

———. "Good Dietary Fat Is Beneficial for Health." *Women's Health Connections* 5.5 (1998): 1–5.

———. "Is Dietary Cholesterol Really Public Enemy #1?" *Women's Health Connections* 6.1 (1998): 1–5.

———. "Protein: The Good Guy With the Bad Reputation." *Women's Health Connections* 5.4 (1998): 1–5.

"Managing Hyperlipidemia in Women." *APGO Educational Series on Women's Health Issues* (July 1999): 13–17.

Managing the Menopausal Patient: Consensus Panel. *Managing the Menopausal Patient: Consensus Guidelines.* Houston, TX: University of Texas—Houston Medical School, 1999.

"Managing the Menopause." *Orlando FL Symposium Proceedings.* Marietta, GA: Reid-Rowell, 1989.

Manson, JoAnn E., Frank B. Hu, Janet W. Rich-Edwards, Graham A. Colditz, Meir J. Stampfer, Walter C. Willett, Frank E. Speizer, and Charles H. Hennekens. "A Prospective Study of Walking as Compared With Vigorous Exercise in the Prevention of Coronary Heart Disease in Women." *The New England Journal of Medicine* 341 (1999): 650–658.

McCord, Holly. "4 Surprising Nutrients Your Bones Are Starving For." *Prevention* (May 2000): 148–149.

Murray, Mary. "Ads Raise Questions About Milk and Bones." *New York Times*, 14 September 1999, F1, F4.

"RDAs for Vitamins." *Harvard Women's Health Watch* (September 1999): 3.

Reavley, Nicola. *The New Encyclopedia of Vitamins, Minerals, Supplements, and Herbs.* New York: M. Evans, 1998. 331–334, 666–667.

Robbins, Jim. "Research Suggests Positive Effects from Living off the Fat of the Sea." *New York Times*, 24 April, F7.

Stengler, Mark. "Lowering Cholesterol Naturally." *Nature's Impact* (February/March 1999): 32–33.

Steward, H. Leighton, Morrison C. Bethea, Sam S. Andrews, and Luis A. Balart. *Sugar Busters!* New York: Ballantine, 1997. 61–65.

"Tone Your Bones." *Prevention* (November 1996): 75–81.

University of Medicine and Dentistry of New Jersey—Robert Wood Johnson Medical School Department of Obstetrics, Gynecology, and Reproductive Sciences. "FemHealth." www.peri-menopause.com, 6 April 2000.

"The Vitamin Controversy." *Mayo Clinic Women's HealthSource* 2.9 (September 1998): 1–2.

Willett, Walter C., William H. Dietz, and Graham A. Colditz. "Guidelines for Healthy Weight." *The New England Journal of Medicine* 341.6 (1999): 427–434.

"Women and Exercise." *ACOG Technical Bulletin* 173 (October 1992): 901–908.

Woods, Jeffrey A. "Exercise and Resistance to Neoplasia." *Canadian Journal of Physiologic Pharmacology* 76 (1998): 581–588.

APPENDIX A
HERBS

Brody, Jane E. "Americans Gamble on Herbs as Medicine." *New York Times*, 9 February 1999, F1, F7.

———. " 'Natural, Drug-Free' Herb May Have Risks of Its Own." *New York Times*, 9 February 1999, F6.

Foster, Steven. "Seven Herbs to See You Through Winter." *Herbs for Health* (January/February 1999): 58–60.

Gazella, Karolyn A. "Menopause: Preparing for a Smooth Transition, Part 2." *Nature's Impact* (October/November 1997): 34–38.

"Herbs and Drugs: Mix and Mismatch." *Consumer Reports on Health* (July 1999): 7.

"HRT vs. Remifemin in Menopause." *American Journal of Natural Medicine* 3.4 (1996): 7–10.

Jancin, Bruce. "Black Cohosh Appears Safe, Effective for Menopause." *Ob. Gyn. News*, 15 June 1999, 16.

Nagourney, Eric. "A Warning Not to Mix Surgery and Herbs." *New York Times*, 6 July 1999, F5.

Taylor, Maida. "Alternatives to Conventional Hormone Replacement." *Menopausal Medicine* 6.3 (1998): 1–6.

University of Medicine and Dentistry of New Jersey—Robert Wood Johnson Medical School Department of Obstetrics, Gynecology, and Reproductive Sciences. *Recognition and Management of the Perimenopausal Patient in Clinical Practice.* Somerville, NJ: EMBRYON, 1998. 12.

APPENDIX B
PHYTOESTROGENS

Anderson, James W., Bryan M. Johnstone, and Margaret E. Cook-Newell. "Meta-Analysis of the Effects of Soy Protein Intake on Serum Lipids." *The New England Journal of Medicine* 333 (1995): 276–282.

Begley, Sharon. "Understanding Perimenopause." *Newsweek Special Edition* (Spring/Summer 1999): 34.

Burros, Marian. "Doubts Cloud Rosy News on Soy." *New York Times*, 26 January 2000, F1, F11.

Carlson, Cornelia. "The Benefits of Flax." *Herbs for Health* (September/October 1998): 63–65.

Gazella, Karolyn A. "Menopause: Preparing for a Smooth Transition, Part 1." *Health Counselor* (August/September 1997): 36–40.

———. "Menopause: Preparing for a Smooth Transition, Part 2." *Nature's Impact* (October/November 1997): 34–38.

Knight, David C., and John A. Eden. "A Review of the Clinical Effects of Phytoestrogens." *Obstetrics & Gynecology* 87.5 (1996): 897–904.

Milligan, Patti Tveit. "Experience the Powerful Benefits of Soy." *Health Counselor* (August/September 1997): 57–59.

"Phytoestrogens: Natural Hormone Replacement Therapy?" *Alternative Therapies in Women's Health* 1.1 (1998): 1–6.

"Supplementing with Soy May Promote Bone and Heart Health." *Mayo Clinic Women's HealthSource* (October 1999): 3.

Taylor, Maida. "Alternatives to Conventional HRT: Phytoestrogens and Botanicals." *Contemporary Ob/Gyn* (June 1999): 27–50.

RESOURCES

GENERAL

Women's Health and Reproductive
   Rights Information Centre
52 Featherstone Street
London EC1Y 8RT
Tel: 020 7251 6333

Women's Resource Centre
76 Wentworth Street
London E1 7SA
Tel: 020 7377 0088

ADDICTIONS

Action on Smoking & Health
(ASH)
(England & Wales)
102 Clifton Street
London EC2A 4HW
Tel: 020 7739 5902

ASH
(Scotland)
8 Frederick Street
Edinburgh EH2 2HB
Tel: 0131 225 4725

NHS Smoking Helpline
Tel: 0800 169 0169

Alcoholics Anonymous
PO Box 1
Stonebow House
York YO1 2NJ
Tel: 01904 644026

CANCER

BACUP
3 Bath Place
Rivington Street
London EC2A 3JR
Tel: 020 7739 2280

Bristol Cancer Help Centre
Grove House
Cornwallis Grove
Clifton, Bristol BS8 4PG
Tel: 0117 980 9500
HELPLINE: 0845 123 2310

The Women's National Cancer
   Control Campaign
1st Floor
Charity House
14–15 Perseverance Works
London E2 8DD
Tel: 020 7729 4688

ADVICE ON H.R.T.

The Menopause Amarant Trust
Tel: 0901 607 0312

BREAST CARE

Breast Care and Mastectomy
  Association of Great Britain
Kiln House
210 New King's Road
London SW6 4NZ
Tel: 020 7384 2984

Glasgow Branch:
46 Gordon Street
Glasgow G1 3PU
Tel: 0141 221 2244

ENDOMETRIOSIS

National Endometriosis Society
50 Westminster Palace Gardens
127 Artillery Row
London SW1P 1RL
Tel: 020 7222 2781

OSTEOPOROSIS

National Osteoporosis Society
Camerton
Bath BA2 0PJ
Tel: 01761 471104
Medical HELPLINE: 0845 4500230

Osteoporosis Screening Services
Freephone: 0800 371989

NUTRITION

Women's Nutritional Advisory
  Service
PO Box 268
Lewes
East Sussex BN7 2QN
Tel: 01273 487366

MIGRAINE

Migraine Action Association
Unit 6 Oakley Hay Lodge
Business Park
Great Folds Road
Great Oakley
Northamptonshire NN18 9AS
Tel: 01536 461 333

Bachmann, Gloria A. et al. "Role of Androgens in the Menopause." *OBG Management* suppl. 10.7 (1998).

Baker, Barbara. "Oral Testosterone Cuts Fat, Raises Lean Muscle Mass." *Ob.Gyn. News*, 1 August 1999, 15.

———. "Testosterone Patch Can Boost Sexual Function." *Ob.Gyn. News*, 1 August 1999, 14.

Begley, Sharon. "Understanding Perimenopause." *Newsweek Special Edition* (Spring/ Summer 1999): 34.

Brody, Jane E. "A Tad of Testosterone Adds Zest to Menopause." *New York Times*, 24 February 1998, F7.

College of Physicians and Surgeons of Columbia University. "Current Clinical Uses of Low-Dose Estrogen Therapy." *Contemporary Ob/Gyn* suppl. (May 1998).

De Lignieres, Bruno. "Oral Micronized Progesterone." *Clinical Therapeutics* 21.1 (1999): 41–60.

Goldman, Erik L. "New Patches, Gels Expected to Flood HRT Market Soon." *Ob.Gyn. News*, 15 February 1999, 1–2.

Holland, Eileen G. "Guide to Oral Contraception Management." *Ob/Gyn Special Edition* 2 (Spring 1999): 57–62.

Johnson, Kate. "Low Testosterone May Underlie Inhibited Libido." *Ob.Gyn. News*, 15 November 1998, 23.

Kaunitz, Andrew M. "Beyond Birth Control." *The Female Patient* 24 (1999): 61–69.

———. "The Role of Androgens in Menopausal Hormone Replacement." *Endocrinology and Metabolism Clinics of North America* 26.2 (1997): 391–397.

Lorrain, Jacques, Gaston Lalumiere, Anne Filion, and Pierre Caron. "Use of Transdermal Estrogen Gel in Postmenopausal Women." *Menopause Management* (January/February 1999): 11–15.

Lourwood, David L. "Guide to Hormone Replacement Therapy." *Ob/Gyn Special Edition* 2 (Spring 1999): 15–20.

McAuliffe, Kathleen. "Words of Caution About a Hot Potato." *New York Times*, 13 June 1999, 15–16.

Oregon Health Sciences University School of Medicine. "Advances in Transdermal Postmenopausal Hormone Therapy." *Ob/Gyn Supplement* (January 1999).

Reichman, Judith. *I'm Not in the Mood.* New York: William Morrow, 1998. 122–123.

Sarrel, Phillip, Barbara Dobay, and Brinda Wiita. "Oestrogen and Estrogen-Androgen Replacement in Postmenopausal Women Dissatisfied With Estrogen-Only Therapy." *Journal of Reproductive Medicine* 43.10 (1998): 847–856.

"Women May Prefer Natural Progesterone Over Synthetic." *Mayo Clinic Women's HealthSource* (August 1999): 3.

Worcester, Sharon. "New Progesterones Offer Good Alternatives." *Ob.Gyn. News*, 1 July 1999, 11.

ACKNOWLEDGMENTS

The idea of writing this book occurred to me at least five years before my co-author and I ever put pen to paper. And for at least five years before *that*, I'd been collecting information about and treating symptoms of perimenopause. Countless people have educated, supported, and trusted me over this time. I'd like to take this opportunity to thank as many of them as possible:

First and foremost, the thousands of patients who have taught me about perimenopause and allowed me to care for them. Without them, this book simply could not have been written.

My colleagues at Mount Sinai Hospital, going back as far as my days as a resident and including those I practice alongside today. I'd especially like to thank those who reviewed specific chapters for accuracy: Lee Ellen Morrone, M.D., Donald Bergman, M.D., Alisan Goldfarb, M.D., Michelle Reichstein, M.D., Richard Smith, M.D., and Richard Firshein, D.O.

The staff of the Mount Sinai Library, who so cheerfully aided our research.

My partners Lee Ellen Morrone, M.D., and Karen Kirsch, M.D., who allowed me the time to pursue my dream of writing this book.

My office staff—Gail Chickory, Mayra Cardi, Tina Fields, Cheryl Fasano, Diana LaRosa, Patti Hughes, and Elsie Gonzalez—for always going the extra mile.

My literary agent, Anne Edelstein, who believed in my idea from the start and found me the perfect collaborator.

My co-author, Linda Kahn—not only a fabulous writer, but a beautiful person who heard my voice and shared my convictions.

All those at Bantam Dell who have contributed to this project, but especially my brilliant editor, Toni Burbank—the one person who is perhaps even more of a perfectionist than I am.

My friends—Marcia Barkin, Meredith Hershey, Diane Platt, and Lisa Ronis—and my siblings—Marie Corio, Ph.D., Sal Corio, Fred Corio, M.D., and Nina Loweth—who have always been there for me.

My parents, who give of themselves every day so that their children could realize their desires.

My children, Max and Marisa, both of whom are wise beyond their years and have always exceeded my expectations.

And Dr. Joseph Blanco, who has always supported me, stood by my side, and encouraged me to write a book that we both believed could make a positive contribution to the world.

LAURA E. CORIO, M.D., is board certified in obstetrics and gynaecology. In addition to her private practice in New York City, she is an attending physician at Mount Sinai Hospital in Manhattan, where she also teaches medical students and residents. She has made numerous media appearances as a medical expert. She lives in New Jersey with her son and daughter.

LINDA G. KAHN is a writer and editor specializing in health and psychology.

Graph on page 91 reprinted from "Menstrual Migraine: Towards a Definition" by E. A. MacGregor. *Cephalalgia* 16:11–12, 1996.

Sample voiding diary on page 116. Source: U.S. Department of Health and Human Services.

Graph on page 128 reprinted from *Maturitas*, Vol 18, 1994, Castelo-Branco et al, " Relationship between skin collagen and bone changes during aging," pages 199–206, copyright © 1994, with permission from Elsevier Science.

Photographs on page 185 reprinted from *J Bone Miner Res* 1986; 1:15–21, with permission of the American Society for Bone and Mineral Research.

Chart on page 206 reprinted from *Therapeutic Options for Menopausal Health*, Charles B. Hammond, M.D., September 1998, with permission of Duke University Medical Center, Office of Continuing Education.

Graph on page 210 reprinted from *Managing Hyperlipidemia in Women*, copyright © 1999, with permission of the Association of Professors of Gynecology and Obstetrics Educational Series on Women's Health Issues.

The list on page 229 reprinted from *HeartStrong Woman: Your Personal Action Plan for Heart Health* by the American College of Obstetricians and Gynecologists.

Chart on page 243. Source: 1987–1988 data, SEER Program of the National Cancer Institute and the American Cancer Society.

Chart on pages 338–339 reprinted from *Sugar Busters* by H. Leighton Steward et al. Copyright © 1999 by Sugar Busters LLC. Reprinted by permission of Ballantine Books, a Division of Random House, Inc.

INDEX

PIATKUS BOOKS

If you have enjoyed reading this book, you may be interested in other titles published by Piatkus. These include:

0 7499 2438 1	10 Days to Better Health	N. Rowley & K. Hartvig	£6.99
0 7499 2320 2	100 Ways to Live to be a 100	Dr R. Henderson	£7.99
0 7499 1968 X	100% Health	Patrick Holford	£10.99
0 7499 1920 5	30-Day Fatburner Diet, The	Patrick Holford	£6.99
0 7499 2362 8	48-Hour Detox	Jane Scrivner	£4.99
0 7499 2534 5	Acupressure	Michael Reed Gach	£14.99
0 7499 2542 6	Arthritis Relief at Your Fingertipes	Michael Reed Gach	£12.99
0 7499 2217 6	Complete Book of Food Combining, The	Kathryn Marsden	£14.99
0 7499 2496 9	Dealing With Depression	Dr Caroline Shreeve	£9.99
0 7499 2448 9	Good Gut Healing	Kathryn Marsden	£10.99
0 7499 2440 3	Holistic Doctor, The	Dr Deborah McManners	£12.99
0 7499 2604 X	Mother-Daughter Wisdom	Dr Christiane Northrup	£10.99
0 7499 2059 9	Natural Solutions to Infertility	Marilyn Glenville	£12.99
0 7499 2211 7	Natural Solutions to PMS	Marilyn Glenville	£10.99
0 7499 2235 4	Natural Health Handbook for Women, The	Marilyn Glenville	£16.99
0 7499 2138 2	Strong Women, Strong Bones	Miriam E. Nelson	£12.99
0 7499 2214 1	Wisdom of the Menopause, The	Dr Christiane Northrup	£10.99
0 7499 1925 6	Women's Bodies, Women's Wisdom	Dr Christiane Northrup	£10.99

All Piatkus titles are available from:

Piatkus Books Ltd, c/o Bookpost, PO Box 29, Douglas, Isle of Man, IM99 1BQ

Telephone (+44) 01624 677 237
Fax (+44) 01624 670 923
Email: bookshop@enterprise.net
Free Postage and Packing in the United Kingdom
Credit Cards accepted. All Cheques payable to Bookpost

Prices and availability are subject to change without prior notice. Allow 14 days for delivery. When placing orders, please state if you do not wish to receive any additional information.